The Anesthesia Drugs Handbook

Compliments of your

GlaxoWellcome

Representative

D0060894

NOTICE

Every effort has been made to ensure that the drug dosage schedules herein
are accurate and in accord with the standards accepted at the time of publication. However, as new research and experience broaden our knowledge,
changes in treatment and drug therapy occur. The medications described do
not necessarily have specific approval by the Food and Drug Administration
for use in the situations and dosages for which they are recommended. This
information is advisory only. The package insert should be consulted for use
and dosage as approved by the FDA for any changes in indications and
dosages and for added warnings and precautions. The ultimate responsibility
lies with the prescribing physician.

This publication is available from State-of-the-Art (S.O.T.A.) Technologies
or Mosby–Year Book in a Windows application for the IBM PC and compat-
ibles. For on-site retrieval of information, the software may be licensed for
use in critical care unit terminals, anesthesia machines, or compatible patient
monitoring systems. Manufacturers of patient monitors and information
terminals should contact S.O.T.A. Technologies for licensing information
(1520 Manhattan Beach Blvd., Suite C, Manhattan Beach, CA 90266, phone
800-9-Medic-9 or internet e mail sota1@aol.com).

The Anesthesia Drugs Handbook

SOTA OMOIGUI M.D.

Assistant Professor of Anesthesiology
Director of Pain Management
Charles R. Drew University of Medicine and
Science
Attending Anesthesiologist
Martin Luther King/Charles Drew Medical
Center
Los Angeles, California

SECOND EDITION

Mosby

St. Louis Baltimore Berlin Boston Carlsbad Chicago London Madrid
Naples New York Philadelphia Sydney Tokyo Toronto

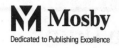

Mosby
Dedicated to Publishing Excellence

A Times Mirror Company

Executive Editor: Susan M. Gay
Developmental Editor: Sandra Clark Brown
Project Manager: Peggy Fagen
Electronic Production Coordinator: Peggy Hill
Manufacturing Supervisor: Theresa Fuchs
Book Designer: Nancy McDonald

SECOND EDITION

Printed in the United States of America
Composition by Mosby Electronic Production
Printing/binding by Malloy

Mosby–Year Book, Inc.
11830 Westline Industrial Drive
St. Louis, MO 63146

ISBN 0-8151-6503-X

96 97 98 99 / 9 8 7 6 5 4 3

CONSULTING EDITORS

Louis Alexander III MD
Attending Anesthesiologist
Cook County Hospital
Chicago, Illinois

Tracy Charles MD
Assistant Professor of Anesthesiology
Director, Division of Obstetric Anesthesia
Martin Luther King/Drew Medical Center
Los Angeles, California

Nowa Omoigui MD, MPH
Senior Fellow, Division of Cardiology
Cleveland Clinic
Cleveland, Ohio

Julie Pippins PharmD
Staff Pharmacist
Memorial Medical Center
Jacksonville, Florida

Shirley Randall MD
Attending Anesthesiologist
Womack Army Hospital
Fayetteville, North Carolina

John Stewart PhD
Professor of Pharmacology
Louisiana State University Medical Center
Shreveport, Louisiana

PREFACE TO THE SECOND EDITION

This second edition is evidence of the rapidly changing field of anesthetic pharmacology and the enormous success of the first edition. Information on all drugs have been updated where applicable, including information on drug storage, current manufacturer, and FDA warnings and guidelines. Expanded dosing information has been provided on many drugs, including the muscle relaxants, narcotics, and local anesthetics. The ACLS protocol has been updated with the addition of the pediatric CPR drugs table in the appendix. New drugs have been added including carboprost, EMLA, enalapril, insulin, ondansetron, rocuronium, and metaraminol. Readers who wish to obtain more information on chronic pain drugs may consult *The Pain Drugs Handbook* (Mosby). Finally, I wish to welcome Dr. Tracy Charles, who joins our team of consulting editors and to thank Drs. Dennis Chambi and Glen P.K. Akiona for their review and valuable suggestions.

Sota Omoigui MD
internet address: sota1@aol.com

PREFACE TO THE FIRST EDITION

The large and rapidly expanding field of anesthetic pharmacology has witnessed a dramatic proliferation in drugs available to the anesthesiologist. These drugs are administered as boluses or infusions by various routes such as intravenous, sublingual, oral, rectal, intranasal, intrapleural, transdermal, intraarticular, inhalational, epidural, caudal, spinal, etc.

The current state of the art requires an intimate familiarity with dosing information and pharmacology for this plethora of new drugs and new indications/routes of administration for old drugs. This may be overwhelming not only to the trainee but also to the seasoned practitioner. In the urgency of the operating rooms or critical care units where there is little room for error, there is a need for this pocket sized compendium that enables the anesthesiologist to identify the best drug, its dose, route of administration, and side effects at a moment's notice.

The Anesthesia Drugs Handbook reviews basic fundamentals of pharmacology and profiles the drugs and inhalational agents commonly used in anesthesia. Rather than providing a comprehensive description, the focus is on selected information required for proper use of each drug. The use of this drug handbook requires a well founded basic knowledge and practical experience which is essential for patient safety.

This handbook has been designed to fit the pocket of your operating room gown or scrub suit. It is hoped that it will make the difference in providing optimal patient care.

Sota Omoigui MD

CONTENTS

Drugs

/

ADENOSINE (ADENOCARD)

Use(s): Treatment of acute paroxysmal supraventricular tachycardia (PSVT); differentiation of supraventricular tachycardia with intraventricular aberrancy from ventricular tachycardia; unmasking of surface ECG delta waves in patients with concealed accessory pathways; afterload reduction in low-output states; controlled hypotension during cerebral aneurysm surgery; pharmacologic stress testing (e.g., with thallium) in coronary artery disease.

Dosing: Treatment/diagnosis of PSVT: rapid IV bolus, 6-12 mg (children 0.05-0.25 mg/kg). May be repeated within 1-2 min ($\times$ 2 doses) if necessary. Single doses >12 mg are not recommended. More effective when administered via a central vein or into the right atrium.

Elimination: Cellular uptake and metabolism (deamination, phosphorylation)

How Supplied: Injection, 3 mg/ml

Storage: Room temperature (15°-30° C). Do not refrigerate; crystallization may occur.

Pharmacology

An endogenous nucleoside with antiarrhythmic activity, adenosine slows conduction through the AV node. It can interrupt the reentry pathways through the AV node and restore normal sinus rhythm in patients with acute PSVT, including that associated with Wolff-Parkinson-White (WPW) syndrome. It decreases peripheral resistance and arterial pressure. Unlike verapamil, systemic hemodynamic effects are minimal and transient. The electrophysiologic effects of adenosine are not blocked by atropine, which indicates a lack of vagal mediation. Adenosine does not convert atrial flutter, atrial fibrillation, or ventricular tachycardia to normal sinus rhythm (with the rare exception of adenosine-sensitive ventricular tachycardia). Modest slowing of ventricular response may occur with atrial flutter or fibrillation.

Pharmacokinetics

Onset: <20 sec
Peak Effect: 20-30 sec
Duration: 3-7 sec
Interaction/Toxicity: Prolonged bradycardia may occur in patients with toxic concentrations of calcium channel blockers; antagonized competitively by methylxanthines (e.g., theophylline, caffeine); potentiated by blockers of nucleoside transport (e.g., dipyridamole); increased heart rate with nicotine; higher degrees of heart block in the presence of carbamazepine.

Guidelines/Precautions

1. Do not confuse this drug with adenosine phosphate, which is used as adjunctive therapy in the treatment of complications associated with varicose veins.
2. Because of the rapid metabolism, it is imperative to administer the dose rapidly over 2-3 sec. If given at a slower rate, a reflex tachycardia may occur as a result of systemic vasodilation. Negative chronotropic and dromotropic effects are seen only with rapid administration.

3. Adenosine may produce a short first-, second-, or third- degree heart block. Do not give additional doses if patients develop a high-level block.
4. It is not effective in patients receiving methylxanthines, which can completely block the electrophysiologic effects.
5. Use with caution in patients capable of rapid AV conduction. Atrial fibrillation or flutter has been observed in patients receiving adenosine.
6. Reduce doses in heart transplant patients. Donor sinus and AV nodes may have increased response to adenosine compared with recipient nodes or control subjects.
7. Significantly lower doses of adenosine should be administered in patients receiving dipyridamole. Initial doses should not exceed 1 mg.
8. Use with caution in patients with asthma. It may produce bronchoconstriction.
9. ECG monitoring is essential to determine conversion to normal sinus rhythm or AV block and detect new arrhythmias.
10. It is contraindicated in patients with second-degree or third-degree AV block or sick sinus syndrome, except where a pacemaker has been placed.

Principal Adverse Reactions

Cardiovascular: Palpitations, chest pain, hypotension, bradycardia, arrhythmias,
Pulmonary: Dyspnea, hyperventilation
CNS: Headache, dizziness, blurred vision, numbness, irritability
GI: Nausea, metallic taste, tightness in throat
Dermatologic: Flushing

ALFENTANIL HCL (ALFENTA)

Use(s): Analgesia, anesthesia

Dosing: Analgesia: IV/IM, 250-500 μg (5-10 μg/kg)

Induction: IV bolus, 50-300 μg/kg; or infusion, 0.5-15 μg/kg/min for $\leq$20 min. Titrate dose to patient response. To avoid chest wall rigidity administer muscle relaxant simultaneously with induction doses.

Anesthesia supplement: IV bolus, 10-100 μg/kg; infusion, 0.05-1.25 μg/kg/min

Sole anesthetic: IV, 500-2000 μg/kg (total dosage); or infusion, 1.25-8 μg/kg/min

Epidural: Bolus, 500-1000 μg (10-20 μg/kg); infusion, 100-250 μg/hr (2-5 μg/kg/hr)

Elimination: Hepatic

How Supplied: Injection, 500 μg/ml

Storage: Room temperature (15°-30° C)

Dilution for Infusion:

IV, 10 mg (20 ml) alfentanil in 250 ml of D_5W or NS (40 μg/ml)

Epidural, 1.5 mg (3 ml) alfentanil in 150 ml local anesthetic or (preservative-free) NS (10 μg/ml)

Pharmacology

A potent opioid analgesic with rapid onset and short duration of action, alfentanil produces a deep level of analgesia and attenuates the hemodynamic response to surgical stress. Like most opioids, it reduces sympathetic tone and may produce bradycardia (probably by stimulation of the vagal nucleus in the medulla), especially in conjunction with nonvagolytic neuromuscular blocking agents (e.g., vecuronium) or in the absence of an anticholinergic. Induction doses produce respiratory depression and decreases in blood pressure secondary to peripheral vasodilation. Alfentanil is associated with more hypotension and bradycardia than either fentanyl or sufentanil. Repeated doses or continuous infusions do not result in a significant cumulation. Alfentanil does not produce any clinically significant changes in cerebral blood flow, cerebral metabolic rate, or intracranial pressure.

Pharmacokinetics

Onset: IV, 1-2 min; IM, <5 min; epidural, 5-15 min
Peak Effect: IV, 1-2 min; IM, <15 min; epidural, 30 min
Duration: IV, 10-15 min; IM, 10-60 min; epidural, 1-2 hr
Interaction/Toxicity: Circulatory and ventilatory depressant effects potentiated by narcotics, sedatives, volatile anesthetics, nitrous oxide; ventilatory depressant effects potentiated by amphetamines, MAO inhibitors, phenothiazines, and tricyclic antidepressants; analgesia enhanced and prolonged by α 2 agonists (e.g., clonidine, epinephrine); serum levels and pharmacologic effects of alfentanil increased with concomitant administration of propofol; addition of epinephrine to epidural alfentanil results in increased side effects (e.g., nausea) and prolonged motor block; reduced clearance and prolonged respiratory depression with concomitant use of erythromycin; muscle rigidity in higher doses sufficient to interfere with ventilation.

Guidelines/Precautions

1. Reduce doses in elderly, hypovolemic, high-risk surgical patients and with concomitant use of sedatives and other narcotics.

2. Narcotic effects are reversed by naloxone (IV, 0.2-0.4 mg or higher).
3. Excessive bradycardia may be treated with atropine.
4. Alfentanil crosses the placental barrier, so use during labor may produce depression of respiration in the neonate. Resuscitation may be required; have naloxone available.
5. Epidural alfentanil may cause delayed respiratory depression (up to 8 hr after single dose), pruritus, nausea and vomiting, urinary retention. Naloxone (IV, 0.2-0.4 mg prn or infusion, 5-10 μg/kg/hr) is effective for prophylaxis and/or treatment. Ventilatory support for respiratory depression must be readily available. Antihistamines (e.g., diphenhydramine, 12.5-25 mg IV/IM q6hr prn) may be used for pruritus. Metoclopramide 10 mg IV q6hr prn may be used for nausea and vomiting. Urinary retention may require straight bladder catheterization.
6. Epidural/intrathecal injections should be avoided when the patient has septicemia, infection at the injection site, or coagulopathy.

Principal Adverse Reactions

Cardiovascular: Bradycardia, hypotension, arrhythmias
Pulmonary: Respiratory depression
CNS: Euphoria, dysphoria, convulsions
GI: Nausea and vomiting, biliary tract spasm, delayed gastric emptying
Eye: Miosis
Musculoskeletal: Muscle rigidity
Other: Pruritus

AMINOCAPROIC ACID (AMICAR)

Use(s): Treatment of life-threatening bleeding disorders secondary to systemic hyperfibrinolysis or urinary fibrinolysis; prophylaxis against recurrent subarachnoid hemorrhage.

Dosing: IV/PO, 4-5 g in 1 hr then 1-1.25 g/hr. Continue for about 8 hr or until bleeding is controlled.
Elimination: Renal
How Supplied:
Injection, 250 mg/ml
Tablets, 500 mg
Oral solution, 250 mg/ml
Storage: Room temperature (15°-30° C)
Dilution for Infusion: 15 g in 500 ml NS (30 mg/ml)

Pharmacology

As an inhibitor of plasminogen activators and to a lesser extent plasmin, this drug is useful in enhancing hemostasis when fibrinolysis contributes to bleeding. In life-threatening situations, fresh whole blood transfusions, fibrinogen infusions, and other emergency measures may be required. Aminocaproic acid should not be used without heparin when there is evidence of active intravascular coagulation.

Pharmacokinetics

Onset: IV, almost immediate; PO, few minutes
Peak Effect: IV, 1-3 hr; PO, < 2 hr
Duration: IV/PO, 3-5 hr
Interaction/Toxicity: Hypotension, bradycardia, arrhythmia from rapid intravenous injection; serious or fatal thrombus formation in disseminated intravascular coagulation.

Guidelines/Precautions

1. Do not use without a definitive diagnosis of hyper-fibrinolysis.
2. Increased risk of hypercoagulability in patients taking estrogens or estrogen-containing oral contraceptives.
3. Injectable form not for use in newborns because of toxicity of preservative (benzyl alcohol).

Principal Adverse Reactions

Cardiovascular: Hypotension, bradycardia
CNS: Dizziness, tinnitus
GI: Nausea, cramps, diarrhea
Musculoskeletal: Myopathy, rhabdomyolysis
GU: Renal failure

AMINOPHYLLINE (AMINOPHYLLINE)

Use(s): Prevention and treatment of bronchial asthma and reversible bronchospasm associated with chronic obstructive pulmonary disease, treatment of post–dural puncture headache.

Dosing: Bronchospasm:
    Loading:
        IV, 5-6 mg/kg (give over 20-30 min)
        PO/rectal, 6 mg/kg
        Each 0.5 mg/kg theophylline (0.6 mg/kg aminophylline) will increase theophylline concentration by 1 μg/ml
    Maintenance:
        Infusion IV, 0.5-1 mg/kg/hr
        PO, 2-4 mg/kg q6-12 hr
    Loading doses in patients receiving theo-

phylline should be based on the serum theophylline levels. If these are not rapidly available, expect each 0.6 mg/kg (ideal body weight) aminophylline (0.5 mg/kg theophylline) to result in 1 μ/ml increase in serum theophylline concentrations. Lower maintenance doses (0.1-0.3 mg/kg/hr) should be used with older patients and patients with cor pulmonale or congestive heart failure. Higher maintenance doses (0.8-1 mg/kg) should be used with children (6 months-16 yr) and young adult smokers.

Post–Dural Puncture Headache: PO (extended release), 225 mg q8hr for 3-5 days

Elimination: Hepatic

How Supplied:

Injection: 1 mg/ml, 2 mg/ml, 25 mg/ml

Tablets: 100 mg, 200 mg

Tablets, extended release: 225 mg

Oral solution: 105 mg/5 ml

Rectal solution: 60 mg/ml

Rectal suppositories: 250 mg, 500 mg

100 mg of aminophylline is equivalent to 78.9 mg anhydrous theophylline.

Storage:

Injection: Room temperature (15°-30° C). Do not permit to freeze. Protect from light.

Suppositories: Refrigerate. Temperature should not exceed 8° C.

Dilution for Infusion:

Loading dose: Dilute in 50 ml D_5W or NS.

Maintenance dose: Dilute 500 mg in 500 ml D_5W or NS (1 mg/ml).

Pharmacology

Aminophylline is converted to theophylline. The exact mechanism of action is unclear. Theophylline, a methylxanthine bronchodilator, may produce its pharmacologic effects by inhibiting phosphodiesterase, thereby increasing the levels of cyclic adenosine monophosphate (cAMP) in bronchial smooth muscle; blocking adenosine receptors; antagonizing of prostaglandin E2; or a direct effect on the mobilization of calcium. It reduces fatigue of diaphragmatic muscles, increases cardiac output, and decreases peripheral vascular resistance. Beneficial effects in alleviating headache after lumbar puncture may be due to blockade of adenosine receptors and increase in cAMP levels in the cells of the choroid plexus, thus enhancing CSF secretion.

Pharmacokinetics

Onset: IV, few minutes; PO, within 30 min
Peak Effect: IV, 1 hour; PO, 1-2 hr
Duration: PO, 4-8 hr
Interaction/Toxicity: Elevated serum levels in patients receiving cimetidine, beta blockers, erythromycin, allopurinol, and oral contraceptive steroids, and in patients with cardiac failure and liver insufficiency; decreased serum levels with phenobarbital, phenytoin, rifampin, and in smokers; aminophylline antagonizes effects of propranolol, potentiates pressor effects of sympathomimetics, and may produce seizures, cardiac dysrhythmias, cardiorespiratory arrest, ventricular dysrhythmia with excessive plasma levels or in patients receiving volatile anesthetics, especially halothane.

Guidelines/Precautions

1. Aminophylline has a very low toxic/therapeutic index. Frequent monitoring of plasma concentrations is essential. Increased toxicity mainly at serum concentration >20 μg/ml, but toxic effects may be seen at therapeutic levels. Treatment of toxicity includes cessation of therapy, supportive and symptomatic treatment.
2. Avoid rapid infusions, which may cause hypotension, arrhythmias, and possibly death.
3. Wait 3 drug half-lives after the last dose of aminophylline is given (i.e., approximately 13 hr in normal individuals) before using halothane to anesthetize an asthmatic patient. Use isoflurane or enflurane in patients who must be given aminophylline or other exogenous sympathomimetic drugs before or during surgery.

Principal Adverse Reactions

Cardiovascular: Palpitations, sinus tachycardia, ventricular arrhythmias
Pulmonary: Tachypnea
CNS: Seizures, headache, irritability
GI: Nausea, vomiting, epigastric pain
Other: Hyperglycemia, syndrome of inappropriate antidiuretic hormone (SIADH)

AMIODARONE (CORDARONE)

Use(s): Treatment of life-threatening ventricular arrhythmias that do not respond to other antiarrhythmics; selective treatment of supraventricular tachyarrhythmias.

Dosing: PO loading, 800-1600 mg/day for 1 to 3 wk
       PO maintenance, 200-600 mg/day
       Therapeutic level, 1.0-2.5 µg/ml
Elimination: Hepatic
How Supplied:
Tablets: 200 mg
Injection: not approved for general clinical use in the
   United States.
Storage: Tablets: Room temperature (15°-30° C). Protect
from light.

Pharmacology

This benzofuran derivative has mixed Class 1C and Class
III antiarrhythmic characteristics. It prolongs action potential duration and increases the refractory period of cardiac
fibers, including accessory pathways. It also causes noncompetitive alpha and beta adrenergic inhibition. Longterm therapy results in dilation of coronary arteries and
increased coronary blood flow.

Pharmacokinetics

Onset: 2-4 days, but may be delayed much longer (e.g., 2
to 3 months)
Peak Effect: Usually 1-3 weeks
Duration: 45 days
Interaction/Toxicity: Amiodarone increases serum levels
of digoxin, potentiates warfarin anticoagulants, and may
cause bradycardia or sinus arrest in patients receiving beta
blockers, calcium antagonists, lidocaine.

Guidelines/Precautions

1. Because of the risk of sinus arrest in patients receiving
   halothane, have available temporary artificial cardiac

(ventricular) pacemakers and sympathomimetics (beta agonists).
2. Thyroid function may be altered.
3. Contraindicated in severe sinus dysfunction causing marked sinus bradycardia, second-degree and third-degree AV block.
4. Discontinue if blurring of vision occurs.
5. Monitor pulmonary toxicity. Perform periodic chest x-rays and pulmonary function tests every 3-6 months.

Principal Adverse Reactions

Cardiovascular: Arrhythmias, congestive heart failure
Pulmonary: Pulmonary inflammation or fibrosis
CNS: Peripheral neuropathy, tremors, involuntary movements
GI: Hepatitis, cirrhosis
Eyes: Corneal deposits
Metabolic: Hyperthyroidism, hypothyroidism
Dermatologic: Photosensitivity

AMRINONE LACTATE (INOCOR)

Use(s): Inotropic agent, short-term management of congestive heart failure.

Dosing: Loading dose: IV, 0.75 mg/kg
Infusion, 2-20 μg/kg/min
Elimination: Renal, hepatic
How Supplied: Injection: 5 mg/ml
Storage: Injection: Room temperature (15°-30° C). Protect from light
Dilution for Infusion: 500 mg in 500 ml NS (1 mg/ml)

Pharmacology

A bipyridine derivative inotropic agent, amrinone is chemically unrelated to cardiac glycosides or catecholamines. The drug inhibits phosphodiesterase and increases intracellular cyclic AMP, which potentiates delivery of calcium ions to the myocardial contractile system. This produces a dose-dependent positive inotropic effect. Peripheral vasodilation is due to direct vascular smooth muscle relaxation and may result in occasional hypotension. In congestive heart failure, the inotropic and vasodilatory effects may result in substantial increases in cardiac output. Therapeutic response to amrinone is not prevented by alpha or beta adrenergic blockade, depletion of catecholamines, or inhibition of the sodium-potassium adenosine triphosphatase (ATPase) ion transport system.

Pharmacokinetics

Onset: Within 5 min
Peak Effect: 10 min
Duration: 30 min-2 hr
Interaction/Toxicity: Excessive hypotension with concomitant use of disopyramide; chemical reaction with dextrose-containing solutions; thrombocytopenia, hepatic dysfunction with chronic therapy; potentiates inotropic, chronotropic, and arrhythmogenic response to catecholamines and theophylline.

Guidelines/Precautions

1. Use with caution in hypotensive patients.
2. Avoid exposure of ampule to light.
3. Do not mix in solutions containing dextrose or furosemide.

4. Contains metabisulfite. Contraindicated in patients hypersensitive to bisulfites.
5. May aggravate outflow tract obstruction in patients with aortic or pulmonary valvular disease or obstructive cardiomyopathy.

Principal Adverse Reactions

Cardiovascular: Arrhythmia, hypotension
Hematologic: Thrombocytopenia
GI: Abdominal pain, hepatic dysfunction
Other: Hypersensitivity reactions

ATENOLOL (TENORMIN)

Use(s): Antihypertensive; antianginal; treatment of acute myocardial infarction, acute alcohol withdrawal; migraine prophylaxis

Dosing: Hypertension/angina: PO, 50-200 mg once daily
Acute myocardial infarction: IV, 5 mg over 5 min and 5 mg 10 min later, then PO, 100 mg once daily or 50 mg twice daily. Dilute IV dose in D_5W or NS.
Alcohol withdrawal/migraine prophylaxis: PO, 50-100 mg once daily.

Elimination: Renal
How Supplied:
Tablets: 50 mg, 100 mg
Injection: 5 mg/10 ml
Storage: Injection/tablets: Room temperature (15°-30° C). Protect from light

Pharmacology

Atenolol is a cardioselective beta-blocking agent without membrane-stabilizing or intrinsic sympathomimetic (agonist) activities. The cardioselectivity is relative, and in high doses the drug blocks both beta-1 and beta-2 receptors. It decreases myocardial contractility, heart rate, and blood pressure, which leads to a reduction in myocardial oxygen requirements.

Pharmacokinetics

Onset: PO, <1 hr; IV, < 5 min
Peak Effect: PO, 2-4 hr; IV, 5 min
Duration: PO, 24 hr; IV, 12 hr
Interaction/Toxicity: Hypotensive effects of atenolol potentiated by volatile anesthetics, catecholamine-depleting drugs (e.g., reserpine), and calcium channel blockers; atenolol may unmask negative inotropic effects of ketamine, prolong the elevation of plasma potassium after the administration of succinylcholine, and mask the tachycardia associated with hypoglycemia.

Guidelines/Precautions

1. The drug should be discontinued slowly, especially in patients subject to myocardial ischemia.
2. Use with caution in asthma, heart failure, and AV block greater than first degree.
3. More water soluble and more dependent on renal clearance mechanisms than most other beta blockers.
4. Manifestations of excessive vagal tone and myocardial depression (profound bradycardia, hypotension) may be corrected with IV atropine (1-2 mg), IV isoproterenol (0.02- 0.15 μg/kg/min), IV glucagon (1-5 mg), or a transvenous cardiac pacemaker.

Principal Adverse Reactions

Cardiovascular: Hypotension, bradyarrhythmias, rebound angina
Pulmonary: Bronchospasm, dyspnea, cough
CNS: Fatigue, depression, disorientation
GI: Nausea, vomiting, pancreatitis
Hematologic: Thrombocytopenic purpura
Musculoskeletal: Arthralgia

ATRACURIUM BESYLATE (TRACRIUM)

Use(s): Skeletal muscle relaxation

Dosing: Intubation: IV, 0.3-0.5 mg/kg
  Maintenance:
    IV, 0.1-0.2 mg/kg (10%-50% of intubating dose)
    Infusion: 2-15 μg/kg/min
  Pretreatment/priming: IV, 10% of intubating dose
    given 3-5 min before depolarizer/nondepolariz-
    er relaxant dose
Elimination: Plasma (Hoffman elimination), hepatic, renal
How Supplied: Injection: 10 mg/ml
Storage: Refrigerate (2°-8° C). Do not permit to freeze. Upon removal from refrigeration to room temperature, use within 14 days even if rerefrigerated.
Dilution for Infusion: 20 mg in 100 ml D_5W or NS (0.2 mg/ml); 50 mg in 100 ml D_5W or NS (0.5 mg/ ml)

Pharmacology

Atracurium is a nondepolarizing skeletal muscle relaxant. It competes for cholinergic receptors at the motor end plate. The duration of neuromuscular blockade is one third that of pancuronium at equipotent doses. It undergoes rapid metabolism via temperature-and pH-dependent Hoffman elimination and nonspecific enzymatic ester hydrolysis. The primary metabolite is laudanosine, a cerebral stimulant excreted primarily in the urine. Repeated doses or continuous infusion have less cumulative effect on recovery rate than other muscle relaxants. Blood laudanosine concentrations may approach convulsant ranges (5.1 μg/ml) with prolonged infusions. Histamine release and hemodynamic changes are minimal within the recommended dose range and when administered slowly. Higher doses (>0.5 mg/kg) may lead to moderate histamine release, decreased arterial pressure, and increased heart rate.

Pharmacokinetics

Onset: <3 min
Peak Effect: 3-5 min
Duration: 20-35 min
Interaction/Toxicity: Neuromuscular blockade potentiated by aminoglycoside, antibiotics, local anesthetics, loop diuretics, magnesium, lithium, ganglionic blocking drugs, hypothermia, hypokalemia, respiratory acidosis, and prior administration of succinylcholine; dosage requirements decreased (about 30%-45%) and duration of neuromuscular blockade prolonged (up to 25%) by volatile anesthetics; pretreatment doses of atracurium decrease fasciculations but reduce intensity and shorten duration of succinylcholine neuromuscular blockade; priming doses decrease the time to onset of maximal blockade by about 30-60 sec; enhanced neuromuscular blockade will occur in patients with myasthenia gravis or inadequate adrenocortical function; effects antagonized by anticholinesterases such as neostigmine, edrophonium, pyridostigmine; increased resistance or reversal of effects with use of theophylline and in patients with burn injury and paresis.

Guidelines/Precautions

1. Monitor response with peripheral nerve stimulator to minimize risk of overdosage.
2. Use with caution in patients with history of bronchial asthma and anaphylactoid reactions.
3. Reverse effects with anticholinesterases such as neostigmine, edrophonium, or pyridostigmine bromide in conjunction with atropine or glycopyrrolate.
4. Pretreatment doses may induce a degree of neuromuscular blockade sufficient to cause hypoventilation in some patients.

Principal Adverse Reactions

Cardiovascular: Hypotension, vasodilation, sinus tachycardia, sinus bradycardia
Pulmonary: Hypoventilation, apnea, bronchospasm, laryngospasm, dyspnea
Musculoskeletal: Inadequate block, prolonged block
Dermatologic: Rash, urticaria

ATROPINE SULFATE (ATROPINE SULFATE)

Use(s): Treatment of sinus bradycardia/CPR, premedication (vagolysis), reversal of neuromuscular blockade (blockade of muscarinic effects of anticholinesterases), adjunctive therapy in treatment of bronchospasm and peptic ulcer

Dosing: Sinus bradycardia/CPR:
Adults, IV/IM/SC, 0.5-1.0 mg; repeat q3-5 min as indicated; maximum dose 40 μg/kg
Children, IV/IM/SC, 10-20 μg/kg (minimum dose 0.1 mg)

Premedication:

Adults:

IV/IM, 0.4-1.0 mg

PO, 0.4-0.6 mg q4-6 h

Children:

IV, 10-20 μg/kg (minimum dose 0.1 mg)

PO, 30 μg/kg q4-6 h. High-potency injectate solutions (>0.3 mg/ml) may be diluted in 3-5 ml apple juice or carbonated cola beverage.

Reversal of neuromuscular blockade: IV, 0.015 mg/kg with anticholinesterase neostigmine (IV, 0.05 mg/kg) or edrophonium (IV 0.5-1 mg/kg).

Bronchodilation: inhalation:

Adults, 0.025 mg/kg q4-6 hr

Children, 0.05 mg/kg q4-6 hr

Maximum dose 2.5 mg. Dilute to 2-3 ml with NS and deliver by compressed air nebulizer.

Elimination: Hepatic, renal

How Supplied:

Injection: 0.05 mg/ml, 0.1 mg/ml, 0.3 mg/ml, 0.4 mg/ml, 0.5 mg/ml, 0.8 mg/ml, 1 mg/ml

Inhalation solution: 0.2%, 0.5%

Tablets: 0.4 mg, 0.6 mg

Storage: Injection/tablets: Room temperature (15°-30° C).

Pharmacology

Atropine competitively antagonizes the action of acetylcholine at the muscarinic receptor. It decreases salivary, bronchial, and gastric secretions, and relaxes bronchial smooth muscle. Gastrointestinal tone and motility are reduced. Lower esophageal sphincter pressure decreases, and intraocular pressure (IOP) increases (because of pupillary dilation). At doses used for premedication, this increase in IOP is not clinically significant. Large doses may increase body temperature by preventing sweat secretion. Peripheral vagal blockade of the sinus and AV node increases heart rate. Transient decreases in heart rate by small doses (<0.5 mg in adults) are due to a weak peripheral muscarinic cholinergic agonist effect. Atropine is a tertiary amine and therefore crosses the blood-brain barrier. In high doses it stimulates and then depresses the medullary and higher cerebral centers.

Pharmacokinetics

Onset:
IV, 45-60 sec; intratracheal, 10-20 sec; IM, 5-40 min; PO, 30 min-2 hr; inhalation, 3-5 min
Peak Effect: IV, 2 min; inhalation, 1-2 hr
Duration:
IV/IM: vagal blockade, 1-2 hr; antisialogogue effect, 4 hr
Inhalation: vagal blockade, 3-6 hr
Interaction/Toxicity: Additive anticholinergic effects with antihistamines, phenothiazines, tricyclic antidepressants, procainamide, quinidine, MAO inhibitors, benzodiazepines, antipsychotics; increase in IOP enhanced by nitrates, nitrites, alkalinizing agents, disopyramide, corticosteroids, haloperidol; potentiates sympathomimetics; antagonizes anticholinesterases and metoclopramide; may produce central anticholinergic syndrome (hallucinations, delirium, coma).

Guidelines/Precautions

1. Use with caution in patients with tachyarrhythmias, congestive heart failure, acute myocardial ischemia or infarction, fever, esophageal reflux, GI infections.

2. Contraindicated in patients with obstructive uropathy or obstructive disease of the GI tract.
3. If intravenous access is not available during cardiopulmonary resuscitation, the drug may be diluted 1:1 in sterile NS and injected via an endotracheal tube. The absorption rate, duration, and pharmacologic effects of intratracheal drug administration compare favorably with the IV route.
4. May accumulate and produce systemic side effects with multiple dosing by inhalation, especially in the elderly.
5. Treat toxicity with sedation (benzodiazepines) and administration of physostigmine.
6. Infants, small children, and elderly patients are more susceptible to the systemic effects of atropine (e.g., rapid and irregular pulse, fever, excitement, agitation).

Principal Adverse Reactions

Cardiovascular: Tachycardia (high doses), bradycardia (low doses), palpitations
Pulmonary: Respiratory depression
CNS: Confusion, hallucinations, drowsiness, excitement, agitation
GU: Urinary hesitancy, retention
GI: Gastroesophageal reflux
Eyes: Mydriasis, blurred vision, increased intraocular pressure
Dermatologic: Urticaria
Other: Decreased sweating, allergic reaction

BENZOCAINE (AMERICAINE, HURRICAINE, RHULICAINE, SOLARCAINE, DERMOPLAST)

Use(s): Topical anesthesia

Dosing: Topical
Elimination: Plasma cholinesterase
How Supplied: Aerosol, cream, ointment 0.5%-20%
Storage: Aerosol, cream, ointment: Room temperature (15°-30° C); do not expose aerosol to heat or temperatures >40° C; protect cream and ointment from light.

Pharmacology

An ester of benzoic acid with a rapid onset of action and short duration, benzocaine stabilizes neuronal membranes by inhibiting ionic fluxes required for initiation and conduction of impulses. There is virtually no systemic absorption.

Pharmacokinetics

Onset: 15-30 sec
Peak Effect: 1 min
Duration: 12-15 min
Interaction/Toxicity: Metabolite (para-amino benzoic acid) inhibits action of sulfonamides and aminosalicylic acid.

Guidelines/Precautions

1. Do not use in the eyes or areas with secondary bacterial infection.
2. Not for injection.
3. Not for prolonged use.

Principal Adverse Reactions

Cardiovascular: Hypotension
Pulmonary: Respiratory depression
CNS: Seizures
Dermatologic: Urticaria, pruritus, anaphylactoid reactions (rare)
Other: Methemoglobinemia

BRETYLIUM TOSYLATE (BRETYLOL)

Use(s): Treatment of ventricular fibrillation and arrhythmias, treatment of sympathetic mediated pain

Dosing: Arrhythmias

  IV loading/IM—ventricular tachycardia: 5-10 mg/kg over 15 min; may be repeated in 1 to 2 hr.

  IV loading—ventricular fibrillation: 5-10 mg/kg over 1 min (q15-30min to maximum 30 mg/kg;)

  Infusion: 1-2 mg/min

  Therapeutic level: 0.5-1.0 μg/ml.

 Sympathetic Mediated Pain:

  IV regional sympathetic block: 1-2 mg/kg; dilute in 40-50 ml of 0.5% lidocaine or NS (upper extremity) or 50-60 ml of 0.5% lidocaine or NS (lower extremity).

  Methylprednisolone (80 mg) may be added to solution to decrease postmanipulation edema. Administer 500 ml of fluid immediately after tourniquet release to prevent orthostasis.

Elimination: Renal
How Supplied: Injection: 50 mg/ml
Storage: Injection: Room temperature (15°-30° C).
Dilution for Infusion: 2 g in 500 ml D$_5$W or NS (4 mg/ml)

Pharmacology

A class III antiarrhythmic agent, bretylium initially releases norepinephrine from sympathetic ganglia and postganglionic adrenergic neurons. This initial action may account for increased heart rate, irritability, and blood pressure. Subsequently there is inhibition of release of norepinephrine in response to sympathetic nerve stimulation. The adrenergic blockade depends on uptake of bretylium by adrenergic neurons and may lead to orthostatic hypotension and bradycardia. Cardiac performance is not significantly changed, but pulmonary artery pressure may be increased. Bretylium increases ventricular fibrillation threshold and suppresses ventricular dysrhythmias. The electrophysiologic effects include an increase in action potential duration and effective refractory period, an increase in ventricular conduction velocity, and a decrease in the disparity between normal and damaged cells. In high concentrations, bretylium has local anesthetic and neuromuscular blocking properties. It alleviates peripheral manifestations of sympathetic mediated pain (reflex sympathetic dystrophy and causalgia) by adrenergic blockade and decrease in sensitivity of peripheral nociceptors.

Pharmacokinetics

Onset:
IV: antifibrillatory, few minutes
IV/IM: suppression of ventricular arrhythmia, 20 min-2 hr

Peak Effect:
IV: antifibrillatory, 20 min-2 hr
IV/IM: suppression of ventricular arrhythmia, 6-9 hr
Duration:
IV/IM (antiarrhythmic effect): 6-24 hr
IV Regional (pain relief in reflex sympathetic dystrophy): 3-10 weeks

Interaction/Toxicity: Initial release of norepinephrine may worsen arrhythmias caused by cardiac glycoside toxicity; resistance to antiadrenergic effects is seen in patients receiving tricyclic antidepressants (which block the uptake of bretylium).

Guidelines/Precautions

1. Use with caution in patients with pheochromocytoma, aortic stenosis, and pulmonary hypertension. Contraindicated in patients with allergy to corn products, who may manifest cross allergy to bretylium.
2. Severe hypotension should be treated with appropriate fluid therapy and vasopressor agents such as dopamine or norepinephrine.
3. In intravenous regional blocks, when normal saline is used as the diluent, the cuff may be deflated cautiously after 10 min. If a local anesthetic is used as the diluent (e.g., lidocaine 0.5%), the cuff should be deflated after 40 min and no less than 20 min. Between 20-40 min, the cuff may be deflated, reinflated immediately, and finally deflated after a minute to reduce the sudden absorption of local anesthetic into the systemic circulation.

Principal Adverse Reactions

Cardiovascular: Hypotension, transitory hypertension and arrhythmias, anginal attacks

Pulmonary: Shortness of breath
CNS: Dizziness, syncope
GI: Nausea, vomiting, diarrhea, abdominal pain
Other: Rash, hiccups

BUPIVACAINE HCL (MARCAINE, SENSORCAINE)

Use(s): Regional anesthesia

Dosing: Infiltration/peripheral nerve block: <150 mg (0.25%-0.5% solution)

Intravenous regional:

Upper extremities, 100-125 mg (40-50 ml of 0.25% solution).

Lower extremities, 125-150 mg (100-120 ml of 0.125% solution).

Do not add epinephrine for intravenous regional block. If desired, add fentanyl 50 μg to enhance the block and/or muscle relaxant (pretreatment doses only, e.g., pancuronium 0.5 mg).

Caudal: 37.5-150 mg (15-30 ml of 0.25% or 0.5% solution); children, 0.4-0.7-1.0 ml/kg (L2-T10-T7 level of anesthesia)

Brachial plexus block: 75-250 mg (30-50 ml of 0.375%-0.5% solution); children, 0.5-0.75 ml/kg. With high doses (>2 mg/kg), add epinephrine 1:200,000 to decrease systemic toxicity (in the absence of any contraindications). Regional blockade may be potentiated by the addition of tetracaine, 0.5-1 mg/kg, or fentanyl, 1-2 μg/kg, or morphine, 0.05-0.1 mg/kg.

Stellate ganglion block: 10-20 ml of 0.25% (25-50 mg) solution with or without epinephrine 1:200,000.

Epidural:

Bolus, 50-150 mg (0.25%-0.75% solution); children, 1.5-2.5 mg/kg (0.25%-0.5% solution)

Infusion: 6-12 ml/hr (0.0625%-0.125% solution with or without epidural narcotics; children, 0.2-0.35 ml/kg/hr

Rate of onset and potency of local anesthetic action may be enhanced by carbonation. (Add 0.1 ml of 8.4% sodium bicarbonate with 20 ml of 0.25 bupivacaine. Do not use if there is precipitation.)

Spinal: bolus/infusion, 7-15 mg (0.75% solution); children, 0.5 mg/kg with minimum of 1 mg

Intrapleural:

Bolus, 100 mg (20 ml of 0.25%-0.5% solution (0.4 ml/kg);

Infusion, 5-7 ml/hr (0.125 mls/kg/hr) (0.125%-0.25% solution)

Intraarticular: <100 mg (20-40 ml of 0.25% solution); ifdesired add morphine 0.5-1 mg

Maximum safe dose: 2 mg/kg without epinephrine, 2-3 mg/kg with epinephrine.

Solutions containing preservatives should not be used for epidural or caudal block. Except where contraindicated, vasoconstrictor drugs may be added to increase effect and prolong local or regional anesthesia. For dosage/route guidelines, see epinephrine or phenylephrine. Do not use vasoconstrictor drugs for IV regional anesthesia or local anesthesia of end organs (digits, penis, nose, ears).

Elimination: Hepatic, pulmonary

How Supplied:

Injection, 0.25%, 0.5%, 0.75% with and without epinephrine 1:200,000

Injection, for spinal: 0.75% with 8.25% dextrose

Storage: Injection: Room temperature (15°-30° C). Solutions containing epinephrine should be protected from light.

Dilution for Infusion: Epidural use only; 20 ml of 0.25% in 20 ml (preservative-free) NS (0.125% solution) or 10 ml of 0.25% solution in 30 ml (preservative-free) NS (0.0625% solution)

Pharmacology

This amino amide local anesthetic stabilizes neuronal membranes by inhibiting ionic fluxes required for the initiation and conduction of impulses. The progression of anesthesia is related to the diameter, myelination, and conduction velocity of affected nerve fibers, with order of loss of function being: (1) autonomic, (2) pain, (3) temperature, (4) touch, (5) proprioception, and (6) skeletal muscle tone. The onset of action is reasonably rapid, and duration is significantly longer than with any other commonly used local anesthetic. Addition of epinephrine improves the quality of analgesia but only marginally increases duration of effect of bupivacaine concentrations ≥0.5%. Hypotension results from loss of sympathetic tone as in spinal or epidural anesthesia. Compared with other amides (e.g., lidocaine or mepivacaine), intravascular injection of bupivacaine is associated with more cardiotoxicity. This is due to slower recovery from bupivacaine-induced cardiac sodium channel blockade and a greater depression of myocardial contractility and cardiac conduction. At high plasma levels bupivacaine produces uterine vasoconstriction and decrease in uterine blood flow. Such plasma levels are seen in paracervical blocks but not with epidural or spinal blocks.

Pharmacokinetics

Onset: Infiltration, 2-10 min; epidural, 4-17 min; spinal <1 min

Peak Effect: Infiltration/epidural, 30-45 min; spinal, 15 min

Duration: Infiltration/epidural/spinal, 200-400 min (prolonged with epinephrine); intrapleural, 12-48 hr

Interaction/Toxicity: Seizures, respiratory and circulatory depression at high plasma levels; reduced clearance with concomitant use of beta-blocking agents and cimetidine; benzodiazepines, barbiturates, and volatile anesthetics increase seizure threshold; reduced dose requirements in pregnant patients; duration of anesthesia prolonged by vasoconstrictor agents (e.g., epinephrine), alpha-2 agonists (e.g. clonidine), and narcotics (e.g., fentanyl); alkalinization increases rate of onset and potency of local or regional anesthesia; prior use of epidural chloroprocaine antagonizes the effects of epidural bupivacaine.

Guidelines/Precautions

1. Bupivacaine is not recommended for obstetric paracervical block. The drug may cause fetal bradycardia or death.
2. Use very cautiously for IV regional anesthesia. High plasma concentrations may occur after tourniquet release and result in refractory cardiac arrest and death.

3. Concentrations above 0.5% are associated with toxic reactions and refractory cardiac arrest. Such concentrations are contraindicated for obstetric epidural analgesia or anesthesia.

4. Cauda equina syndrome with permanent neurologic deficit may occur in patients receiving >15 mg of a 0.75% bupivacaine solution with a continuous spinal technique.

5. Intravenous access is essential during major regional block.

6. Use with caution in patients with hypovolemia, severe congestive heart failure, shock, and all forms of heart block.

7. In intravenous regional blocks, deflate the cuff after 40 min and no less than 20 min. Between 20-40 min, the cuff can be deflated, reinflated immediately, and finally deflated after 1 min to reduce the sudden absorption of anesthetic into the systemic circulation.

8. Contraindicated in patients with hypersensitivity to amide-type local anesthetics.

9. The recommended volumes for brachial plexus block are consistent with available data on plasma levels (subtoxic) after brachial plexus block. The risks of systemic toxicity may be decreased by adding epinephrine to the local anesthetic and avoiding IV injection, which may result in an immediate toxic reaction.

10. Toxic plasma levels (e.g., from accidental intravascular injection) may cause cardiopulmonary collapse and seizures. Premonitory signs and symptoms manifest as numbness of the tongue and circumoral tissues, metallic taste, restlessness, tinnitus, and tremors. Support of circulation (IV fluids, vasopressors, IV sodium bicarbonate 1-2 mEq/kg to treat cardiac toxicity [sodium

channel blockade], IV bretylium 5 mg/kg, DC cardioversion/defibrillation for ventricular arrhythmias) and securing a patent airway (ventilate with 100% oxygen) are paramount. Thiopental (0.5-2 mg/kg IV), midazolam (0.02-0.04 mg/kg IV), or diazepam (0.1 mg/kg IV) may be used for prophylaxis and/or treatment of seizures.

11. The level of sympathetic blockade (bradycardia with block above T5) determines the degree of hypotension (often heralded by nausea and vomiting) after epidural or intrathecal bupivacaine (or other local anesthetic). Fluid hydration (10-20 ml/kg NS or lactated Ringer's solution), vasopressor agents (e.g., ephedrine), and left uterine displacement in pregnant patients may be used for prophylaxis and/or treatment. Administer atropine to treat bradycardia.

12. Epidural, caudal, or intrathecal injections should be avoided when the patient has hypovolemic shock, septicemia, infection at the injection site, or coagulopathy.

13. Monitor for hypoventilation with release of the cuff when a muscle relaxant is added to the local anesthetic solution for intravenous regional blockade.

Principal Adverse Reactions

Cardiovascular: Hypotension, arrhythmias, cardiac arrest
Pulmonary: Respiratory impairment, arrest
CNS: Seizures, tinnitus, blurred vision
Allergic: Urticaria, angioneurotic edema, anaphylactoid symptoms
Epidural/Caudal/Spinal: High spinal, hypotension, urinary retention, lower extremity weakness and paralysis, loss of sphincter control, headache, backache, cranial nerve palsies, slowing of labor

BUTORPHANOL TARTRATE (STADOL)

Use(s): Analgesia

Dosing: IM, 1 to 4 mg (0.02-0.08 mg/kg) q3-4hr
IV, 0.5 to 2 mg (0.01-0.04 mg/kg) q3-4hr
Nasal spray, 1-2 mg (1-2 sprays q3-4 hr)
Patient controlled analgesia: IV bolus, 0.2-0.3 mg
(4-6 μg/kg); lockout interval, 5-15 min
Epidural bolus, 1-2 mg (0.02-0.04 mg/kg)
Elimination: Hepatic/renal
How Supplied: Injection: 1 mg/ml, 2 mg/ml
Storage: Injection: Room temperature (15°-30° C). Protect from light.
Dilution for Infusion: Epidural bolus, Dilute 1-2 mg in 10 ml local anesthetic or (preservative-free) NS.

Pharmacology

A synthetic benzomorphan derivative, butorphanol tartrate is a potent opioid agonist-antagonist (partial agonist) with analgesic potency 3.5-7 times that of morphine or 30-40 times that of meperidine. Butorphanol has a ceiling effect for respiratory depression and analgesia at high doses (>30-60 μg/kg). Respiratory depression and psychotomimetic effects of butorphanol may be reversed by naloxone. Analgesic doses increase systemic blood pressure, pulmonary artery blood pressure, and cardiac output. Analgesia is not adequate for the performance of surgery. Usefulness of epidural butorphanol is limited by dose-dependent increase in sedation secondary to vascular uptake and activation of kappa receptors in the central nervous system.

Pharmacokinetics

Onset: IV, 1-5 min; IM, 10 min; nasal, < 15 min
Peak Effect: IV, 5-10 min; IM, 30-60 min; nasal, 1-2 hr
Duration: IV, 2-4 hr; IM/epidural, 3-4 hr; nasal, 4-5 hr
Interaction/Toxicity: Decreases effectiveness of parenteral and epidural/spinal opioid agonists; may precipitate withdrawal in opioid-dependent patients; additive effects with phenothiazines, droperidol, barbiturates, and other tranquilizers

Guidelines/Precautions

1. Slight increase in systolic blood pressure when used for premedication.
2. May cause respiratory depression.
3. Use with caution in patients who have been chronically receiving opiate agonists. Butorphanol may precipitate withdrawal symptoms as a result of opiate antagonist effect.
4. Crosses the placental barrier, so use during labor may produce respiratory depression in the neonate. Resuscitation may be required; have naloxone available.
5. Drug increases cardiac work and should be used with caution in patients with ischemic disease.
6. Undesirable side effects of epidural butorphanol include delayed respiratory depression, pruritus, nausea and vomiting, urinary retention. Naloxone (IV, 0.2-0.4 mg prn or infusion, 5-10 μg/kg/hr) is effective for prophylaxis and/or treatment. Ventilatory support for respiratory depression must be readily available. Antihistamines (e.g., diphenhydramine, 12.5-25 mg IV/IM q6hr prn) may be used in treating pruritus. Metoclopramide (10 mg IV q6hr prn) may be used in treating nausea and

vomiting. Urinary retention may require straight bladder catheterization.

7. Epidural/intrathecal injections should be avoided when the patient has septicemia, infection at the injection site, or coagulopathy.

Principal Adverse Reactions

Cardiovascular: Hypertension, hypotension, palpitations
Pulmonary: Respiratory depression
CNS: Euphoria, hallucinations, sedation, headache
GI: Nausea, vomiting
Eye: Miosis
Autonomic: Flushing, dry mouth, sensitivity to cold

CALCIUM CHLORIDE (CALCIUM CHLORIDE)

Use(s): Electrolyte replacement, positive inotrope, treatment of hyperkalemia (with ECG changes), hypermagnesemia, and calcium antagonist overdose

Dosing: IV, 500-1000 mg (10 mg/kg) 2%-10% solution.
Do not exceed rate of 1 ml/min.
Maintain serum calcium levels at 8.5-10 mg/dl.
Elimination: GI, renal
How Supplied: Injection, 10% solution
Storage: Injection: room temperature (15°-30° C)

Pharmacology

Calcium is essential for maintenance of the functional integrity of nervous, muscular, and skeletal systems, cell membrane, and capillary permeability. It is also essential for contraction of cardiac, smooth, and skeletal muscles, renal function, respiration, and blood coagulation. Increase in cardiac output follows an increase in myocardial contractility and a decrease in peripheral vascular resistance and is associated with a decreased heart rate. 10% Calcium chloride is more irritating to the veins and provides three times more calcium (270 mg/13.5 mEq/g) than an equal volume of 10% calcium gluconate (90 mg/4.5 mEq/g).

Pharmacokinetics

Onset: <30 sec (electrolyte replacement and inotropic effects)
Peak Effect: <1 min (electrolyte replacement and inotropic effects)
Duration: 10-20 minutes (inotropic effects)
Interaction/Toxicity: May precipitate arrhythmias in digitalized patients; antagonizes effects of verapamil and other calcium channel blockers, magnesium; sloughing and necrosis with extravasation, IM or SC injection; complexes with tetracycline antibiotics when mixed; chemically incompatible in parenteral admixtures of carbonates, phosphates, sulfates, or tartrates.

Guidelines/Precautions

1. IV injection should be given slowly and through a large vein to minimize venous irritation.
2. Treat extravasation by discontinuing calcium and local infiltration with 1% procaine HCL and hyaluronidase.
3. Hypercalcemia is more dangerous than hypocalcemia. ECG monitoring and frequent determinations of serum calcium concentrations should be done.
4. Rapid IV injection may cause arrhythmias, hypotension, or hypertension.
5. Inadvertent systemic overloading with calcium ions can produce an acute hypercalcemic syndrome characterized

by a markedly elevated plasma calcium level, weakness, lethargy, intractable nausea and vomiting, coma and sudden death. Treat by immediate discontinuation of calcium, administration of normal saline infusions (up to 6 L/24 hr), and IV furosemide (20-40 mg every 2-4 hr). Fluid therapy can be monitored with a CVP catheter.

6. Chloride salt is acidifying and should not be used when acidosis coincides with hypocalcemia.

7. Hypocalcemia may develop after rapid transfusion of citrated blood (>2 ml/kg/min) or large volumes of colloid solution. Administer IV calcium 1.35 mEq/27 mg (adults) or 0.45 mEq/9 mg (children) after every 100 ml of citrated blood.

Principal Adverse Reactions

Cardiovascular: Hypertension, hypotension, bradycardia, arrhythmias, cardiac arrest.
CNS: Lethargy, coma
Dermatologic: Sloughing, necrosis, abscess formation
Metabolic: Hypercalcemia

CALCIUM GLUCONATE (CALCIUM GLUCONATE)

Use(s): Electrolyte replacement, positive inotrope, treatment of hyperkalemia (with ECG changes), hypermagnesemia, and calcium antagonist overdose.

Dosing: IV, 500-2000 mg (30 mg/kg) (10% solution). Do not exceed rate of 1 ml/min.
PO, 500-2000 mg as required.
Maintain serum calcium levels at 8.5-10 mg/dl.
Elimination: G1, renal

How Supplied:

Injection, 10% solution

Tablets, 500 mg (45 mg calcium), 650 mg (58.5 mg calcium), 1 g (90 mg calcium)

Storage: Injection: room temperature (15°-30° C)

Pharmacology

Calcium is essential for maintenance of the functional integrity of nervous, muscular, and skeletal systems, cell membrane, and capillary permeability. It is also essential for contraction of cardiac, smooth, and skeletal muscles, renal function, respiration, and blood coagulation. Increase in cardiac output follows an increase in myocardial contractility; a decrease in peripheral vascular resistance is associated with a decreased heart rate. 10% Calcium gluconate is less irritating to the veins and provides 3 times less calcium (90 mg/4.5 mEq/g) than an equal volume of 10% calcium chloride (270 mg/13.5 mEq/g).

Pharmacokinetics

Onset: IV <30 sec (electrolyte replacement and inotropic effects)

Peak Effect: IV <1 min (electrolyte replacement and inotropic effects)

Duration of Action: IV 10-20 min (inotropic effects)

Interaction/Toxicity: May precipitate arrhythmias in digitalized patients; antagonizes effects of verapamil and other calcium channel blockers, magnesium; sloughing and necrosis with extravasation, IM or SC injection; complexes with tetracycline antibiotics when mixed; chemically incompatible in parenteral admixtures of carbonates, phosphates, sulfates, or tartrates; rapid IV injection may cause peripheral vasodilation and hypotension.

Guidelines/Precautions

1. IV injection should be done slowly and through a large vein to minimize venous irritation.
2. Treat extravasation by discontinuing calcium and local infiltration with 1% procaine HCL and hyaluronidase.
3. Hypercalcemia is more dangerous than hypocalcemia. ECG monitoring and frequent determinations of serum calcium concentrations should be done.
4. Rapid IV injection may cause arrhythmias, hypotension, or hypertension.
5. Inadvertent systemic overloading with calcium ions can produce an acute hypercalcemic syndrome characterized by a markedly elevated plasma calcium level, weakness, lethargy, intractable nausea and vomiting, coma, and sudden death. Treat by immediate discontinuation of calcium, administration of normal saline infusions (up to 6 L/24 hr), and IV furosemide (20-40 mg every 2-4 hr). Fluid therapy can be monitored with a CVP catheter.
6. Hypocalcemia may develop after rapid transfusion of citrated blood (>2 ml/kg/min) or large volumes of colloid solution. Administer IV calcium 1.35 mEq/27 mg (adults) or 0.45 mEq/9 mg (children) after every 100 ml of citrated blood.

Principal Adverse Reactions

Cardiovascular: Hypertension, hypotension, bradycardia, arrhythmias, cardiac arrest
CNS: Lethargy, coma
Dermatologic: Sloughing, necrosis, abscess formation
Metabolic: Hypercalcemia

CAPTOPRIL (CAPOTEN)

Use(s): Antihypertensive; treatment of congestive heart failure (CHF); prevention of post MI ventricular remodeling

Dosing: Hypertension: PO, 6.25-50 mg bid or tid. Sublingual (chewed), 25-50 mg

CHF: PO, 25-100 mg tid to maximum of 450 mg/day

Use initial low doses (6.25 mg) in hypertension or CHF, when added to a diuretic, or in patients with salt depletion, renal impairment.

Elimination: Renal, hepatic

How Supplied: Tablets, 12.5 mg, 25 mg, 37.5 mg, 50 mg, 100 mg

Pharmacology

Captopril inhibits angiotensin converting enzyme (ACE), thereby blocking the conversion of angiotensin I to angiotensin II. Angiotensin II is a potent vasoconstrictor and acts to release aldosterone. Thus captopril lowers total peripheral vascular resistance and blood pressure and inhibits water and salt retention normally produced by aldosterone. It lowers both preload and afterload. ACE also is responsible for the metabolism of bradykinin, a potent vasodilatory autacoid. Bradykinin levels in tissue increase after captopril. Cerebral blood flow and intracranial pressure are increased.

Pharmacokinetics

Onset: PO/SL, <15 minutes

Peak Effect: PO, 60-90 min; SL <60 minutes

Duration: PO/SL, 2-6 hr

Interaction/Toxicity: Additive hypotensive effects with diuretics, vasodilators, beta blockers, calcium channel blockers, volatile anesthetics; elevates serum potassium levels, which may be significant with renal insufficiency and use of potassium-sparing diuretics such as spironolactone, triamterene, or amiloride; antihypertensive effect antagonized by indomethacin and other nonsteroidal antiinflammatory drugs.

Guidelines/Precautions

1. May be associated with angioedema, bone marrow suppression, and proteinuria. Emergency therapy for angioedema with airway obstruction should include SC epinephrine 1:1000 (0.5-1.0 mg).
2. Immune-based side effects (taste disturbances, rashes, neutropenia), seldom serious provided the total daily dose is <150 mg, are found largely in patients with collagen vascular disease or receiving other drugs likely to alter the immune response (e.g., procainamide, tocainide, hydralazine, acebutolol, probenicid). All patients should have a pre-captopril renal evaluation, tests for antinuclear antibodies, a full blood count, and a screen of all other medications (check for potassium- retaining diuretics).
3. May cause profound first-dose hypotension, particularly in patients who are volume-depleted or when used concomitantly with agents that reduce vascular volume. Treat hypotension with volume expansion.
4. Should not be used with potassium-sparing diuretics because of the possibility of hyperkalemia.
5. May be associated with a persistent, dry cough (and on occasion, bronchospasm) resistant to normal antitus-

sives but that may respond to a decrease in dose or to inhaled cromolyn therapy.

6. Use with caution in hypertensive patients with renal disease. Increases in BUN and serum creatinine may develop after reduction of blood pressure. Monitor renal function during the first few weeks of therapy.

7. In patients with CHF, whose renal function may depend on the renin-angiotensin-aldosterone system, treatment with captopril may be associated with oliguria or progressive azotemia and, rarely, with acute renal failure or death.

8. Use in pregnancy associated with increased incidence of cranial facial dysplasias, other fetal abnormalities.

Principal Adverse Reactions

Cardiovascular: Hypotension, palpitations, tachycardia
Pulmonary: Cough, dyspnea, bronchospasm
CNS: Dizziness, fatigue
GI: Abdominal pain, dysgeusia, peptic ulcer
Dermatologic: Rash, pruritus
Renal: Elevation of BUN and creatinine, proteinuria, renal failure
Hematologic: Neutropenia, thrombocytopenia, hemolytic anemia, eosinophilia
Other: Angioedema, lymphadenopathy

CARBOPROST TROMETHAMINE (HEMABATE)

Use(s): Treatment of postpartum hemorrhage caused by uterine atony

Dosing: Deep IM, 250 μg. Dose may be repeated at 15-90 min intervals if necessary. Maximum dose 2 mg (8 doses).

Elimination: Renal, hepatic
How Supplied: Injection, 250 μg/ml
Storage: Refrigerate (2°-4° C)

Pharmacology

Carboprost, an oxytocic, is the tromethamine salt of the methyl analog of naturally occurring prostaglandin F2 alpha. The drug stimulates uterine contractions at all stages of pregnancy (in contrast to oxytocin). Use of carboprost after failure of conventional methods of management (oxytocin, uterine massage, ergot preparations, such as methylergonovine) may result in satisfactory control of life-threatening postpartum hemorrhage.

Pharmacokinetics

Onset: <5 min
Peak Effect: 15-60 min
Duration: >60 min
Interaction/Toxicity: May augment the activity of other oxytocic agents.

Guidelines/Precautions

1. Contraindicated in patients with acute pelvic inflammatory disease.
2. Use with caution in patients with asthma; hypertension; cardiovascular, pulmonary, renal, or hepatic disease; anemia; jaundice; diabetes; epilepsy.
3. Contains benzyl alcohol, which has been reported to be associated with a fatal "grasping syndrome" in premature infants.
4. Use may be associated with transient pyrexia, which may be due to the effect of carboprost on hypothalamic thermoregulation.

Principal Adverse Reactions

Cardiovascular: Hypertension, palpitations, tachycardia
Pulmonary: Cough, respiratory distress, pulmonary edema, bronchospasm
CNS: Headache, drowsiness, tinnitus, blurred vision, vertigo
GI: Epigastric pain, nausea, vomiting
Uterus: Uterine perforation, retained placental fragment, uterine sacculation
Dermatologic: Rash
Hematologic: Leukocytosis

CHLORDIAZEPOXIDE HCL (LIBRIUM)

Use(s): Premedication, sedative/hypnotic, treatment of acute alcohol withdrawal

Dosing: Premedication:
        PO, 5-10 mg (0.2 mg/kg).
        IM, 50-100 mg (1-2 mg/kg).
        Withdrawal symptoms: IM/IV/PO, 50 - 100 mg (IM or IV: dilute in supplied diluent, 5 ml NS or sterile water). Repeat every 2-4 hr if necessary. Maximum daily dose 300 mg. Do not use intramuscular diluent for intravenous administration.
Elimination: Hepatic
How Supplied:
Injection, 100 mg (5 ml dry filled ampule containing 100 mg chlordiazepoxide and a 2 ml ampule of special intramuscular diluent. Solution is unstable. Prepare just before use. Discard unused portions).
Tablets, 5 mg, 10 mg, 25 mg.

Storage:

Injection, refrigerate diluent (2°-8° C). Injection should be
  prepared immediately before use. Discard unused portion.
Tablets, protect from light.

Pharmacology

This benzodiazepine increases gamma-aminobutyric acid
(GABA) neurotransmission in the CNS. The drug exerts
antianxiety, sedative, appetite-stimulating, and weak analgesic effects. Chlordiazepoxide may possess some peripheral anticholinergic activity. It has minimal depressant
effects on ventilation and circulation in the absence of
other CNS depressant drugs. Recovery may be prolonged.

Pharmacokinetics

Onset: IV, 1-5 min; IM/PO, 15-30 min
Peak Effect: IV, 5 min; IM/PO, 45 min
Duration: IV, 15 min-1 hr; IM/PO, 2-6 hr
Interaction/Toxicity: Potentiates CNS and circulatory-
depressant effect of narcotics, alcohol, sedative-hypnotics,
phenothiazines, MAO inhibitors; reduces requirements for
volatile anesthetics; elimination decreased by cimetidine,
propranolol; effects antagonized by flumazenil.

Guidelines/Precautions

1. Reduce dosage in elderly, hypovolemic, high-risk surgical patients and with concomitant use of narcotics and
   other sedatives.
2. Paradoxic reactions (excitement, stimulation) may occur
   in hyperactive aggressive children and psychiatric
   patients.

3. Treat overdosage with supportive measures and flumazenil (slow IV, 0.2-1 mg).

Principal Adverse Reactions

Cardiovascular: Hypotension, tachycardia
Pulmonary: Hypoventilation, apnea
CNS: Drowsiness, ataxia, confusion
Hematologic: Agranulocytosis
Other: Hepatic dysfunction

CHLOROPROCAINE HCL (NESACAINE)

Use(s): Regional anesthesia

Dosing: Infiltration/peripheral nerve block : <40 ml (1%-2% solution)

Epidural:

Bolus, 200-750 mg (10-25 ml of a 2% or 3% solution). Approximately 1.5-2 ml/kg for each segment to be anesthetized). Repeat doses at 40-60 min intervals.

Infusion, 20-30 ml/hr (0.5%-1% solution).

Caudal: 10-25 ml of a 2% or 3% solution. Children 0.4-0.7-1.0 ml/kg. (L2-T10-T7 level of anesthesia). Repeat doses at 40-60 min intervals.

Rate of onset and potency of local anesthetic action may be enhanced by carbonation. (Add 1 ml of 8.4% sodium bicarbonate with 30 ml of 2%-3% chloroprocaine. Do not use if there is precipitation.)

Maximum safe dose: 10 mg/kg (without epinephrine), 15 mg/kg (with epinephrine).

Use only preservative-free solution for epidural or caudal anesthesia. Except where contraindicated, vasoconstrictive drugs may be added to increase effect and prolong local or regional anesthesia. For dosage/route guidelines, see Epinephrine, Dosing; or Phenylephrine, Dosing. Do not use vasoconstrictive drugs for local anesthesia of end organs (digits, penis, nose, ears).

Elimination: Plasma cholinesterase

How Supplied: 1% and 2% preservative-containing solution; 2% and 3% preservative-free solutions.

Storage: Room temperature (15°-30° C). Protect from light.

Dilution for infusion: Epidural use only, 12.5 ml (2%) in 37.5 ml (preservative-free) NS (0.5% solution)

Pharmacology

Chloroprocaine is a benzoic acid ester and short-acting local anesthetic. It stabilizes the neuronal membrane and prevents the initiation and transmission of impulses. It is rapidly hydrolyzed by plasma pseudocholinesterase with one of the metabolites being para-aminobenzoic acid. Epinephrine prolongs the duration of action by reducing the rate of absorption and plasma concentration. Toxic blood concentrations produce decreased myocardial contractility and peripheral vasodilation, resulting in decreased arterial pressure and cardiac output. It is ineffective for topical anesthesia. Chloroprocaine is not recommended for IV regional anesthesia because of the high incidence of thrombophlebitis. Epidural chloroprocaine may decrease the duration of analgesia of epidural narcotics, possibly because of a specific antagonism of mu-receptor-mediated analgesia.

Pharmacokinetics

Onset: Infiltration/epidural, 6-12 min
Peak Effect: Infiltration/epidural, 10-20 min
Duration: Infiltration/epidural 30-60 min (prolonged with epinephrine)
Interaction/Toxicity: Prolongs the effect of succinyl-choline; metabolite (PABA) inhibits the action of sulfon-amides and aminosalicylic acid; toxicity is enhanced by cimetidine, anticholinesterases (which inhibit degradation); high plasma levels are associated with seizures, respiratory and circulatory depression; benzodiazepines, barbiturates, and volatile anesthetics increase seizure threshold; duration of local or regional anesthesia is prolonged by vasoconstric-tor agents, e.g., epinephrine; alkalinization increases rate of onset and potency of local or regional anesthesia; epidural chloroprocaine antagonizes the analgesic effect of epidural bupivacaine, narcotics, and alpha-2 agonists.

Guidelines/Precautions

1. Do not use for spinal anesthesia.
2. Use with caution in patients with severe disturbances of cardiac rhythm, shock, or heart block.
3. Reduce doses in obstetric, elderly, hypovolemic, high-risk patients, and those with increased intraabdominal pressure.
4. Potential for allergic reaction with repeated use.
5. Contraindicated in patients with hypersensitivity to chloroprocaine or ester-type local anesthetics and patients with allergy to suntan lotion (contains PABA derivatives).
6. Occasional cases of severe back pain have occurred after epidural anesthesia with chloroprocaine. Con-

tributing factors include use of a disodium edetate
(EDTA)-containing formulation of chloroprocaine,
large volume (>20 ml), and low pH of the commercial
solution (pH may be increased with carbonation).

7. Toxic plasma levels, e.g., from accidental intravascular injection, may cause cardiopulmonary collapse
and seizures. Premonitory signs and symptoms manifest as numbness of the tongue and circumoral tissues,
metallic taste, restlessness, tinnitus, and tremors. Support of circulation (IV fluids, vasopressors, IV sodium
bicarbonate 1-2 mEq/kg to treat cardiac toxicity [sodi-
um channel blockade], IV bretylium 5 mg/kg, DC
cardioversion/defibrillation for ventricular arrhythmias) and securing a patent airway (ventilate with
100% oxygen) are paramount. Thiopental (0.5-2
mg/kg IV), midazolam (0.02-0.04 mg/kg IV), or
diazepam (0.1 mg/kg IV) may be used for prophylaxis
and/or treatment.

8. The level of sympathetic blockade (bradycardia with
block above T5) determines the degree of hypotension
(often heralded by nausea and vomiting) after epidural
administration of chloroprocaine. Fluid hydration
(10-20 ml/kg NS or lactated Ringer's solution), vasopressor agents, e.g., ephedrine, and left uterine displacement in pregnant patients may be used for prophylaxis and/or treatment. Administer atropine to treat
bradycardia.

9. Epidural, caudal, or intrathecal injections should be
avoided when the patient has hypovolemic shock, septicemia, infection at the injection site, or coagulopathy.

10. Persistent neurologic damage or prolonged sensory or
motor deficits have been reported after accidental spinal

anesthesia with large doses of sodium bisulfite and/or methyl paraben-containing chloroprocaine solutions.

Principal Adverse Reactions

Cardiovascular: Hypotension, arrhythmias, bradycardia
Pulmonary: Respiratory depression, arrest
CNS: Seizures, tinnitus, tremors
Allergic: Urticaria, pruritus, angioneurotic edema
Epidural/Caudal/Spinal: High spinal; arachnoiditis; backache; loss of perineal sensation and sexual function; permanent motor, sensory, and/or autonomic (sphincter control); deficit of lower segments; slowing of labor.

CHLORPROMAZINE HCL (THORAZINE)

Use(s): Antipsychotic, premedication, antiemetic, and relief of hiccups.

Dosing: Premedication:
PO, 25-50 mg (0.5-1 mg/kg)
IM, 12.5-25 mg (0.25-0.5 mg/kg)
Emesis/Hiccups:
PO/IM, 10-50 mg (0.25-0.55 mg/kg) 3 or 4 times daily
Maximum IM dosage for children: 40 mg/day (<5 years of age), 75 mg/day (5-12 years of age);
Rectal, 50-100 mg (1.1 mg/kg)
IV, 25-50 mg (0.25-0.55 mg/kg). Dilute to 1 mg/ml with NS. Give at rate of 1 mg/min.
Observe for hypotension with parenteral administration.

Elimination: Hepatic
How Supplied:
Tablets: 10 mg, 25 mg, 50 mg, 100 mg, 200 mg
Oral solution: 2 mg/ml
Oral concentrate: 30 mg/ml, 100 mg/ml
Rectal suppositories: 25mg and 100 mg
Injection: 25 mg/ml
Storage: Injection/tablets: room temperature (15°-30° C).
Protect from light.

Pharmacology

Chlorpromazine is a phenothiazine tranquilizer with strong antiemetic, antiadrenergic, anticholinergic, and sedative effects. The drug has weak antiserotonergic, antihistaminic, and ganglion-blocking activity. The neuroleptic actions are most likely due to antagonism of dopamine as a synaptic neurotransmitter in the basal ganglia and limbic portions of the forebrain. Moderate extrapyramidal side effects are evidence of interference with the normal actions of dopamine.

Pharmacokinetics

Onset: IV/IM, within 30 min; PO, 30-60 min
Peak Effect: PO, 2-3 hr
Duration: PO, 4-6 hr; IM, 3-4 hr
Interaction/Toxicity: Potentiates depressant effects of barbiturates, narcotics, anesthetics; has additive anticholinergic effects with atropine, glycopyrrolate, and other anticholinergics; decreases hepatic metabolism and increases serum levels and pharmacologic/toxic effects of tricyclic antidepressants; decreases neuronal uptake and antihypertensive effects of guanethidine; decreases alpha adrenergic effects

of epinephrine, leaving unopposed beta activity; may potentiate neuromuscular blockade in conjunction with polypeptide antibiotics; interferes with metabolism of Dilantin and
may precipitate toxicity; lithium reduces bioavailability;
mephentermine, epinephrine, thiazide diuretics potentiate
perphenazine-induced hypotension; concomitant administration of propranolol increases plasma levels of both drugs.

Guidelines/Precautions

1. May suppress laryngeal reflex with possible aspiration
   of vomitus.
2. May lower seizure threshold.
3. Use cautiously in geriatric patients, patients with glaucoma, prostatic hypertrophy and seizure disorders, and
   children with acute illnesses (e.g. chickenpox, measles).
4. Neuroleptic malignant syndrome, a rare but potentially
   fatal side effect, may manifest with hyperpyrexia, muscle rigidity, altered mental status, and evidence of autonomic instability (irregular pulse or blood pressure,
   tachycardia, diaphoresis, arrhythmias). Discontinue
   chlorpromazine, treat symptomatically and with dantrolene or bromocriptine (PO 2.5-10 mg tid).
5. Extrapyramidal reactions may consist of dystonic reactions, feelings of motor restlessness (akathisia), and
   parkinsonian signs and symptoms. Dystonic reactions
   occur more frequently in children, especially those with
   acute infections, whereas parkinsonian symptoms predominate in geriatric patients. Therapy should include
   discontinuation of chlorpromazine or reduction in
   dosage and treatment with an anticholinergic antiparkinsonian agent (e.g., benztropine, trihexyphenidyl) or with
   diphenhydramine (IV/PO 25 mg). Maintenance of an
   adequate airway should be instituted if necessary.

6. Do not use epinephrine to treat chlorpromazine-associated hypotension. Phenothiazines cause a reversal of epinephrine's vasopressor effects and a further lowering of blood pressure. Treat the drug-induced hypotension with norepinephrine or phenylephrine.

Principal Adverse Reactions

Cardiovascular: Hypotension, tachycardia
CNS: Extrapyramidal reactions, seizures, syncope, drowsiness
Allergic: Urticaria, photosensitivity
Hematologic: Agranulocytosis, hemolytic anemia
Other: Neuroleptic malignant syndrome

CIMETIDINE (TAGAMET)

Use(s): Treatment of peptic ulcer, pathologic hypersecretory states; prophylaxis against acid pulmonary aspiration, stress ulcers, upper GI bleeding in critically ill patients.

Dosing: PO, 300 mg (7.5 mg/kg) q6-8hr; alternately 400-1600 mg at bedtime
Slow IV/IM, 300 mg (7.5 mg/kg) q6-8hr. Dilute IV dose in 20 ml D_5W or NS (15 mg/ml) and infuse over 2 min
Infusion, 50 mg/hr
Elimination: Renal, hepatic
How Supplied:
Tablets, 200 mg, 300 mg, 400 mg, 800 mg
Oral solution, 60 mg/ml
Injection, 150 mg/ml
Storage: Injection/tablets, room temperature (15°-30° C).

Protect from light. Do not refrigerate because precipitation (of injection) may occur.

Dilution for Infusion: 250 mg in 50 ml D_5W or NS (concentration, 5 mg/ml, rate 10 ml/hr)

Pharmacology

Cimetidine is a competitive histamine H_2 receptor antagonist that blocks the effects of histamine, pentagastrin, and acetylcholine on gastric acid secretion. It has no significant effect on gastric emptying time, volume, lower esophageal sphincter tone, or pancreatic secretions. Like ranitidine, it will not reduce the pH of gastric fluid already present in the stomach, but it will increase the pH of fluid produced thereafter.

Pharmacokinetics

Onset: PO/IV, < 45 min
Peak Effect: PO/IV, 60-90 min
Duration: PO, 6-8 hr; IV, 4-4.5 hr
Interaction/Toxicity: May inhibit metabolism of benzodiazepines, caffeine, calcium channel blockers, carbamazepine, chloroquine, labetalol, lidocaine, metoprolol, metronidazole, pentoxifylline, phenytoin, propranolol, quinidine, quinine, sulfonylureas, theophyllines, triamterene, tricyclic antidepressants, coumarin anticoagulants; decreases renal tubular secretion of procainamide; may decrease serum concentrations of digoxin; may decrease effects of tocainide; increases the neuromuscular blocking effects of succinylcholine and nondepolarizing muscle relaxants; absorption of cimetidine may be decreased by antacids, anticholinergics, metoclopramide.

Guidelines/Precautions

1. Rapid IV administration may produce hypotension, bradycardia, or heart block.
2. Use with caution in elderly patients because it may produce central nervous system dysfunction (e.g., confusion, agitation, seizures).
3. May increase airway resistance in patients with bronchial asthma, reflecting loss of H_2-receptor-mediated bronchodilation, leaving unopposed H_1-receptor-mediated bronchoconstriction.

Principal Adverse Reactions

Cardiovascular: Bradycardia, arrhythmias
CNS: Dizziness, somnolence, confusion, disorientation, seizures
GI: Diarrhea
Dermatologic: Rash
Musculoskeletal: Arthralgia
Endocrine: Gynecomastia
Hematologic: Agranulocytosis, aplastic anemia, thrombocytopenia
Renal: Minor reversible elevations of serum creatinine

CLONIDINE HCL (CATAPRES)

Use(s): Antihypertensive, premedication, treatment of opioid/alcohol withdrawal states, supplementation of anesthesia; epidural/spinal analgesia; prolongation of duration of action of local anesthetics.

Dosing: Premedication: PO, 3-5 μg/kg
Antihypertensive: PO, 0.05-0.1 mg 3 or 4 times daily

Detoxification: PO, 0.1-0.3 mg 3 or 4 times daily. Titrate to patient response and tolerance.

Hypertensive crisis: IV, 0.15-0.3 mg over 5 min

Supplementation of anesthesia:

IV bolus, 2-4 μg/kg over 5 min

Infusion, 1-2 μg/kg/hr

Sublingual, 0.2-0.4 mg/day

Transdermal, 0.1-0.3 mg/24 hr; replace systems every 7 days

Epidural analgesia:

Bolus, 150-500 μg (2-10 μg/kg), Dilute in 10 ml (preservative-free) NS or local anesthetic.

Infusion, 10-40 μg/hr (0.2-0.8 μg/kg/hr)

Spinal analgesia: Bolus, 15-150 μg (0.3-3 μg/kg)

Brachial plexus block: Add 25-150 μg (0.5-3 μg/kg) clonidine to 40 ml local anesthetic.

Elimination: Renal, hepatic

How Supplied:

Tablets, 0.1 mg, 0.2 mg, or 0.3 mg

Transdermal therapeutic system, releases 0.1, 0.2, 0.3 mg/24 hr

Parenteral form currently is not available for general clinical use in the United States.

Storage: Transdermal system/tablets, temperature below 30° C. Protect from light.

Dilution for Infusion: Epidural, 200 μg in 100 ml local anesthetic or (preservative-free) NS solution (2 μg/ml)

Pharmacology

Clonidine is a selective agonist at the alpha-2 adrenoceptor with a ratio of 200:1 (alpha-2:alpha-1). It inhibits central sympathetic outflow through activation of alpha-2 adrenergic receptors in the medullary vasomotor center. Clonidine decreases blood pressure, heart rate, and cardiac output, and produces a dose-dependent sedation. Unlike opioids, it produces minor respiratory depression with a ceiling effect, and unlike benzodiazepines, does not enhance opioid-induced repiratory depression. Direct stimulation of peripheral alpha-1 adrenergic receptors results in transient vaso-constriction. Rebound hypertension occurs when therapy is discontinued abruptly. Clonidine suppresses signs and symptoms of opioid withdrawal by replacing opioid-mediated inhibition with alpha-2–mediated inhibition of central nervous system sympathetic activity. It acts on alpha-2 adrenoceptors located in the dorsal horn neurones of the spinal cord. Local effects may include inhibition of the release of nociceptive neurotransmitters such as substance P (presynaptic first-order neurones) and decrease in the rate of depolarization (postsynaptic second-order neurones). These effects, which are separate from opiate-mediated analgesia, are not inhibited by opiate antagonists, e.g., naloxone, but are blocked by alpha-2 antagonist drugs, e.g., phentolamine. As an anesthetic adjunct, clonidine attenuates the hemodynamic response to intubation, reduces requirements for opioids and volatile anesthetics, prolongs regional block, and enhances postoperative analgesia.

Pharmacokinetics

Onset:
PO, 30-60 min (hypotensive effect)
IV, <5 min (hypotensive effect)
Epidural/spinal, (analgesia) <15 min
Transdermal (hypotensive effect), <2 days
Peak Effect:
PO, 2-4 hr (hypotensive effect)

Transdermal, 2-3 days (hypotensive effect)
IV, 30-60 min (hypotensive effect)
Duration:
PO, 8 hr (hypotensive effect)
IV, >4 hr (hypotensive effect)
Epidural/spinal (analgesia and sedation), 3-4 hr
Transdermal (hypotensive effect), 7 days
Interaction/Toxicity: Potentiates effects of opioids, alcohol, barbiturates, sedatives; augments pressor response to intravenous ephedrine; decreases the requirements for volatile anesthetics (MAC reduced by 50%); has decreased effects with alpha-2 antagonists, tricyclic antidepressants; addition of clonidine to epidural or spinal anesthetics or narcotics prolongs duration of sensory and motor block and may be accompanied by hypotension and bradycardia; addition of clonidine to local anesthetics results in prolonged anesthesia and analgesia.

Guidelines/Precautions

1. When discontinuing clonidine therapy, rebound hypertension may be minimized by tapered withdrawal of the drug over 2-4 days. Discontinuation for 6 hr or more before surgery may result in perioperative hypertension.
2. Use with caution in patients with severe coronary insufficiency, recent myocardial infarction, cerebrovascular disease, chronic renal failure, Raynaud's disease, thromboangiitis obliterans, or a history of mental depression.
3. Epidural or spinal clonidine (>10 μg/kg) may produce dose-dependent maternal and fetal bradycardia.
4. Epidural, caudal, or intrathecal injections should be avoided when the patient has septicemia, infection at the injection site, or coagulopathy.

5. Clonidine transdermal system is contraindicated in patients with known hypersensitivity to clonidine or to any ingredient or component in the administration system.

6. Signs and symptoms of overdosage include somnolence, hypotension, transient hypertension, cardiac arrhythmias, respiratory depression, and seizures. Symptomatic and supportive measures should be instituted. Alpha adrenergic blockers, e.g., tolazoline (IV 10 mg) or phentolamine (IV 5 mg) may reverse the cardiovascular, sedative, and analgesic effects.

Principal Adverse Reactions

Cardiovascular: Hypotension, bradycardia, rebound hypertension with drug withdrawal, congestive heart failure, AV block

Pulmonary: Mild ventilatory depression, upper respiratory tract obstruction

CNS: Sedation, depression, anxiety

GU: Impotence, urinary retention

GI: Nausea, vomiting, parotid pain

Dermatologic: Rash, angioneurotic edema

COCAINE HCL (COCAINE HCL)

Use(s): Topical anesthesia and vasoconstriction (mucous membranes only)

Dosing: Topical, 1 mg/kg (1%-4% solution)
Nasal, 1-2 ml each nostril (1%-10% solution).
Concentrations greater than 4% are not advisable and increase potential for systemic toxic reactions. Maximum safe dose 1.5 mg/kg.

Elimination: Plasma cholinesterase, hepatic
How Supplied:
Cocaine solvets, soluble tablets 135 mg with lactose
Topical solution, 4% and 10%
Powder, 5 g, 25 g
Storage: Tablets/topical solution, room temperature (15°-30° C). Protect from light.

Pharmacology

A naturally occurring alkaloid and a topical anesthetic, cocaine stabilizes the neuronal membrane, preventing the initiation and transmission of nerve impulses. Sympathetically mediated vasoconstriction occurs secondary to a block in the uptake of catecholamines at adrenergic nerve endings. Small doses initially produce bradycardia and a decrease in arterial pressure by central vagal stimulation, but after moderate doses blood pressure and heart rate increase. Cocaine produces uterine vasoconstriction and may significantly decrease uterine blood flow. It stimulates the central nervous system, including the vomiting center, and produces euphoria.

Pharmacokinetics

Onset: <1 min
Peak Effect: 2-5 min
Duration: 30-120 min
Interaction/Toxicity: Causes sloughing of corneal epithelium and raises intraocular pressure; potentiates arrhythmogenic effects of sympathomimetics; increases MAC for volatile anesthetics; concomitant use with halothane may be associated with tachycardia, hypertension, and arrhythmias.

Guidelines/Precautions

1. Not for intraocular or intravenous use.
2. Sensitizes the heart to catecholamines. Concomitant use with epinephrine or ketamine is dangerous and unnecessary.
3. In some patients, even small doses of 0.4 mg/kg may cause hypertension, ventricular fibrillation, and cardiac arrest.
4. Treat tachycardia with a cardioselective beta blocker, e.g., esmolol IV 10-40 mg, or with a calcium channel blocker, e.g., verapamil IV 2.5-10 mg or nifedipine SL 10 mg. Use of a nonselective beta blocker may result in paradoxic hypertension caused by blocking of beta-2 vasodilating effects and unopposed alpha vasoconstricting effects of accumulated catecholamines.
5. Treat sodium-channel-blockade–induced QRS prolongation with sodium bicarbonate IV 1-2 mEq/kg.
6. Use with caution in patients with severely traumatized mucosa and sepsis in the region of proposed application.
7. Cocaine is detoxified by plasma and liver cholinesterases. Persons with cholinesterase deficiencies may be at increased risk for sudden death.
8. High addiction potential.

Principal Adverse Reactions

Cardiovascular: Hypertension, bradycardia and tachyarrhythmias, ventricular fibrillation
Pulmonary: Tachypnea, respiratory failure
CNS: Euphoria, excitement, seizures
Eyes: Sloughing of corneal epithelium

COUMARIN DERIVATIVE - WARFARIN SODIUM (COUMADIN, PANWARFIN, SOFARIN, CARFIN)

Use(s): Prophylaxis and/or treatment of venous thrombosis, pulmonary embolism; prophylaxis and/or treatment of thromboembolism in patients with atrial fibrillation, dilated cardiomyopathy, prosthetic heart valves; adjunct in prophylaxis of systemic embolism after myocardial infarction.

Dosing: Initial dose: PO/IV/IM, 10-15 mg

Daily dose: PO, 2-10 mg.

Adjust according to prothrombin time response, 1.2-2 times control. Preferably for standardized reporting, adjust dosing to INR (International Normalized Ratio) of 2-3 for low-intensity anticoagulation and INR of 4-5 for high-intensity anticoagulation.

Elimination: Renal, hepatic
How Supplied:
Tablets, 1 mg, 2 mg, 2.5 mg, 5 mg, 7.5 mg, 10 mg
Injection, 50 mg vial with 2 ml diluent
Storage: Injection/tablets, temperature below 40° C. Protect from light.

Pharmacology

4-Hydroxy coumarin and its derivatives (warfarin sodium, dicumarol) depress synthesis in the liver of vitamin K–dependent clotting factors II, VII, IX, and X. Warfarin sodium inhibits thrombus formation when stasis is induced. It does not have a direct effect on an established thrombus but may prevent further extension.

Pharmacokinetics

Onset: IV/IM/PO, 8-12 hr
Peak Effect: IV/IM/PO, 1-5 days
Duration: IV/IM/PO, 2-10 days
Interaction/Toxicity: Risks of hemorrhage increased with concomitant use of platelet aggregation inhibitors such as aspirin, phenylbutazone, other NSAIDS; enhanced anticoagulant effect with phenylbutazone, disulfiram, cimetidine, and clofibrate; decreased effect with alcohol, antihistamines, and barbiturates.

Guidelines/Precautions

1. The oral anticoagulants have a great potential for clinically significant drug reactions. Patients should not take any drugs, including nonprescription products, without the advice of a physician or pharmacist.
2. Periodic determination of prothrombin time is essential. Monitor PT daily during the initiation of therapy, with the addition or discontinuation of an interacting drug, and every 4-6 weeks after the patient is stabilized.
3. Contraindicated when risk of hemorrhage is greater than potential clinical benefits.
4. Regional anesthesia is contraindicated.
5. Use is not recommended during pregnancy, and heparin should be substituted if anticoagulation is required. Warfarin-induced embryopathies may occur in the 6th-12th week of pregnancy. CNS and ocular fetal anomalies may develop at any time during pregnancy. Only the inactive form of warfarin is secreted in milk, and postpartum administration poses no hazard.
6. Effects are counteracted by administration of vitamin K (PO 2.5-10 mg with mild or no bleeding; IV 5-50 mg

with frank bleeding), fresh whole blood, or fresh frozen plasma (15 ml/kg).

7. Anticoagulant therapy with warfarin sodium may enhance the release of atheroma plaque emboli, which may cause the "purple toes syndrome." Discontinuing therapy is recommended. The condition has been reported to be reversible.

8. The International Normalized Ratio (INR) takes into account the variability of each laboratory's source and preparation of tissue thromboplastin used in determining the prothrombin time ratio (patient's PT divided by control PT). The INR standardizes the prothrombin time ratio (PTR) by using an intrinsic sensitivity index (ISI), which is a measure of the ISI responsiveness of the tissue thromboplastin. (INR = PTR).

Principal Adverse Reactions

Hematologic: Agranulocytosis, eosinophilia, leukopenia, hemorrhage from any organ
GI: Nausea, vomiting
Dermatologic: Necrosis of skin, urticaria, dermatitis
Other: "Purple toes syndrome," neuropathy, nephropathy

CYCLOSPORINE A (SANDIMMUNE)

Use(s): Immunosuppression for organ transplantation; treatment of chronic allograft rejection in patients previously treated with other immunosuppressive agents, e.g., azathioprine; treatment of severe autoimmune disease resistant to corticosteroids and other therapy.

Dosing: Organ transplantation:
            Preoperative PO, 15 mg/kg (range 6-18 mg/kg)

IV infusion, 0.5-6 mg/kg (over 2-6 hr)

Administer as single dose 4-12 hr before transplantation

Postoperative PO, 15 mg/kg (range 6-18 mg/kg) once daily for 1-2 wk. Taper by 5% per week (over 6-8 wk) to:

Maintenance PO, 4-10 mg/kg

Postoperative IV infusion, 0.5-6 mg/kg once daily (give over 2-6 hr). Switch to oral administration as soon as possible after surgery.

Patients receiving IV cyclosporine should be closely monitored for allergic reactions or anaphylaxis. Appropriate equipment for resuscitation should be readily available.

Trough blood or plasma concentrations (at 24 hours) of 250-800 or 50-300 ng/ml, respectively, as determined by radioimmunoassay (RIA), minimize the frequency of graft rejection and cyclosporine-induced adverse effects.

Concomitant corticosteroid/azathioprine therapy is recommended.

Prednisone PO, 2 mg/kg daily for 4 days tapered to 1 mg/kg/day by 1 wk, 0.6 mg/kg/day by 2 wk, 0.3 mg/kg/day by 1 month, 0.15 mg/kg/day by 2 months and thereafter as a maintenance dose. Adjustments in dosage of prednisone must be made according to the clinical situation.

Azathioprine PO, 1-2 mg/kg/day

Acute allograft rejection: methylprednisolone 0.5-1 g daily for 3 days. Maximum dose 6 g. If

rejection continues discontinue cyclosporine and
continue with azathioprine and corticosteroids.

NOTE: Numerous protocols exist and change continuously.

Elimination: Hepatic

How Supplied:

Capsules (liquid filled), 25 mg, 100 mg

Oral solution, 100 mg/ml

Injection (concentrate for infusion), 50 mg/ml

Storage:

Injection, temperature below 30° C. Protect from freezing
and light.

Oral solution, temperature below 30° C. Avoid refrigeration, which may cause coalescence and separation of the
oral solution.

Dilution for Infusion: 50 mg in 50 ml NS or D_5W
(1 mg/ml)

Pharmacology

A cyclic polypeptide antibiotic, cyclosporine is a potent
immunosuppressive agent produced by the fungus species
Tolypocladium inflatum Gams. It inhibits cell-mediated
immune responses such as allograft rejection, delayed
hypersensitivity (e.g., tuberculin-induced), experimental
allergic encephalomyelitis, Freund's adjuvant-induced
arthritis, and graft-vs.-host disease. Cyclosporine also may
inhibit humoral immune responses. It prolongs survival of
allogenic transplants involving skin, heart, kidney, pancreas, bone marrow, small intestine, and lung. Unlike other
currently available immunosuppressive agents, cyclosporine lacks clinically important myelosuppressive activity.
Bone marrow cell counts (i.e., granulocytes, monocytes,
stem cells) show only slight reductions in cell numbers

with normal or enhanced stem cell proliferation. Cyclosporine produces dose-dependent and reversible hepatotoxic and nephrotoxic effects. Increased plasma renin activity may contribute to the development of hypertension. The clinical importance of its antimalarial, antineoplastic, and antischistosomal activity has not been determined.

Pharmacokinetics

Onset: PO, variable
Peak Effect: PO, 3.5 hr (peak blood levels)
Duration: Half-life 10-40 hr
Interaction/Toxicity: Additive nephrotoxic effects with concomitant use of other nephrotoxic drugs, e.g., acyclovir, indomethacin, disopyramide, aminoglycoside antibiotics, amphotericin B; increased plasma concentrations of cyclosporine and elevated serum creatinine with ketoconazole, erythromycin, methotrexate, methylprednisolone, verapamil, diltiazem, acetazolamide, diclofenac; increased creatinine clearance with concomitant administration of cimetidine and ranitidine; decreased plasma concentrations of cyclosporine with warfarin, rifampin, phenytoin, phenobarbital, sulfamethazine, and trimethoprim. Cyclosporine may interfere with the activity of warfarin and the elimination of methotrexate; may prolong neuromuscular blockade of nondepolarizing muscle relaxants, e.g., atracurium, vecuronium; concomitant administration with furosemide may result in hyperuricemia and gout; concomitant administration with potassium-sparing diuretics, e.g., spironolactone, may result in hyperkalemia; GI absorption is increased by oral metoclopramide; increased incidence of gingival hyperplasia with calcium channel blockers, especially nifedipine; cyclosporine increases serum levels of

digoxin, and combined therapy may result in digoxin, toxicity; concomitant administration with disulfiram may result in an Antabuse-type reaction (caused by the alcohol content of the oral and intravenous formulations of cyclosporine).

Guidelines/Precautions

1. Use only under the supervision of a physician experienced in immunosuppressive therapy and management of organ-transplant patients.
2. Cyclosporine increases susceptibility to infections and lymphoma, especially with concomitant administration of other immunosuppressive agents.
3. Because of the risk of anaphylaxis, IV cyclosporine should be reserved for patients unable to tolerate the oral formulation of the drug.
4. Periodic monitoring of renal function, hepatic function, and blood or plasma cyclosporine concentrations are especially important.
5. Increased BUN and serum creatinine do not necessarily indicate that organ rejection has occurred. In patients with renal allografts, acute episodes of allograft rejection must be differentiated from nephrotoxic effects of cyclosporine. Increased serum creatinine concentrations without the usual symptoms of allograft rejection (e.g., fever, graft tenderness, or enlargement) imply cyclosporine-induced nephrotoxicity.
6. If severe, intractable renal allograft rejection occurs, it is preferable to allow the kidney to be rejected and removed than to increase cyclosporine dosage to a high level in an attempt to reverse the rejection episode.
7. Increased frequency of seizures in children may be related to concomitant hypertension or high-dose corticosteroid therapy.

Principal Adverse Reactions

Cardiovascular: Hypertension, chest pain, myocardial infarction

CNS: Headache, tremors, seizures, paresthesia, confusion, anxiety, depression, neurotoxic syndrome (cortical blindness, quadriplegia, seizures, and/or coma) possibly associated with low serum cholesterol

GI: Nausea, vomiting, anorexia, diarrhea, constipation, peptic ulcer, hiccups, abdominal discomfort

Hepatic: Abnormal liver function tests

GU: Increased BUN and serum creatinine, hyperkalemia, fluid retention

Metabolic: Hyperchloremic hyperkalemic metabolic acidosis

Infectious Complications: Pneumonia; septicemia; abscesses; urinary tract, viral, local, systemic fungal, skin, and wound infections

Hematologic: Leukopenia, anemia, thrombocytopenia, lymphoma

Allergic: Anaphylaxis

Dermatologic: Flushing, hirsutism, gingival hyperplasia

Other: Hyperlipidemia, hyperglycemia, hypomagnesemia, conjunctivitis, tinnitus, fever, pancreatitis, benign fibroadenoma, gynecomastia, sinusitis, aseptic necrosis, weight loss, night sweats

DANTROLENE SODIUM (DANTRIUM)

Use(s): Treatment or prevention of malignant hyperthermia; treatment of hypermetabolic states associated with neuroleptic malignant syndrome (NMS), tetanus, amphotericin-B–induced rigors, toxic reactions to L-asparaginase, and MAOI overdose; relief of spasticity from upper motor neuron disease.

Dosing: Malignant hyperthermia:

> Treatment:
>> IV push, 1-2 mg/kg every 5-10 min (maximum of 10 mg/kg, dose may be repeated), then
>>
>> PO, 4-8 mg/kg/day in 3 divided doses for up to 3 days after the crisis
>
> Prophylaxis:
>> Infusion, 2.5 mg/kg over 15-30 min just before induction of anesthesia and/or
>>
>> PO, 4-8 mg/kg/day in 3 divided doses for 1-2 days, last dose 3 hr before anesthesia
>
> Appropriate supportive measures (outlined below) should be instituted in conjunction with drug treatment.
>
> Chronic spasticity: PO, 25 mg once daily. Titrate upward to 100 mg 2 or 4 times daily.
>
> Neuroleptic malignant syndrome/hypermetabolic states:
>> IV, 1-2.5 mg/kg q6hr for up to 2 days or
>>
>> PO, 4-10 mg/kg/day in 2-3 divided doses for 1-2 days

Elimination: Hepatic, renal

How Supplied:

Vials, 20 mg dantrolene and 3000 mg mannitol to be reconstituted in 60 ml sterile water

Capsules, 25 mg, 50 mg, and 100 mg

Storage:

Powder for injection, temperature below 30° C. Protect from light. Use within 6 hr of reconstitution.

Capsules, room temperature (15°-30° C). Do not permit to freeze.

Pharmacology

Dantrolene is a direct-acting skeletal muscle relaxant. It inhibits the release of calcium from the sarcoplasmic reticulum. Neuromuscular transmission and electrical properties of the skeletal muscle membrane are not altered. It attenuates or reverses the physiologic, metabolic, and biochemical changes associated with malignant hyperthermia crisis, neuroleptic malignant syndrome, and other hypermetabolic states. Skeletal muscle weakness may interfere with ventilation and protective pharyngeal reflexes.

Pharmacokinetics

Onset: PO, 1-2 hr; IV, <5 min
Peak Effect: PO, 4-6 hr; IV, 1 hr
Duration: PO, 8-9 hr; IV, 3 hr
Interaction/Toxicity: Combination with calcium channel blockers may produce hyperkalemia and cardiovascular collapse; hepatitis with long-term use.

Guidelines/Precautions

1. Avoid combination with calcium channel blockers during management of malignant hyperthermia or other hypermetabolic states. May cause ventricular fibrillation and cardiovascular collapse in association with marked hyperkalemia.
2. Other supportive measures must be continued in the management of malignant hyperthermia or other hypermetabolic states. These include discontinuing the suspect triggering agents, attending to increased oxygen requirements, managing the metabolic acidosis, instituting cooling, and monitoring the urinary output and electrolyte balance. (See Appendix A: Malignant Hyperthermia Protocol.)

3. After a malignant hyperthermia crisis, oral or IV dantrolene should be used for up to 3 days to prevent a recurrence.
4. Monitor liver function if therapy exceeds 45 days.
5. Greater risk of hepatotoxicity in women over 35, especially if taking concurrent medications such as estrogens.

Principal Adverse Reactions

Cardiovascular: Tachycardia, labile blood pressure
CNS: Drowsiness, dizziness, seizures
GU: Hematuria, urinary frequency, incontinence
GI: Diarrhea, constipation
Hepatic: Fatal or nonfatal hepatitis
Dermatologic: Rash, pruritus
Musculoskeletal: Myalgia, backache

DESMOPRESSIN ACETATE (DDAVP, STIMATE)

Use(s): Maintenance of hemostasis after cardiopulmonary bypass; treatment of neurogenic diabetes insipidus, hemophilia A (with factor VIII levels greater than 5%), von Willebrand's disease (type I with factor VIII levels greater than 5%), and primary nocturnal enuresis

Dosing: Diabetes insipidus:

SC/IV: 2-4 μg daily in two divided doses. The morning and evening doses should be separately adjusted for an adequate diurnal rhythm of water turnover.

Intranasal: 10-40 μg (0.1-0.4 ml) daily in 1-3 divided doses. If there is nasal congestion or poor nasal absorption, switch to injection form and use one tenth of the intranasal dose.

Hemophilia A/von Willebrand's disease, hemo-
stasis following cardiopulmonary bypass:
IV, 0.3 μg/kg (dilute in 50 ml sterile saline.
Give over 30 min)
If plasma factor VIII level is <5%, do not rely on
desmopressin.

Elimination: Renal
How Supplied:
Intranasal, 0.1 mg/ml
Injection, 4 μg/ml
Storage:
Injection, refrigerate (4° C). Do not permit to freeze.
Nasal solution, refrigerate (2°-8° C). Stable at room tem-
perature (22° C) for 3 weeks in unopened sterile bottle.

Pharmacology

Desmopressin is a synthetic analog of 8-arginine vasopressin, the natural human posterior pituitary hormone
(ADH). Compared with vasopressin, desmopressin has
greater antidiuretic potency, possesses little pressor activity,
is relatively free of oxytocic activity, and has a longer duration of action (due to slower enzymatic inactivation).
Intranasal desmopressin is preferable to the other vasopressin analogs for chronic treatment in patients with mild
to moderate neurogenic diabetes insipidus. Desmopressin is
ineffective in treating nephrogenic diabetes insipidus
(which is treated with thiazide diuretics, amiloride and
inhibitors of prostaglandin synthesis. The drug increases the
cyclic AMP content of cells in the renal tubules and collect-
ing ducts, which increases cellular permeability to water. As
a consequence, the urine becomes more concentrated.
Desmopressin also releases von Willebrand's factor, necessary for adequate activity of factor VIII and optimal func-

tion of platelets. Vasoconstrictor effects may produce an increase in systemic and pulmonary arterial blood pressure.

Pharmacokinetics

Onset:
IV (increase in plasma factor VIII activity), 15-30 min
Intranasal (antidiuretic effects), <1 hr
Peak Effect:
IV (increase in plasma factor VIII activity), 90 min-3 hr
Intranasal (antidiuretic effects), 1-5 hr
Duration:
IV (increase in plasma factor VIII activity), 6-20 hr
Intranasal (antidiuretic effects), 8-20 hr
Interaction/Toxicity: Water intoxication and hyponatremia; elevation of blood pressure, antidiuretic effect potentiated by chlorpropamide, carbamazepine, clofibrate, tricyclic antidepressants, phenformin, urea, and fludrocortisone; antidiuretic effect decreased by demeclocycline, heparin, alcohol, and lithium.

Guidelines/Precautions

1. Monitor fluid intake.
2. Severe allergic reaction may occur with repeated use.
3. Use with caution in patients with hypertension and coronary artery disease.
4. Do not use in patients with type IIB or platelet-type (pseudo) von Willebrand's disease. May cause platelet aggregation and thrombocytopenia.
5. Patients should be weighed daily to check for edema.

Principal Adverse Reactions

Cardiovascular: Coronary ischemia, hypertension
CNS: Headache

GI: Abdominal pain, nausea
Dermatologic: flushing, erythema
Other: Water intoxication, hyponatremia, rhinitis

DEXAMETHASONE (DECADRON, HEXADROL)

Use(s): Treatment of inflammatory diseases, cerebral edema, aspiration pneumonitis, bronchial asthma, myofascial pain with trigger points, allergic reactions; prevention of rejection in organ transplantation; replacement therapy for adrenocortical insufficiency

Dosing: Inflammatory diseases:

Dexamethasone phosphate, intraarticular/intratissue, 1-16 mg. May repeat at 1-3 wk

Dexamethasone acetate,IM/intraarticular/intratissue, 4-16 mg. May repeat at 1-3 wk

Dexamethasone phosphate, IV/IM, 0.5-25 mg/day

Cerebral edema: dexamethasone phosphate, IV, 10 mg then IM 4 mg every 6 hours or PO 1-3 mg 3 times daily. Taper off over 5-7 days.

Recurrent/inoperable brain tumors (relief of increased ICP): dexamethasone phosphate, IV/IM, 2mg 2 or 3 times daily

Myofascial pain (with trigger point): dexamethasone phosphate, intratissue, 1-4 mg (dilute in 10 ml local anesthetic). May repeat at 1-3 wk.

Bronchospasm: dexamethasone phosphate, inhalation, 300 μg (3 inhalations) 3 or 4 times daily

Taper off dexamethasone dose if used for more than a few days. Avoid concomitant NSAIA use.

Elimination: Hepatic
How Supplied:

Injection, dexamethasone phosphate (IV/IM), 4 mg/ml, 10 mg/ml, 20 mg/ml

Injection, dexamethasone phosphate (IV use only), 20 mg/ml, 24 mg/ml

Injection, dexamethasone acetate (IM use only), 8 mg/ml, 16 mg/ml

Tablets, dexamethasone, 0.25 mg, 0.5 mg, 0.75 mg, 1.5 mg, 4 mg, 6 mg

Oral solution, dexamethasone, 0.1 mg/ml

Aerosol, dexamethasone phosphate, 100 μg/metered spray

Storage: Injection/tablets/oral solution, room temperature (15°-30° C). Do not permit to freeze. Protect from light.
Aerosol: temperature below 40° C

Pharmacology

A fluorinated derivative of prednisolone with potent antiinflammatory effect. 0.75 Mg is equivalent to 20 mg cortisol. Dexamethasone may decrease the number and activity of inflammatory cells, enhance the effects of beta adrenergic drugs on cyclic-AMP production, and inhibit bronchoconstrictor mechanisms. At equipotent doses, dexamethasone lacks the sodium-retaining property of hydrocortisone. It may suppress the hypothalamic-pituitary-adrenal (HPA) axis.

Pharmacokinetics

Onset: Antiinflammatory effects, IV/IM, few min
Peak Effect: Antiinflammatory effects, IV/IM, 12-24 hr
Duration: Antiinflammatory effects/HPA suppression, IV/IM, 36-54 hr

Interaction/Toxicity: Clearance enhanced by phenytoin, phenobarbital, rifampin, ephedrine; altered response to coumarin anticoagulants; increases requirements of insulin; interacts with anticholinesterase agents (e.g., neostigmine) to produce severe weakness in patients with myasthenia gravis; potassium-wasting effects enhanced with potassium-depleting diuretics (e.g., thiazides, furosemide); diminishes response to toxoids and live or inactivated vaccines; increased risk of GI bleeding with concomitant NSAIA.

Guidelines/Precautions

1. Induced adrenocortical insufficiency may occur with rapid withdrawal of dexamethasone .
2. Use with caution in patients with hypertension, congestive heart failure, thromboembolytic tendencies, hypothyroidism, cirrhosis, myasthenia gravis, peptic ulcer, diverticulitis, nonspecific ulcerative colitis, fresh intestinal anastomosis, psychosis, seizure disorders, and systemic fungal and viral infections.
3. Administration of live virus vaccines (i.e., smallpox) is contraindicated in patients receiving immunosuppresive doses.

Principal Adverse Reactions

Cardiovascular: Arrhythmias, hypertension, congestive heart failure in susceptible patients
CNS: Seizures, increased intracranial pressure, steroid psychosis
Dermatologic: Impaired wound healing, petechiae, erythema
Eye: Increased intraocular pressure, subcapsular cataracts
Metabolic: Fluid retention, sodium retention, potassium depletion

Endocrine: Secondary adrenocortical and pituitary unresponsiveness during stress, growth suppression, increased requirements for insulin

Musculoskeletal: Myopathy, weakness, osteoporosis

Other: Thromboembolism, diminished response to toxoids and live or inactivated vaccines, increased susceptibility to and masked symptoms of infection

---

DIAZEPAM (VALIUM)

Use(s): Premedication, amnesia, sedative/hypnotic, induction agent, skeletal muscle relaxant, anticonvulsant, treatment of acute alcohol withdrawal and panic attacks

Dosing: Premedication/sedation: IV/IM/PO/rectal, 2-10 mg (0.1-0.2 mg/kg)

Induction, IV, 0.3-0.5 mg/kg

Anticonvulsant:

IV, 0.05-0.2 mg/kg q 10-15 min; maximum dose 30 mg

PO/rectal, 2-10 mg 2 to 4 times daily

PO extended release, 15-30 mg once daily

Withdrawal:

IV, 5-10 mg (0.15-0.2 mg/kg) q3-4hr

PO, 5-10 mg 3 or 4 times daily

PO extended release, 15-30 mg once daily

Elimination: Hepatic

How Supplied:

Tablets, 2 mg, 5 mg, 10 mg

Capsule sustained release, 15 mg

Oral solution, 5 mg/5 ml, 5 mg/ml

Injection, 5 mg/ml

Storage: Injection/tablets/oral solution, room temperature (15°-30° C). Protect from light.

Pharmacology

This benzodiazepine derivative acts on the limbic system, thalamus, and hypothalamus, inducing calming effects. Diazepam exerts antianxiety and skeletal-muscle-relaxing effects by increasing the availability of the glycine inhibitory neurotransmitter, whereas the sedative action reflects the ability of benzodiazepines to facilitate actions of the inhibitory neurotransmitter gamma amino butyric acid (GABA). The site of action for production of anterograde amnesia has not been confirmed. With a diazepam induction, the awake alpha rhythm changes to a beta rhythm on the EEG. Alpha activity returns after 30 min. Diazepam has no peripheral autonomic blocking action. It has minimal effects on ventilation and circulation in the absence of other CNS depressant drugs. IV diazepam is considered the drug of choice in termination of status epilepticus or acute seizure episodes resulting from drug overdosage and poisons. Because of the short-lived effect, other agents should be used for long-term seizure control.

Pharmacokinetics

Onset: IV, <2 min; rectal, <10 min;
PO, 15 min-1 hr (shorter in children)
Peak Effect: IV, 3-4 min; PO, 1 hr
Duration: IV, 15 min-1 hr; PO, 2-6 hr
Interaction/Toxicity: Sedative and circulatory depressant effect potentiated by opioids, alcohol, and other CNS depressants; elimination reduced by cimetidine; reduces requirements for volatile anesthetics; thrombophlebitis results with intravenous administration; clearance and dosage requirements are decreased in old age; effects antagonized by flumazenil; may cause neonatal hypothermia; interacts with plastic containers; and administration sets significantly decreasing bioavailability.

Guidelines/Precautions

1. Contraindicated in acute narrow angle or open angle glaucoma unless patients are receiving appropriate therapy.
2. Reduce dose in elderly/high-risk or hypovolemic patients, in patients with limited pulmonary reserve, and with concomitant use of narcotics and other sedatives.
3. Inject slowly through large veins to reduce thrombophlebitis.
4. Return of drowsiness may occur 6-8 hr after dose because of enterohepatic recirculation.
5. Treat overdose with supportive measures and flumazenil (slow IV 0.2-1 mg).
6. IM route is painful and results in slow, erratic absorption.
7. Do not mix or dilute with other solutions or drugs.

Principal Adverse Reactions

Cardiovascular: Bradycardia, hypotension
Pulmonary: Respiratory depression
CNS: Drowsiness, ataxia, confusion, depression, paradoxic excitement
GU: Incontinence
Dermatologic: Skin rash
Other: Venous thrombosis and phlebitis at site of injection, dry mouth

DIGOXIN (LANOXIN, LANOXICAPS)

Use(s): Inotropic agent; treatment of heart failure and supraventricular arrhythmias

Dosing: Adults:

Loading dose, IV or PO, 0.5 to 1 mg in divided doses. Give 50% of loading dose as first dose, then 25% fractions at 4-8 hr intervals until an adequate therapeutic response is obtained, toxic effects occur, or the total digitalizing dose has been administered. Monitor clinical response before each additional dose.

Maintenance dose: IV or PO, 0.125 to 0.5 mg daily. Dosages should be individualized and reduced in patients with impaired renal function. (Maintenance dose of 0.125-0.25 mg IV/PO with creatinine clearance of 10-79 ml/min.)

Elderly adults (> 65), 0.125 mg PO daily as maintenance dose. Frail or small patients may require less.

Children over 2 yr:

  PO loading 0.02 to 0.06 mg/kg divided q8h for 24 hr.

  IV loading 0.015 to 0.035 mg/kg divided q8h for 24 hr.

  Maintenance: 25%-35% loading dose PO/IV daily divided q12h.

Children 1 mo to 2 yr:

  PO loading 0.035 to 0.06 mg/kg divided q8hr for 24 hr.

  IV loading, 0.03 to 0.05 mg/kg divided q8hr for 24 hr.

  Maintenance: 25%-35% loading dose PO/IV daily divided q12hr.

Full-term neonates:

  PO loading, 0.025 to 0.035 mg/kg divided q8hr for 24 hr.

  IV loading, 0.02 to 0.03 mg/kg divided q8hr for 24 hr.

        Maintenance: 25%-35% loading dose PO/IV daily divided q12hr.

    Premature neonates:

        PO loading, 0.02 to 0.03 mg/kg divided q8hr for 24 hr.

        IV loading, 0.015 to 0.025 mg/kg divided q8hr for 24 hr.

        Maintenance: 25%-35% loading dose PO/IV daily divided q12hr.

    Therapeutic drug levels are 0.5-2 ng/ml in adults and 1.1-1.7 ng/ml in neonates and infants. Higher levels may be required for heart-rate control in atrial fibrillation.

Note: Therapeutic levels do not exclude toxicity.

Elimination: Renal

How Supplied:

Tablets, 0.125 mg, 0.25 mg, 0.5 mg

Capsules (lanoxicaps): 0.05 mg, 0.1 mg, 0.2 mg

Oral solution, 0.05 mg/ml

Injection, 0.1 mg/ml, 0.25 mg/ml

Storage: Injection/tablets/capsules/oral solution: room temperature (15°-30° C). Protect from light.

Pharmacology

This glycoside composed of a sugar and a cardenolide has a direct inotropic effect via inhibition of the sodium-potassium adenosine triphosphatase (ATPase) ion transport system. It has an indirect vagomimetic effect with decreased activity of the SA node and prolonged conduction through the AV node. Digoxin increases contractility and decreases myocardial oxygen consumption in the failing heart.

Pharmacokinetics

Onset: IV, 5-30 min; PO, 30 min-2 hr
Peak Effect: IV, 1-4 hr; PO, 2-6 hr
Duration: IV/PO, 3-4 days (digitalized patients)
Interaction/Toxicity: Enhanced toxicity in hypokalemia, hypomagnesemia, hypercalcemia; increased serum levels with calcium channel blockers (e.g., verapamil, nifedipine, diltiazem), esmolol, quinidine, amiodarone, flecainide, captopril, benzodiazepines, anticholinergics, oral aminoglycosides, erythromycin; resistance in atrial fibrillation associated with hypermetabolism, e.g., hyperthyroidism; succinylcholine may cause arrhythmias in digitalized patients; overdosage may cause complete heart block, A-V dissociation, ventricular tachycardias or fibrillation.

Guidelines/Precautions

1. Dosage requirements are decreased in patients with impaired renal function and the elderly.
2. Monitor serum potassium and digoxin levels. To allow for equilibration of digoxin between serum and tissue, determine serum digoxin levels at least 6 hr after an IV dose and 6 hr after an oral dose.
3. Contraindicated in ventricular fibrillation.
4. Use of synchronized cardioversion in a digitalis toxic patient should avoided because it may initiate ventricular fibrillation.
5. Steady-state levels may take as long as 7 days to be achieved.
6. Use with succinylcholine may precipitate arrhythmias.

7. Use caution when switching from standard tablets to Lanoxicaps because of increased bioavailability of the latter.
8. Digoxin toxicity may manifest with anorexia, nausea, vomiting, cardiac arrhythmias, headache, drowsiness, hyperkalemia, normokalemia, or hypokalemia. Discontinue digoxin, monitor serum electrolytes and glycoside concentration, and initiate supportive and symptomatic treatment. Digoxin immune Fab is a specific antidote. Give in approximate equimolar quantities as total dose of glycoside absorbed. Empirical dose of 800 mg (20 40-mg vials) of digoxin immune Fab is adequate to treat most life-threatening toxicity in adults and children. Small children should be monitored closely for fluid overload when this large dose is used.

Principal Adverse Reactions

Cardiovascular: Wide range of arrhythmias, AV block
CNS: Headache, psychosis, confusion
GI: Nausea, vomiting, diarrhea
Other: Gynecomastia

DIPHENHYDRAMINE HCL (BENADRYL)

Use(s): Antiemetic; antivertigo; treatment of allergic reactions; adjuvant use in the treatment of anaphylaxis, symptomatic treatment of drug-induced extrapyramidal reactions

Dosing: PO, 25-50 mg (0.3-0.5 mg/kg) every 6-8 hr
IV/IM, 10-50 mg (0.2 - 0.5 mg/kg); maximum daily dose is 400 mg

Elimination: Hepatic
How Supplied:
Tablets, 25 mg, 50 mg
Capsules, 25 mg, 50 mg
Oral solution, 12.5 mg per 5 ml
Injection, 10 mg/ml, 50 mg/ml
Storage: Injection/tablets/capsules/oral solution: Room temperature (15°-30° C). Do not permit to freeze. Protect from light.

Pharmacology

This is a histamine H_1-receptor antagonist with anticholinergic and sedative effects. It partially inhibits vasodilator effects of histamine on peripheral vascular smooth muscle. Diphenhydramine should be employed in anaphylactic reactions as adjunctive therapy only after epinephrine and other life-saving measures.

Pharmacokinetics

Onset: IV, few min; PO <15 min
Peak Effect: IV, 1-3 hr; PO, 2 hr
Duration: IV/PO, <7 hr
Interaction/Toxicity: Anticholinergic effects potentiated by MAO inhibitors; additive sedative effect with alcohol, hypnotics, sedatives, and tranquilizers

Guidelines/Precautions

1. Children are at an increased risk for experiencing paradoxic CNS stimulant effects (restlesssness, insomnia, tremors, euphoria, seizures).
2. Use with caution in patients with narrow-angle glaucoma, increased intraocular pressure, seizure disorders,

bowel or bladder neck obstruction, lower respiratory diseases including asthma.
3. Contraindicated in newborn or premature infants

Principal Adverse Reactions

Cardiovascular: Hypotension, palpitation, extrasystoles
Pulmonary: Wheezing, tightness of chest
CNS: Sedation, confusion, blurred vision, tinnitus, tremors, seizures
GU: Urinary frequency, urinary retention

DOBUTAMINE HCL (DOBUTREX)

Use(s): Inotrope; pharmacologic stress testing in coronary artery disease

Dosing: Infusion, 0.5-30 μg/kg/min
Elimination: Hepatic
How Supplied: Injection, 12.5 mg/ml
Storage: Injection: Room temperature (15°-30° C). Solutions diluted for IV infusion should be used within 24 hr.
Dilution for Infusion: 500 mg in 500 ml D_5W or NS (1 mg/ml)

Pharmacology

A beta-1 adrenergic agonist that increases myocardial rate and force of contraction. In therapeutic doses, it has mild beta-2 and alpha-1 adrenergic receptor agonist effects and decreases peripheral and pulmonary vascular resistance. Systolic blood pressure may be increased because of the augmented cardiac output. Unlike dopamine, dobutamine does not stimulate release of endogenous norepinephrine and does not act on dopaminergic receptors. Dobutamine facilitates atrioventricular conduction, and patients with atrial fibrillation may be at risk of developing a rapid ventricular response. However, the arrythmogenic effects are less than that of dopamine, isoproterenol, or other catecholamines. Dobutamine increases vascular resistance and decreases uterine blood flow.

Pharmacokinetics

Onset: 1-2 min
Peak Effect: 1-10 min
Duration of Action: <10 min
Interaction/Toxicity: Less effective with beta blockers; use with nitroprusside results in higher cardiac output and lower pulmonary wedge pressure; bretylium potentiates effects of dobutamine and may result in arrhythmias; inactivated in alkaline solutions; increased risk of supraventricular and ventricular arrhythmias with use of volatile anesthetics.

Guidelines/Precautions

1. Arrhythmias and hypertension result at high doses. Risk of dangerous arrhythmias is higher with use of volatile anesthetics.
2. Contraindicated in idiopathic hypertrophic subaortic stenosis (IHSS).
3. Do not mix with sodium bicarbonate, furosemide, or other alkaline solutions.
4. In patients with atrial fibrillation and rapid ventricular rate, a digitalis preparation should be instituted before commencing therapy with dobutamine.
5. Correct hypovolemia as fully as possible before or during treatment.

6. Commercially available formulations may contain sulfites, which may cause allergic-type reactions (wheezing, anaphylaxis) in susceptible populations.

Principal Adverse Reactions

Cardiovascular: Hypertension, tachycardia, arrhythmias, angina
Pulmonary: Shortness of breath
CNS: Headache
Other: Phlebitis at injection site

DOPAMINE HCL (INTROPIN)

Use(s): Inotropic agent, vasoconstrictor, diuresis in cardiac or acute renal failure

Dosing: Infusion, 1 to 50 μg/kg/min
Elimination: Hepatic
How Supplied: Injection:
Parenteral concentrate for infusion, 40, 80, and 160 mg/ml
Premixed solution in 5% dextrose 80 mg/100 ml, 160 mg/100 ml, 320 mg/100 ml
Storage: Room temperature (15°-30° C). Protect from light. IV infusion prepared from concentrate should be used within 24 hr.
Dilution for Infusion: 400 mg in 250 ml D_5W or NS (1600 μg/ml)

Pharmacology

A naturally occurring catecholamine that acts directly on alpha, beta-1, and dopaminergic receptors and indirectly by releasing norepinephrine from its storage sites. At low doses (1-3 μg/kg/min) it specifically increases blood flow to the renal, mesenteric, coronary, and cerebral beds by activating the dopamine receptors. A rise in glomerular filtration rate and increased sodium excretion accompanies the increase in renal blood flow. Infusion of dopamine at 2-10 μg/kg/min stimulates beta-1 adrenergic receptors in the heart, causing an increase in myocardial contractility, stroke volume, and cardiac output. Higher doses above 10 μg/kg/min stimulate alpha adrenergic receptors, causing increased peripheral vascular resistance, decreased renal blood flow, and increased potential for arrhythmias. Dopamine increases uterine vascular resistance and decreases uterine blood flow.

Pharmacokinetics

Onset: 2-4 min
Peak Effect: 2-10 min
Duration: Less than 10 min
Interaction/Toxicity: Increased risk of supraventricular and ventricular arrhythmias with use of volatile anesthetics; possible necrosis in patients with occlusive vascular disease; inactivated in alkaline solutions such as sodium bicarbonate, furosemide; concomitant use with phenytoin may cause seizures, severe hypotension, and bradycardia.

Guidelines/Precautions

1. Dopamine should not be administered to patients with pheochromocytoma or in the presence of uncorrected tacharrhythmias or ventricular fibrillation.
2. Use with caution and monitor carefully in patients with occlusive vascular disease (e.g., Raynaud's disease). Compromise in circulation may manifest by a change in color or temperature of the extremities. Decrease or discontinue the dopamine infusion and if necessary admin-

ister IV phentolamine (5-10 mg in 10 mls NS) or IV chlorpromazine (10 mg).

3. Infuse into large vein. Extravasation may cause sloughing and necrosis. Treat by local infiltration of phentolamine (5-10 mg in 10 ml NS).

4. Correct hypovolemia as fully as possible before or during treatment.

5. Commercially available formulations may contain sulfites, which may cause allergic type reactions (wheezing, anaphylaxis) in susceptible populations.

Principal Adverse Reactions

Cardiovascular: Arrhythmias, angina, AV block, hypotension, hypertension, vasoconstriction
Pulmonary: Dyspnea
CNS: Headache, anxiety
GI: Nausea and vomiting
Dermatologic: Piloerection
Other: Gangrene of extremities with prolonged period of high doses.

DOXACURIUM CHLORIDE (NUROMAX)

Use(s): Skeletal muscle relaxation

Dosing: Intubating: IV, 0.05-0.08 mg/kg
  Maintenance: IV, 0.005-0.04 mg/kg (10%-50% of intubating dose)
  Pretreatment/priming: IV, 10% of intubating dose given 3-5 min before depolarizer/nondepolarizer relaxant dose
Elimination: Renal
How Supplied: Injection, 1 mg/ml

Storage: Room temperature (15°-25° C). Do not permit to freeze.

Pharmacology

A long-acting, nondepolarizing neuromuscular blocking agent. It binds competitively to cholinergic receptors on the motor end plate and antagonizes the action of acetylcholine, resulting in a block of neuromuscular transmission. Doxacurium is 2.5 to 3 times more potent than Pancuronium. The time of onset and duration are similar to those of pancuronium at comparable doses. The drug has no clinically significant hemodynamic effects. Histamine release rarely occurs.

Pharmacokinetics

Onset: <4 min
Peak Effect: 3-9 min
Duration: 30-160 min
Interaction/Toxicity: Neuromuscular blockade potentiated by aminoglycoside, antibiotics, local anesthetics, loop diuretics, magnesium, lithium, ganglionic blocking drugs, hypothermia, hypokalemia, respiratory acidosis, and prior administration of succinylcholine; dosage requirements decreased (about 30%-45%) and duration of neuromuscular blockade prolonged (up to 25%) by volatile anesthetics; recurrent paralysis with quinidine, enhanced neuromuscular blockade in patients with myasthenia gravis or inadequate adrenocortical function; effects antagonized by anticholinesterases such as neostigmine, edrophonium, pyridostigmine; pretreatment doses of doxacurium decrease fasciculations but reduce intensity and shorten duration of succinylcholine neuromuscular blockade; priming doses

decrease the time to onset of maximal blockade by about 30-60 sec; increased resistance or reversal of effects with use of carbamazepine and phenytoin, and in patients with burn injury and paresis; incompatible with alkaline solutions with a pH >8.5, such as barbiturate solutions.

Guidelines/Precautions

1. Monitor response with peripheral nerve stimulator to minimize risk of overdosage.
2. Reverse effects with anticholinesterases such as neostigmine, edrophonium, or pyridostigmine bromide in conjunction with atropine or glycopyrrolate. Neostigmine (0.05 mg/kg) is more effective than edrophonium (1 mg/kg) in antagonizing moderate to deep levels of neuromuscular block.
3. Pretreatment doses may induce a degree of neuromuscular blockade sufficient to cause hypoventilation in some patients.

Principal Adverse Reactions

Cardiovascular: Hypotension, flushing, ventricular fibrillation, myocardial infarction
Pulmonary: Hypoventilation, apnea, bronchospasm
CNS: Depression
GU: Anuria
Dermatologic: Rash, urticaria
Musculoskeletal: Inadequate block, prolonged block

DOXAPRAM HCL (DOPRAM)

Use(s): Respiratory stimulant

Dosing: Slow IV, 0.5-1.5 mg/kg, repeat in 5 min, maximum dose, 2 mg/kg

Infusion, 5 mg/min until satisfactory respiratory
response is obtained, then 1-3 mg/min, maximum dose, 4 mg/kg

Elimination: Hepatic
How Supplied: Injection, 20 mg/ml
Storage: Room temperature (15°-40° C). Do not permit to
freeze.
Dilution for Infusion: 250 mg in 250 ml D$_5$W or NS
(1 mg/ml)

Pharmacology

A respiratory stimulant with action mediated through the
peripheral carotid chemoreceptors. As dosage level is
increased, the central respiratory centers in the medulla are
stimulated, with progressive stimulation of other parts of
the brain and spinal cord. Stimulant action is manifested by
an increase in tidal volume associated with a slight increase
in respiratory rate. Doxapram may produce a pressor
response caused by release of catecholamines and
improved cardiac output. This is more marked in hypovolemic patients. Although opiate-induced respiratory
depression is antagonized, the analgesic effect is not affected. Stimulation of respiration is short-lived and is useful
only in patients with drug-induced postanesthesia respiratory depression or apnea other than that caused by muscle-
relaxant drugs.

Pharmacokinetics

Onset: 20-40 sec
Peak Effect: 1-2 min
Duration: 5-12 min
Interaction/Toxicity: Additive pressor effect in patients
receiving sympathomimetics or MAO inhibitors; may mask

residual effects of muscle relaxants; increased risk of arrhythmias in patients receiving volatile anesthetics; precipitate formation with alkaline solutions such as thiopental, bicarbonate, aminophylline.

Guidelines/Precautions

1. Because of the benzyl alcohol content, do not use doxapram in newborns.
2. Contraindicated in patients with epilepsy, convulsive disorders, mechanical disorders of ventilation (such as mechanical obstruction, muscle paresis, flail chest, pneumothorax, acute bronchial asthma, pulmonary fibrosis, conditions resulting in restriction of chest walls, muscles of respiration, or alveolar expansion). Also contraindicated in patients with evidence of head injury or cerebral vascular accident and in those with significant cardiovascular impairment, severe hypertension, or known hypersensitivity to the drug.
3. It is neither an antagonist to muscle relaxants nor a specific narcotic antagonist. Adequacy of airway and oxygenation must be assured before administration.
4. Maintain close observation of patient for 1 hr after patient has been fully alert, as narcosis may recur.
5. Do not use in conjunction with mechanical ventilation.
6. Use with caution in patients with hypermetabolic states.
7. Because of myocardial sensitization to catecholamines, delay administration for at least 10 min after discontinuation of volatile anesthetics.

Principal Adverse Reactions

Cardiovascular: Hypertension, chest pain, tachycardia, bradycardia, arrhythmias

Pulmonary: Cough, tachycardia, laryngospasm, bronchospasm, hiccough

CNS: Seizures, hyperactivity, headache, disorientation, clonus, pupillary dilation

GU: Urinary retention, spontaneous voiding, proteinuria

GI: Nausea, vomiting, desire to defecate

Hematologic: Decreased hemoglobin, and hematocrit, and red blood cell count; leukopenia

DROPERIDOL (INAPSINE)

Use(s): Antiemetic, premedication, neuroleptic, reduction of side effects and potentiation of epidural opioid analgesia

Dosing: Antiemetic: IV, 0.625-2.5 mg (15 μg/kg)

Premedication: IV/IM, 2.5-10 mg

Neuroleptanesthesia: IV, 0.2 mg/kg with fentanyl 4 μg/kg

Epidural: 1.25-2.5 mg (preservative-free) with epidural opioid and diluted with normal saline or local anesthetic

Elimination: Hepatic, renal

How Supplied:

Injection, 2.5 mg/ml

Combination with fentanyl citrate (Innovar) injection, droperidol 2.5 mg/ml with fentanyl citrate 50 μg/ml

Storage: Room temperature (15°-30° Celsius). Protect from light.

Pharmacology

A butyrophenone derivative, chemically related to haloperidol, droperidol interferes with CNS transmission at dopamine, noradrenaline, serotonin, and gamma-amino butyric acid synaptic sites. Droperidol produces marked tranquilization and sedation, inducing a state of mental detachment and indifference while maintaining a state of reflex alertness. Antiemetic effects are due to receptor blockade in the chemoreceptor trigger zone. The drug has an alpha-1 adrenergic antagonist action, which may produce a decrease in systemic vascular resistance and blood pressure. Independent of alpha adrenergic blockade, droperidol prolongs the duration of the refractory period and decreases the rate of upstoke of the action potential. The threshold is increased (up to 2 times) for epinephrine-induced or halothane-associated ventricular arrhythmias. Droperidol is combined with fentanyl to produce neuroleptanalgesia, a state of tranquilization, amnesia, detachment, and analgesia. Droperidol does not produce any clinically significant changes in cerebral blood flow, cerebral metabolic rate, or intracranial pressure. Epidural droperidol may decrease epidural opioid side effects (e.g., nausea, vomiting, pruritus, urinary retention) and enhance analgesia because of the alpha-agonist and dopamine-antagonist activity at spinal and supraspinal levels.

Pharmacokinetics

Onset: IM/IV, 3-10 min
Peak Effect: IM/IV, 30 min
Duration of Action: IM/IV, 2-4 hr
Interaction/Toxicity: Potentiates other CNS depressants; reduces pressor and arrhythmogenic effects of epinephrine; increases threshold for halothane and epinephrine-associated arrhythmias; may induce extrapyramidal symptoms.

Guidelines/Precautions

1. Rule out hypotension as a cause or result of emesis before administering droperidol.
2. Contraindicated in patients with Parkinson's disease. Extrapyramidal reactions may consist of dystonic reac-

tions, feelings of motor restlessness (akathisia), and parkinsonian signs and symptoms. Therapy should include discontinuation of droperidol or reduction in dosage, and treatment with an anticholinergic antiparkinsonian agent (e.g., benztropine, trihexyphenidyl) or with diphenhydramine (IV/PO 25 mg). Maintenance of an adequate airway should be instituted if necessary.

3. Prolonged central nervous system depression may occur with neuroleptanalgesia.
4. When administered preoperatively, patients may express fear of death and refuse a previously accepted operative procedure.

Principal Adverse Reactions

Cardiovascular: Hypotension, tachycardia
Pulmonary: Laryngospasm, bronchospasm
CNS: Extrapyramidal symptoms, drowsiness, hyperactivity

D-TUBOCURARINE CHLORIDE (TUBOCURARINE CHLORIDE)

Use(s): Skeletal muscle relaxation

Dosing: Intubating: IV, 0.3-0.6 mg/kg
Maintenance: IV, 0.05-0.3 mg/kg (10%-50% of intubating dose)
Infusion: 1-6 μg/kg/min
Pretreatment/priming: IV, 10% of intubating dose given 3-5 min before depolarizer/nondepolarizer relaxant dose
Elimination: Renal, hepatic
How Supplied: Injection: 3 mg/ml

Storage: Room temperature (15°-30° C). Do not permit to freeze.

Dilution for Infusion: 15 mg in 100 ml D_5W (0.15 mg/ml)

Pharmacology

D-Tubocurarine is an intermediate-acting, nondepolarizing neuromuscular blocking agent. It competes for cholinergic receptors at the motor end plate. The hypotension associated with clinical doses is secondary to autonomic ganglion blockade and release of histamine. Repeated doses may have a cumulative effect.

Pharmacokinetics

Onset: <2 min
Peak Effect: 2-6 min
Duration: 25-90 min
Interaction/Toxicity: Effects potentiated by volatile anesthetics, aminoglycoside antibiotics, local anesthetics, diuretics, magnesium, lithium, ganglionic blocking drugs, respiratory acidosis, hypokalemia; enhanced neuromuscular blockade will occur in patients with myasthenia gravis or inadequate adrenocortical function; effects antagonized by anticholinesterases such as neostigmine, edrophonium, pyridostigmine; resistance with concomitant use of phenytoin and in patients with burn injury and paresis; pretreatment doses of d-tubocurarine decrease fasciculations but reduce intensity and shorten duration of succinylcholine neuromuscular blockade; priming doses decrease the time to onset of maximal blockade by about 30-60 sec; increased resistance or reversal of effects with use of theophylline and in patients with burn injury and paresis; reduces MAC requirement for volatile anesthetics.

Guidelines/Precautions

1. Monitor response with peripheral nerve stimulator to minimize risk of overdosage.
2. Use with caution in patients with history of bronchial asthma and anaphylactoid reactions.
3. Reverse effects with anticholinesterases such as neostigmine, edrophonium, or pyridostigmine bromide in conjunction with atropine or glycopyrrolate.
4. Pretreatment doses may induce a degree of neuromuscular blockade sufficient to cause hypoventilation in some patients.

Principal Adverse Reactions

Cardovascular: Hypotension, vasodilation, sinus tachycardia, sinus bradycardia
Pulmonary: Hypoventilation, apnea, bronchospasm, laryngospasm, dyspnea
Musculoskeletal: Inadequate block, prolonged block
Dermatologic: Rash, urticaria

EDROPHONIUM CHLORIDE (TENSILON, ENLON, REVERSOL)

Use(s): Reversal of nondepolarizing muscle relaxants, diagnostic assessment of myasthenia gravis, differential diagnosis and treatment of supraventricular tachyarrhythmias

Dosing: Reverse neuromuscular blockade: slow IV, 0.5-1.0 mg/kg. Maximum dose 40 mg (with atropine 0.015 mg/kg or glycopyrrolate 0.01 mg/kg)
Assessment of myasthenia/cholinergic crisis:

Slow IV, 1 mg q1-2min until change in symptoms. Maximum dose 10 mg.

IM, 10 mg

Supraventricular tacharrhythmias:

Slow IV, 2 mg q 1-2 min until decrease in heart rate. Maximal dose 10 mg (have atropine available).

Infusion, 0.25-2 mg/min (use undiluted injectate solution).

Elimination: Hepatic, renal
How Supplied: Injection: 10 mg/ml
Storage: Room temperature (15°-30° C).

Pharmacology

This short-acting quaternary ammonium anticholinesterase agent inhibits the hydrolysis of acetylcholine by competitively binding acetylcholinesterase. The buildup of acetylcholine facilitates the transmission of impulses across the neuromuscular junction. In myasthenia gravis there is improved skeletal muscle tone in conditions of low acetylcholine and increased skeletal muscle weakness in conditions of cholinergic crisis. Cholinergic stimulation may be useful in terminating supraventricular tachyarrhythmias. Edrophonium may be more effective in converting supraventricular tachyarrhythmias to normal sinus rhythm when underlying organic heart disease is not present. When used for reversal of neuromuscular blockade, the muscarinic cholinergic effects (bradycardia, salivation) are prevented by concurrent use of atropine or glycopyrrolate.

Pharmacokinetics

Onset: IV, 30-60 sec; IM, 2-10 minutes
Peak Effect: IV, 1-5 min

Duration: IV, 5-20 min; IM, 10-40 min

Interaction/Toxicity: Does not antagonize and may prolong the phase 1 block of depolarizing muscle relaxants such as succinylcholine; antagonizes the effects of nondepolarizing muscle relaxants such as tubocurarine, atracurium, vecuronium, pancuronium; antagonism of neuromuscular blockade is reduced by aminoglycoside antibiotics, corticosteroids, magnesium, hypothermia, hypokalemia, respiratory and metabolic acidosis.

Guidelines/Precautions

1. Contraindicated in patients with peritonitis or mechanical obstruction of the intestines or urinary tract.
2. Use with caution in patients with bradycardia, bronchial asthma, cardiac arrhythmias, or peptic ulcer.
3. Edrophonium overdosage may induce a cholinergic crisis characterized by nausea, vomiting, bradycardia or tachycardia, excessive salivation and sweating, bronchospasm, weakness, and paralysis.
4. Treatment of a cholinergic crisis includes discontinuation of edrophonium and administration of atropine (10 μg/kg IV q3-10min until muscarinic symptoms disappear) and, if necessary, pralidoxime (15 mg/kg IV over 2 min) for reversal of nicotinic symptoms.
5. Because of the brief duration of action of edrophonium, neostigmine or pyridostigmine are generally preferred for reversal of the effects of nondepolarizing muscle relaxants.

Principal Adverse Reactions

Cardiovascular: Bradycardia, tachycardia, AV block, nodal rhythm, hypotension

Pulmonary: Increased oral, pharyngeal, and bronchial secretions; bronchospasm, respiratory depression
CNS: Seizures, dysarthria, headaches
Eye: Lacrimation, miosis, visual changes
GI: Nausea, emesis, flatulence, increased peristalsis
Dermatologic: Rash, urticaria
Allergic: Allergic reactions, anaphylaxis

EUTECTIC MIXTURE OF LIDOCAINE AND PRILOCAINE (EMLA)

Use(s): Topical anesthesia

Dosing: Minor dermal procedures (e.g., IV cannulation):
Topical: apply 2.5 g of EMLA cream (half the 5 g tube) over 20-25 sq cm of intact skin and cover with occlusive dressing for at least 45 min
Major dermal procedures (e.g., split-thickness skin graft): Topical: apply 2 g of EMLA cream per 10 sq cm of intact skin and cover with occlusive dressing for at least 2 hr
Maximum recommended dose: 60 g
Maximum recommended area of application on normal intact skin:
<10 kg, 100 sq cm
10-20 kg, 600 sq cm
>20 kg, 2000 sq cm
Maximum recommended duration of application: 4 hr
Estimated mean absorption of lidocaine: 0.045 mg/sq cm/hr
Estimated mean absorption of prilocaine: 0.075 mg/sq cm/hr

Smaller areas of treatment are recommended in debilitated patients, small children, and patients with impaired elimination.

Elimination: Hepatic (lidocaine), hepatic and renal (prilocaine)

How Supplied: Cream: lidocaine 2.5% (25 mg/g) and prilocaine 2.5% (25 mg/g)

Storage: Room temperature (15°-30° C). Protect from light.

Pharmacology

EMLA cream is a eutectic mixture of amide local anesthetics, lidocaine 2.5%, and prilocaine 2.5% formulated as an oil-in-water emulsion. Both lidocaine and prilocaine stabilize neuronal membranes by inhibiting the ionic fluxes required for the initiation and conduction of impulses, thereby effecting local anesthetic action. At a ratio of 1:1, the melting point of the mixture is 18° C, lower than either compound alone (lidocaine 67° C, prilocaine 37° C). The mixture is an oil at room temperature, and the penetration and subsequent systemic absorption of both prilocaine and lidocaine are enhanced. The amount absorbed is determined by the area over which it is applied and the duration of application under occlusion. The onset, depth, and duration of dermal analgesia depend primarily on the duration of application. Dermal analgesia can be expected to increase for up to 3 hr under occlusive dressing.

Pharmacokinetics

Onset: <20 min
Peak Effect:
Satisfactory dermal analgesia: 45 min (adults), 60 min (children)

Maximum dermal analgesia: 2-3 hr
Duration: 1-5 hr
Interaction/Toxicity: Methemoglobinemia at high doses and with concomitant administration of methemoglobin-inducing agents (e.g., sulfonamides, acetaminophen, acetanilid, aniline dyes, benzocaine, chloroquine, dapsone, naphthalene, nitrates, nitrites, nitrofurantoin, nitroglycerin, sodium nitroprusside, pamaquine, para-aminosalicylic acid, phenacetin, phenobarbital, phenytoin, primaquine and quinine); additive cardiac effects with other antiarrhythmics (e.g., tocainide, maxiletine)

Guidelines/Precautions

1. EMLA cream is not recommended for use on mucous membranes because of the risk of systemic toxicity. EMLA cream should be used with caution in the external auditory canal. Penetration or migration beyond the tympanic membrane into the middle ear may result in ototoxicity.
2. The amount of lidocaine and prilocaine systemically absorbed is directly related to the duration of application and the area over which it is applied.
3. Toxic plasma levels may occur with application of EMLA cream to broken or inflamed skin or to 2000 sq cm or more of skin.
4. EMLA cream should not be used in infants under the age of 1 month. EMLA cream is contraindicated in patients with congenital or idiopathic methemoglobinemia and in infants under the age of 12 months who are receiving treatment with methemoglobin-inducing agents. EMLA cream should be used with caution in patients with glucose-6-phosphate deficiencies, who are more susceptible to methemoglobinemia.

5. Treat methemoglobinemia with methylene blue (IV 1- 2 mg/kg injected over 5 min).
6. Dermal application of EMLA cream may cause a transient local blanching, followed by redness or erythema.
7. EMLA cream should be used with caution in patients who may be more sensitive to the systemic effects of lidocaine and prilocaine, including acutely ill, debilitated, elderly patients or those with severe hepatic disease.
8. Avoid contact of EMLA cream with the eye. If eye contact occurs, immediately wash out the eye with water or saline and protect the eye until sensation returns.
9. The patient should avoid inadvertent trauma to the treated area, or exposure to hot or cold temperatures until complete sensation has returned.

Principal Adverse Reactions

Cardiovascular: Hypotension, bradycardia
Pulmonary: Respiratory depression, bronchospasm
CNS: Euphoria, confusion, tinnitus, seizures, blurred vision
Dermatologic: Blanching, pallor, erythema, edema, urticaria, pruritus, anaphylactoid reactions (rare)
Other: Methemoglobinemia

ENALAPRIL MALEATE (VASOTEC)
ENALAPRILAT (VASOTEC IV)

Use(s): Antihypertensive; treatment of congestive heart failure, prevention of post-MI ventricular remodeling

Dosing: Hypertension:
        PO, 2.5-20 mg once or twice daily
        IV, 0.625-1.25 mg q6hr. Give slowly over 5 min.

CHF:

PO, 2.5-20 mg once or twice daily.

Use initial low doses (2.5 mg) when added to a diuretic or in patients with salt depletion, renal impairment.

Elimination: Renal, hepatic

How Supplied:

Tablets, 2.5 mg, 5 mg, 10 mg, 20 mg

Injection, 1.25 mg/ml

Storage: Injection/tablets: Temperature below 30° C

Pharmacology

Enalapril, an angiotensin-converting enzyme (ACE) inhibitor is the ethyl ester of enalaprilat. A prodrug, enalapril is hydrolyzed to the active form, enalaprilat, in the liver, and therapeutic effects depend on hepatic metabolism. The affinity of enalaprilat for ACE is 200,000 times greater than that of angiotensin 1, and 2 and 17 times that of enalapril and captopril respectively. Enalapril differs from captopril by lack of a sulfhydryl group, which may result in decreased risk of immune-based side effects (e.g., cutaneous reactions, taste disturbances). Enalapril reduces blood pressure by several mechanisms. It inhibits the conversion of angiotensin 1 to the potent vasoconstrictor angiotensin 2 and decreases the inactivation of vasodilatory bradykinins. Natriuresis occurs secondary to decreased secretion of aldosterone by angiotensin 2 and specific renal vasodilation. Systemic vascular resistance is decreased with slight increase or no change in heart rate, stroke volume, or cardiac output. It causes arterial and possibly venous dilation. In patients with CHF, enalapril, usually in conjunction with cardiac glycosides and loop diuretics, decreases total peripheral resistance (arteriolar and venous dilation), mean arterial pressure, PCWP, heart size, and the elevated levels of plasma catecholamines. Stroke volume, cardiac output, and excercise tolerance are increased. Enalapril, like other ACE inhibitors, is a cerebral vasodilator. It increases cerebral blood flow and intracranial pressure.

Pharmacokinetics

Onset: PO, <1 hr; IV, <15 min
Peak Effect: PO, 4-8 hr
Duration: PO, 12-24 hr
Interaction/Toxicity: Additive hypotensive effects with diuretics, vasodilators, beta blockers, calcium channel blockers, volatile anesthetics; elevates serum potassium levels, which may be significant with renal insufficiency and use of potassium-sparing diuretics such as spironolactone, triamterene, or amiloride; may produce hypoglycemia in diabetic patients; antihypertensive effect antagonized by indomethacin and other nonsteroidal antiinflammatory drugs.

Guidelines/Precautions

1. May be associated with angioedema, bone marrow suppression, and proteinuria. Emergency therapy for angioedema with airway obstruction should include SC epinephrine 1:1000 (0.5-1.0 mg).
2. Enalapril is preferable to captopril in patients with collagen vascular disease or during cotherapy with other drugs altering the immune status.
3. May cause profound first-dose hypotension, particularly in those patients who are volume-depleted or when used concomitantly with agents that reduce vascular volume. Treat hypotension with volume expansion.
4. Should not be used with potassium-sparing diuretics because of the possibility of hyperkalemia.

5. May be associated with a persistent, dry cough (and sometimes bronchospasm) resistant to normal antitussives but that may respond to a decrease in dose and/or inhaled cromolyn.
6. Use with caution in hypertensive patients with renal disease. Increases in BUN and serum creatinine may develop after reduction of blood pressure. Monitor renal function during the first few weeks of therapy.
7. In patients with CHF, whose renal function may depend on the renin-angiotensin-aldosterone system, treatment with enalapril may be associated with oliguria or progressive azotemia and, rarely, with acute renal failure or death.
8. Use in pregnancy may be associated with increased incidence of cranial facial dysplasias, other fetal abnormalities.

Principal Adverse Reactions

Cardiovascular: Hypotension, palpitations, tachycardia
Pulmonary: Cough, dyspnea, bronchospasm
CNS: Dizziness, fatigue
GI: Diarrhea, nausea, abdominal pain, dyspepsia
Dermatologic: Rash, pruritus
Renal: Elevation of BUN and creatinine, proteinuria, renal failure
Hematologic: Neutropenia, thrombocytopenia, hemolytic anemia, eosinophilia

---

EPHEDRINE SULFATE (EPHEDRINE SULFATE)

Use(s): Vasopressor, bronchodilator

Dosing: IV, 5-20 mg (100-200 μg/kg)
IM, 25-50 mg
PO, 25 to 50 mg q3-4hr

Elimination: Hepatic, renal
How Supplied:
Injection, 25 mg/ml, 50 mg/ml
Capsules, 25 mg and 50 mg
Oral solution, 20 mg/5 ml
Storage: Injection/capsules/oral solution: Room temperature (15°-30° C). Ephedrine is subject to oxidation. Protect from light. Do not use unless solution is clear.

Pharmacology

This drug is a noncatecholamine sympathomimetic with mixed direct and indirect actions. It is resistant to metabolism by MAO and COMT, resulting in prolonged duration of action. Ephedrine increases cardiac output, blood pressure, and heart rate by alpha and beta adrenergic stimulation. It increases coronary and skeletal blood flow and produces bronchodilation by stimulation of beta-2 receptors. Ephedrine has minimal effects on uterine blood flow. However, it restores uterine blood flow when used to treat epidural or spinal hypotension in pregnant patients.

Pharmacokinetics

Onset: IV, almost immediate; IM, few min
Peak Effect: IV, 2-5 min; IM, <10 min
Duration: IV/IM, 10-60 min
Interaction/Toxicity: Increased risk of arrhythmias with volatile anesthetic agents; potentiated by tricyclic antidepressants; increases MAC of volatile anesthetics

Guidelines/Precautions

1. Tolerance may develop, but temporary cessation of the drug restores its original effectiveness.
2. Use cautiously in patients with hypertension and ischemic heart disease.

3. Unpredictable effect in patients in whom endogenous catecholamines are depleted.
4. May produce an unacceptable degree of CNS stimulation resulting in insomnia.

Principal Adverse Reactions

Cardiovascular: Hypertension, tachycardia, arrhythmias
Pulmonary: Pulmonary edema
CNS: Anxiety, tremors
Metabolic: Hyperglycemia, transient hyperkalemia then hypokalemia
Dermatologic: Necrosis at site of injection

EPINEPHRINE HCL (ADRENALINE, EPINEPHRINE)

Use(s): Inotrope, bronchodilator, prolongation of duration of local anesthetics, treatment of allergic reactions, postintubation and infectious croup, resuscitation

Dosing: Cardiac arrest:

Standard dose: IV bolus, 1 mg or 0.02 mg/kg (10 ml or 0.1 ml/kg of 1:10,000 solution). Administer every 3-5 min as necessary. If no response after second dose, administer high dose.

High dose (acceptable, possibly helpful): IV bolus, 5-10 mg or 0.1-0.2 mg/kg (5-10 ml of a 1:1000 solution) every 3- 5 min as necessary.

If intravenous access is not available, dilute 5-10 mg or 0.1-0.2 mg/kg (5-10 ml of a 1:1000 solution) in an equal volume of sterile NS and inject via an endotracheal tube.

Inotropic support: Infusion, 2-20 μg/min (0.1-1.0 μg/kg/min)

Anaphylaxis/severe asthma:

   Adults: 0.1-0.5 mg SC or IM (0.1-0.5 ml of a 1:1000 solution)

   Children: 0.01 mg/kg SC or IM (0.01 ml/kg of a 1:1000 solution), not to exceed 0.5 mg

   Subcutaneous doses may be repeated at 10-15 min intervals in patients with anaphylactic shock and at 20 min-4 hr intervals in patients with asthma.

Bronchodilator/croup therapy:

   Inhalation: Nebulization with oxygen: 2.25% racemic epinephrine or 1% (1:100) epinephrine. Dilute 1 ml in 3 ml NS. Give 1-3 inhalations and repeat after 5 min if necessary. Administer treatments q2-6hr. Allow no less than 30 min between treatments. (Children 0.5% [1:200] epinephrine or 1.25% racemic epinephrine. Dilute 0.5 ml in 1.5 ml NS. Give q2-6hr.)

   Metered aerosol: 160-250 μg (1 inhalation). Repeat once if necessary after at least 1 min. Subsequent doses should not be administered for at least 4 hr.

   Rebound effect with increasing obstruction may follow an initial clearing of the airway. Monitor patient closely.

Test dose in regional anesthesia (marker for accidental intravascular injection): 10-15 μg (2-3 ml of 1:200,000 epinephrine solution mixed with local anesthetic). Intravascular injections detected by increase in heart rate (>10 beats per minute) within 30-45 sec.

Prolongation of infiltration/plexus/epidural/caudal/intrapleural anesthesia: 1:200,000 to 1:100,000 solution mixed with local anesthetic (0.1 mg epinephrine diluted in 20 ml local anesthetic gives 1:200,000 solution or 5 μg/ml) Maximum dose 250 μg (3-5 μg/kg)

Prolongation of spinal anesthesia: 0.1-0.4 mg (0.1-0.4 ml of a 1:1000 solution) added to anesthetic spinal fluid mixture (Children: 5 μg/kg or epinephrine wash)

Elimination: Enzymatic degradation (hepatic, renal, and GI tract)

How Supplied:

Injection, 0.01 mg/ml (1:100,000), 0.1 mg/ml (1:10,000), 0.5 mg/ml (1:2,000), 1 mg/ml(1:1,000);

Solution for nebulization, 1% epinephrine, 1.25% racemic epinephrine, 2.25% racemic epinephrine;

Aerosol, 160 μg, 200 μg, 220 μg, 250 μg/metered spray

Storage: Injection/solution: Protect from light, extreme heat, and freezing. Preparations should be clear. Do not use injection if it is discolored or contains a precipitate.

Dilution for Infusion: 3 mg in 250 ml D_5W or NS (12 μg/ml)

Pharmacology

An endogenous catecholamine, epinephrine activates both alpha and beta adrenergic receptors. At therapeutic parenteral doses, the prominent effects are on beta adrenergic receptors. There is increased myocardial contractility and heart rate, relaxation of the smooth muscle of the bronchial tree, dilation of skeletal muscle vasculature, and a decrease in total peripheral resistance. At higher doses, alpha adrenergic effects predominate, and there is an increase in total peripheral resistance. Epinephrine increases uterine activity and produces uterine vasoconstriction and decrease in uterine blood flow. Epinephrine decreases the rate of absorption of local anesthetics. It prolongs the duration of anesthesia and decreases the risk of systemic toxicity. Decrease in onset time and improvement in the quality of anesthesia may be due to the alpha-2 adrenergic effects of epinephrine. Analgesic effects of epinephrine at the spinal cord level may partly be due to alpha-2 agonist effects and suppressed activity of wide dynamic range neurons.

Pharmacokinetics

Onset: IV, 30-60 sec SC, 6-15 min; Intratracheal, 5-15 sec; Inhalation 3-5 min
Peak Effect: IV within 3 min
Duration: IV, 5-10 min; Intratracheal, 15-25 min; Inhalation/SC, 1-3 hr
Interaction/Toxicity: Ventricular arrhythmias, (increased risk with use of volatile anesthetics, especially halothane); reduction of renal blood flow and urinary outflow; enhanced effect with tricyclic antidepressants and bretylium; decreases onset time and improves quality of epidural/spinal anesthetics (alpha-2 adrenergic effects)

Guidelines/Precautions

1. Use with digitalis or volatile anesthetics may result in arrhythmias. The 50% effective dose (ED50) of epinephrine in saline per 20-min period needed to produce 3 or more premature ventricular contractions in adults:

1.25 MAC halothane 1.5 μg/kg, 1.25 MAC enflurane 3.5 μg/kg, 1.25 MAC isoflurane 6.5 μg/kg. The ED50 of epinephrine in 0.5% lidocaine: 1.25 MAC halothane 3.7 μg/kg in adults and 7.8-15 μg/kg in children.

2. Use with caution in patients with cardiovascular disease, hypertension, diabetes, and hyperthyroidism.

3. Use with caution for obstetric regional anesthesia, especially in high-risk parturients with uteroplacental insufficiency. The alpha-1 adrenergic effects may decrease uterine blood flow, and the beta-2 adrenergic effects may slow labor and increase the need for oxytocic supplementation.

4. Contraindicated for IV regional anesthesia or local anesthesia of end organs (digits, penis, nose, ears).

5. In cardiopulmonary resuscitation, intratracheal administration may be advantageous in bypassing the sluggish blood flow, hemodilution, and significant degradation in the blood stream attending injection of the drug into a peripheral vein. The absorption rate, duration, and pharmacologic effects of intratracheal drug administration compares favorably with the IV route.

6. Avoid intramuscular injections of epinephrine oil suspension into the buttocks. Gas gangrene may occur because epinephrine reduces oxygen tension of the tissues, encouraging the growth of anaerobic organisms.

Principal Adverse Reactions

Cardiovascular: Hypertension, tachycardia, arrhythmias, angina
Pulmonary: Pulmonary edema
CNS: Anxiety, headache, cerebrovascular hemorrhage
Dermatologic: Necrosis at site of injection

Metabolic: Hyperglycemia, transient hyperkalemia, hypokalemia

---

ERGONOVINE MALEATE (ERGOTRATE)

Use(s): Treatment of postpartum uterine atony and bleeding; involution of the uterus

Dosing: IV/IM, 0.2 mg. May require repeated doses (usually q2-4 hr prn).
PO, 0.2-0.4 mg every 6-12 hr for 48 hr.
Elimination: Hepatic
How Supplied:
Injection, 0.2 mg/ml
Tablets, 0.2 mg
Storage:
Injection: Temperature below 8° C. Stable at room temperature (15-30° C). for 60-90 days. Protect from light.
Tablets: Protect from light.

Pharmacology

This ergot alkaloid stimulates contractions of uterine and vascular smooth muscle. It increases contractile frequency and tone of the uterine musculature. Ergonovine produces vasoconstriction, mainly of capacitance vessels; increased central venous pressure and elevated blood pressure.

Pharmacokinetics

Onset: IV, 40 sec; IM, 7-8 min; PO, 10 min
Peak Effect: IV, <5 min; IM, <1 hr
Duration: IV, 45 min; IM, 3-6 hr
Interaction/Toxicity: Vasoconstriction potentiated by sympathomimetics (e.g., ephedrine, phenylephrine).

Guidelines/Precautions

1. Administration in the second or third stage of labor before delivery of the placenta may lead to captivation of the placenta.
2. Use cautiously in patients with preeclampsia, hypertension, or cardiac disease. The drug may produce severe maternal hypertension, cerebrovascular accidents, and retinal detachment.
3. Avoid in patients with peripheral vascular disease.
4. Uterine contractions may continue for 3 hr or more after injection.
5. Intravenous administration has a higher incidence of side effects and should be used in emergency situations only.
6. Severe cramping is evidence of effectiveness of oral doses but may justify reduction in dosage.

Principal Adverse Reactions

Cardiovascular: Hypertension, tachycardia
CNS: Cerebrovascular accidents, seizures
GI: Nausea and vomiting
Eye: Retinal detachment

ESMOLOL HCL (BREVIBLOC)

Use(s): Treatment of supraventricular tachyarrhythmias, perioperative and intraoperative hypertension

Dosing: SVT:

IV loading: 500 μg/kg (Give over 1 minute)
Infusion, 50-200 μg/kg/min (if needed, repeat loading dose at intervals of 5 min. Titrate

infusion upward in increments of 25-50 μg/kg/min to desired heart rate or patient tolerance (e.g., decreased blood pressure). Infusion doses above 200 μg/kg/min provide little added benefit.

Hypertension:

IV, 25-100 mg (0.5-2 mg/kg); may repeat q5min if necessary. May be administered 2 min before laryngoscopy to attenuate the pressor response to intubation.

Infusion, 50-300 μg/kg/min. Titrate to blood pressure response.

Elimination: Esterases (in cytosol of red blood cells)
How Supplied: Injection, 10 mg/ml, 250 mg/ml
Storage: Room temperature (15°-30° C).
Dilution for Infusion: 5 g in 500 ml D_5W (10 mg/ml); 10 mg/ml vials do not need to be diluted

Pharmacology

A cardioselective beta blocker with rapid onset and short duration of action. The drug is hydrolyzed by red blood cell esterases. It produces negative inotropic and chronotropic effects. At high doses, selectivity for beta-1 adrenergic receptors usually diminishes and inhibition of beta-2 receptors of bronchial and vascular smooth muscle will occur.

Pharmacokinetics

Onset: 1-2 min
Peak Effect: 5 min
Duration: 10-20 min
Interaction/Toxicity: Potentiates myocardial depression produced by inhaled or injected anesthetics; increases

serum levels of digoxin; esmolol serum levels increased with concomitant use of morphine, warfarin sodium; prolongs succinylcholine neuromuscular blockade; may unmask the direct negative inotropic effect of ketamine; incompatible with sodium bicarbonate.

Guidelines/Precautions

1. Use with caution in patients with AV heart block or cardiac failure not caused by tachycardia and in patients with chronic obstructive airway disease.
2. May mask signs of hypoglycemia in diabetes mellitus.
3. Excessive myocardial depression may be treated with IV atropine (1-2 mg), IV isoproterenol (0.02-0.15 μg/kg/min), IV glucagon (1-5 mg), or a transvenous cardiac pacemaker.
4. May enhance the actions of nondepolarizing neuromuscular blocking agents such as tubocurarine, gallamine, metocurine, and pancuronium.
5. After achieving adequate heart rate and blood pressure control, transfer to an alternative antiarrhythmic or antihypertensive such as propranolol, verapamil, or digoxin. Reduce infusion rate of esmolol by 50% , half an hour after the first dose of alternative agent. Discontinue esmolol after second dose if pressure and rate control have been attained.

Principal Adverse Reactions

Cardiovascular: Hypotension, bradycardia
Pulmonary: Bronchospasm
CNS: Confusion, depression
GU: Urinary retention
GI: Nausea, vomiting
Dermatologic: Erythema, edema at infusion site

ETHACRYNIC ACID (EDECRIN)

Use(s): Diuretic; treatment of hypertension, increased intracranial pressure, edema associated with congestive heart failure, hepatic cirrhosis, and nephrotic syndrome; differential diagnosis of acute oliguria

Dosing: Slow IV, 0.5-1 mg/kg
PO, 50-200 mg/day (children, 25 mg/day initial dose and adjust in increments of 25 mg)
Elimination: Renal
How Supplied:
Powder for injection, 50 mg/vial in 50 ml vials for reconstitution
Tablets, 25 mg, 50 mg
Storage: Powder for injection/tablets: Room temperature (15°-30° C). Protect from light. Reconstituted solutions should be used within 24 hr of preparation.

Pharmacology

This loop diuretic inhibits reabsorption of sodium and chloride ions, primarily in the medullary portion of the ascending limb of the loop of Henle. It inhibits reabsorption of sodium to a greater proportion than most other diuretics and may be effective in patients with significant degrees of renal insufficiency.

Pharmacokinetics

Onset: IV, <5 min; PO, 30 min
Peak Effect: IV, 15-30 min; PO, 2 hr
Duration: IV, 2 hr; PO, 6-8 hr
Interaction/Toxicity: Potassium loss increases likelihood of digitalis toxicity and enhances effects of muscle relaxants;

additive effects with other diuretics; potentiates carbonic anhydrase inhibitors; coadministration of aminoglycosides and cisplatin may increase potential for ototoxicity.

Guidelines/Precautions

1. Do not use to treat acute oliguria because of decreased intravascular volume.
2. Requires periodic monitoring of fluids and electrolytes.
3. Use with caution in patients with hearing impairment or cirrhosis.
4. May predispose patients to digitalis glycoside toxicity because of hypokalemia.
5. Do not give SC or IM because of pain and irritation at site.

Principal Adverse Reactions

Cardiovascular: Hypotension
CNS: Headaches, confusion
GI: Anorexia, malaise, diarrhea, abdominal discomfort, bleeding
Metabolic: Hyperuricemia
Special Senses: Deafness, tinnitus, vertigo, blurred vision
Other: Rash, fever, chills, hematuria

ETIDOCAINE HCL (DURANEST)

Use(s): Regional anesthesia

Dosing: Infiltration/peripheral nerve block: 50-400 mg (1% solution);
Epidural:
Bolus, 100-300 mg (10-20 ml of 1%-1.5% solution)
Infusion, 6-12 ml/hr (0.25%-0.5% solution with or without epidural narcotics)

Caudal, 100-300 mg (10-30 ml of 1% solution); children, 0.4-0.7-1.0 ml/kg for L2-T10-T7 level of anesthesia.

Maximum safe dose: 3 mg/kg without epinephrine; 4 mg/kg with epinephrine

Solutions containing preservatives should not be used for epidural or caudal block. Except where contraindicated, vasoconstrictor drugs may be added to increase effect and prolong local or regional anesthesia. For dosage/route guidelines, see Epinephrine, Dosing or Phenylephrine, Dosing. Do not use vasoconstrictor drugs for local anesthesia of end organs (digits, penis, nose, ears).

Elimination: Hepatic

How Supplied: Injection, 1% solution with or without, epinephrine, 1:200,000; 1.5% solution with epinephrine, 1:200,000

Storage: Room temperature (15°-40° C). Do not permit to freeze.

Pharmacology

An aminoamide and a long acting local anesthetic, etidocaine stabilizes neuronal membrane by inhibiting the ionic fluxes required for the initiation and conduction of impulses. Etidocaine produces a profound degree of motor blockade and abdominal muscle relaxation when used for peridural analgesia. Toxic blood levels may cause seizures and cardiovascular collapse secondary to a decrease in peripheral vascular resistance and direct myocardial depression. High plasma levels (as occur in paracervical blocks) produce uterine vasoconstriction and decrease in uterine blood flow. Vasoconstrictor agents decrease rate of absorption and prolong duration of action.

Pharmacokinetics

Onset:
Infiltration, 3-5 min
Epidural, 5-15 min
Peak Effect:
Infiltration, 5-15 min
Epidural, 15-20 min
Duration:
Infiltration, 2-3 hr; with epinephrine, 3-7 hr:
Epidural 3-5 hr
Interaction/Toxicity: Reduced clearance with concomitant use of beta blocking agents, cimetidine; seizures, respiratory and circulatory depression at high plasma levels; benzodiazepines, barbiturates, and volatile anesthetics increase seizure threshold; duration of local or regional anesthesia prolonged by vasoconstrictor agents (e.g., epinephrine), alpha-2 agonists (e.g., clonidine), and narcotics (e.g., fentanyl); alkalinization increases rate of onset and potency of local or regional anesthesia.

Guidelines/Precautions

1. Do not use for spinal anesthesia.
2. Because of profound motor blockade, not recommended for epidural anesthesia in normal delivery.
3. Use with caution in patients with hypovolemia, severe congestive heart failure, shock, and all forms of heart block. The increased cardiac toxicity of etidocaine (compared with lidocaine or mepivacaine) results from a greater decrease in myocardial contractility and depression of cardiac conduction.
4. Contraindicated in patients with hypersensitivity to amide-type local anesthetics.

5. Benzodiazepines increase seizure threshold.
6. Use for paracervical block may be associated with fetal bradycardia.
7. Toxic plasma levels (e.g., from accidental intravascular injection) may cause cardiopulmonary collapse and seizures. Premonitory signs and symptoms manifest as numbness of the tongue and circumoral tissues, metallic taste, restlessness, tinnitus, and tremors. Support of circulation (IV fluids, vasopressors, IV sodium bicarbonate 1-2 mEq/kg to treat cardiac toxicity [sodium channel blockade], IV bretylium 5 mg/kg, DC cardioversion/defibrillation for ventricular arrhythmias) and securing a patent airway (ventilate with 100% oxygen) are paramount. Thiopental (0.5-2 mg/kg IV), midazolam (0.02-0.04 mg/kg IV), or diazepam (0.1 mg/kg IV) may be used for prophylaxis and/or treatment of seizures.
8. The level of sympathetic blockade (bradycardia with block above T5) determines the degree of hypotension (often heralded by nausea and vomiting) after epidural or intrathecal etidocaine. Fluid hydration (10-20 ml/kg NS or lactated Ringer's solution), vasopressor agents (e.g., ephedrine), and left uterine displacement in pregnant patients may be used for prophylaxis and/or treatment. Administer atropine to treat bradycardia.
9. Epidural or caudal injections should be avoided when the patient has hypovolemic shock, septicemia, infection at the injection site, or coagulopathy.

Principal Adverse Reactions

Cardiovascular: Bradycardia, hypotension
Pulmonary: Respiratory depression
CNS: Euphoria, tinnitus, seizures
Allergic: Urticaria, edema, anaphylactoid symptoms

Epidural/Caudal: High spinal, loss of bladder and bowel control, loss of perineal sensation and sexual function, persistent motor sensory and/or autonomic (sphincter control) deficit

ETOMIDATE (AMIDATE)

Use(s): Induction and supplementation of anesthesia

Dosing: IV induction, 0.1-0.4 mg/kg
         Infusion, 0.25-1 mg/min (5-20 μg/kg/min)
Elimination: Hepatic
How Supplied: Injection: 2 mg/ml
Storage: Room temperature (15°-30° C).

Pharmacology

Etomidate is a nonbarbiturate hypnotic without analgesic activity. Therapeutic doses have minimal effect on myocardial metabolism, cardiac output, and peripheral or pulmonary circulation. Etomidate effects on the EEG include an initial increase in the alpha amplitude followed by a progressive decrease in activity with periods of burst suppression at high doses. Myoclonic movements occur in about one third of patients during induction and are due to disinhibition of subcortical suppression of extrapyramidal activity. Etomidate (more than thiopental or propofol) may elicit alterations in somatosensory evoked potentials. Etomidate lowers cerebral metabolism, cerebral blood flow, and intracranial pressure. Because of its minimal effect on systemic blood pressure, it is more successful than thiopental or propofol in maintaining cerebral perfusion pressure. Intraocular pressure is decreased. Adrenocortical suppression, which may occur after a single induction dose, lasts 4-8 hr and is due to etomidate-induced inhibition of 11-beta hydroxylase. Etomidate does not release histamine.

Pharmacokinetics

Onset: 30-60 sec
Peak Effect: 1 min
Duration of Action: 3-10 min
Interaction/Toxicity: Cardiovascular and CNS depressant effects potentiated by other sedatives, narcotics, and volatile anesthetics; venous pain and myoclonus on rapid injection

Guidelines/Precautions

1. Use with caution in patients with focal epilepsy.
2. Use large veins. Pain is more likely if injected into small veins.
3. Myoclonus is reduced by premedication with benzodiazepine or opioid.

Principal Adverse Reactions

Cardiovascular: Hypotension, hypertension, arrhythmias
Pulmonary: Hyperventilation, hypoventilation, laryngospasm, hiccups
CNS: Myoclonus, tonic movements, eye movements
GI: Nausea or vomiting
Endocrine: Adrenocortical suppression
Other: Thrombophlebitis

FAMOTIDINE (PEPCID)

Use(s): Peptic ulcer disease; pathologic hypersecretory states; prophylaxis against acid pulmonary aspiration, stress ulcers, or allergic reactions

Dosing: IV, 20 mg q12hr (dilute in 10 ml NS/inject over 2 min)
          PO, 20 mg twice daily or 20-40 mg at bedtime
Elimination: Renal

How Supplied:

Tablets, 20 mg, 40 mg
Powder for oral suspension, 40 mg per 5 ml when reconstituted
Injection, 10 mg/ml

Storage:

Powder for injection/tablets, temperature below 40° C. Protect from light. Reconstituted solutions should be stored below 30° C and used within 30 days of preparation.
Injection, refrigerate (2°-8° C).

Pharmacology

This competitive inhibitor of histamine H2 receptors suppresses acid concentration and volume of gastric secretion. Gastric emptying and exocrine pancreatic functions are not affected. It does not have any cumulative effect with repeated doses.

Pharmacokinetics

Onset: PO, within 1 hr; IV, <30 min
Peak Effect: PO, 1-4 hr; IV, 30 min-3 hr
Duration of Action: PO/IV, 10-12 hr
Interaction/Toxicity: Bioavailability enhanced by food and decreased by antacids

Guidelines/Precautions

1. Reduce dosage in patients with renal impairment.

Principal Adverse Reactions

Cardiovascular: Palpitations, hypotension
Pulmonary: Bronchospasm
CNS: Tinnitus, fatigue, dizziness, depression, paresthesia, headache
GI: Nausea, vomiting, diarrhea
Musculoskeletal: Musculoskeletal pain, arthralgia
Hematologic: Thrombocytopenia

FENTANYL (SUBLIMAZE)

Use(s): Analgesia, anesthesia

Dosing: Analgesia:

IV/IM, 25-100 μg (0.7-2 μg/kg);

Oral transmucosal, 200-400 μg (5-15 μg/kg) every 4-6 hr. Oralets should be sucked and not chewed.

Induction:

IV bolus, 5-40 μg/kg or

Infusion, 0.25-2 μg/kg/min for ≤20 min. Titrate dose to patient response. To avoid chest wall rigidity administer muscle relaxant simultaneously with induction doses.

Anesthesia Supplement:

IV, 2-20 μg/kg

Infusion, 0.025-0.25 μg/kg/min

Sole anesthetic:

IV, 50-150 μg/kg (average total dosage—titrate to effect) or

Infusion, 0.25-0.5 μg/kg/min

Epidural:

Bolus, 50-100 μg (1-2 μg/kg); dilute in 10 ml (preservative-free) NS or local anesthetic

Infusion, 25-60 μg/hr (0.5-0.7 μg/kg/hr)

Spinal: bolus, 5-20 μg (0.1-0.4 μg/kg)

IV regional block: Add 50 μg (1 μg/kg) fentanyl to local anesthetic (see lidocaine, prilocaine, or bupivacaine for dosing and volume)

Brachial plexus block: Add 50-100 μg (1-2 μg/kg) fentanyl to 40 ml (0.5-0.75 ml/kg) local anesthetic

Patient controlled analgesia:
IV:
Bolus, 15-75 μg (0.3-1.5 μg/kg)
Infusion, 15-100 μg/hr (0.3-2 μg/kg/hr)
Lockout interval 3-10 min
Epidural:
Bolus, 4-8 μg (0.08-0.16 μg/kg)
Infusion, 6 μg/hr (0.12 μg/kg)
Lockout interval 10 min
Transdermal system:
Initial: 25-50 μg/hr
Maintenance: 25-100 μg/hr.
Base dose on prior 24 hr analgesic requirements. 60 mg IM morphine dose = 360 mg PO morphine dose = 100-200 μg/hr transdermal fentanyl dose. Doses >50 μg/hr should be used only in patients who are already receiving and have developed some tolerance to opioids.

Each transdermal application provides 72 hr of reliable analgesic delivery. Therapeutic concentrations are not achieved until 12 to 24 hr after initial application. Initial dosage may be increased after 3 days. Further titration should be evaluated after 2 applications (6 days) on the new dose. To maintain adequate pain control, add short-acting opioids prn for breakthrough pain.

Elimination: Hepatic, pulmonary
How Supplied:
Injection, 50 μg/ml
Transdermal: 25 μg/hr, 50 μg/hr, 75 μg/hr, 100 μg/hr
Transmucosal oralets, 200 μg, 300 μg, 400 μg

Storage:

Injection: Room temperature (15°-30° C). Protect from light.

Transdermal Systems: Temperature below 30° C.

Dilution for Infusion:

IV, 500 μg in 100 ml NS (5 μg/ml)

Epidural bolus, 50-100 μg in 15-20 ml local anesthetic or (preservative-free) NS

Epidural infusion, 100-500 μg in 100 ml local anesthetic or (preservative-free) NS (1-5 μg/ml)

Pharmacology

This phenylpiperidine derivative is a potent opioid agonist. As an analgesic, fentanyl is 75-125 times more potent than morphine. The rapid onset and short duration of action reflect the greater lipid solubility of fentanyl compared with morphine. Depression of ventilation is dose-dependent and may last longer than the analgesia. Cardiovascular stability is maintained even in large doses when used as a sole anesthetic. Cerebral blood flow, cerebral metabolic rate, and intracranial pressure are decreased. Fentanyl (and other opioids) enhance the action of local anesthetics on peripheral nerve block. This is partly due to weak local anesthetic properties (high doses suppress nerve conduction) and effects on opiate receptors in peripheral nerve terminals. Fentanyl is combined with droperidol to produce neuroleptanalgesia.

Pharmacokinetics

Onset:

IV, within 30 sec; IM, < 8 min

Epidural/spinal, 4-10 min

Transdermal, 12-18 hr

Oral transmucosal, 5-15 min

Peak Effect:
IV, 5-15 min; IM, <15 min; epidural/spinal, <30 min; oral transmucosal, 20-30 min
Duration:
IV, 30-60 min; IM, 1-2 hr; epidural/spinal, 1-2 hr; transdermal, 3 days
Oral transmucosal, 1-2 hr
Interaction/Toxicity: Circulatory and ventilatory depressant effects potentiated by narcotics, sedatives, volatile anesthetics, nitrous oxide; ventilatory depressant effects potentiated by amphetamines, MAO inhibitors, phenothiazines, and tricyclic antidepressants; analgesia enhanced and prolonged by alpha-2 agonists (e.g., epinephrine, clonidine); muscle rigidity in higher dose range sufficient to interfere with ventilation; addition of epinephrine to intrathecal/epidural fentanyl results in increased side effects (e.g., nausea) and prolonged motor block.

Guidelines/Precautions

1. In hemodynamically stable patients, analgesic doses may be given 2-4 minutes before laryngoscopy to attenuate the pressor response to intubation. Requirements for induction agents (e.g., sodium thiopental) may be decreased.
2. Reduce doses in elderly, hypovolemic, or high-risk patients and with concomitant use of sedatives and other narcotics. Incremental doses should be determined from effect of initial dose.
3. Narcotic effects are reversed by naloxone (IV 0.2-0.4 mg or higher). Duration of reversal may be shorter than duration of narcotic action.
4. High doses may produce a naloxone-sensitive increased muscle tone and rigidity.

5. Crosses the placental barrier; usage in labor may produce depression of respiration in the neonate. Resuscitation may be required; have naloxone available.
6. Undesirable side effects of epidural, caudal, or intrathecal fentanyl include delayed respiratory depression (up to 8 hr after single dose), pruritus, nausea and vomiting, urinary retention. Naloxone (IV 0.2-0.4 mg prn or infusion 5-10 μg/kg/hr) is effective for prophylaxis and/or treatment of these side effects. Ventilatory support for respiratory depression must be readily available. Antihistamines (e.g., diphenhydramine 12.5-25 mg IV/IM q6hr prn) may be used in treating pruritus. Metoclopramide (10 mg IV q6hr) may be used in treating nausea and vomiting. Urinary retention that does not respond to naloxone may require straight bladder catheterization.
7. Epidural, caudal, or intrathecal injections should be avoided when the patient has septicemia, infection at the injection site, or coagulopathy.
8. The transmucosal oralets should be removed after consumption or if the patient has shown an adequate sedative/analgesic level or signs of respiratory depression. Remove the drug matrix from the handle with tissue paper and flush down a sink.
9. Accidental dermal exposure to transmucosal oralets should be treated by rinsing the affected area with cool water.
10. Fentanyl transdermal system is contraindicated in the management of acute or postoperative pain, including use in outpatient surgeries. Deaths have been reported with misuse.

Principal Adverse Reactions

Cardiovascular: Hypotension, bradycardia
Pulmonary: Respiratory depression, apnea
CNS: Dizziness, blurred vision, seizures
GI: Nausea, emesis, delayed gastric emptying, biliary tract spasm
Eye: Miosis
Musculoskeletal: Muscle rigidity

FLECAINIDE ACETATE (TAMBOCOR)

Use(s): Treatment of documented life-threatening ventricular arrhythmias such as sustained ventricular tachycardia

Dosing: PO, 100-200 mg every 12 hr; keep trough levels below 0.2-1.0 μg/ml
Elimination: Renal, hepatic
How Supplied: Tablets,100 mg (IV not available for general clinical use in the United States)
Storage: Tablets: Room temperature (15°-30° C). Protect from light.

Pharmacology

A fluorinated analog of procainamide, flecainide is a class 1C antiarrhythmic. It produces dose-related decrease in intracardiac conduction in all parts of the heart, with the greatest effect on the His-Purkinje system (H-V conduction). This results in QRS complex widening and prolonged QT interval. Pacing threshold is increased by flecainide. Although it does not usually alter heart rate, it usually exerts a moderate negative inotropic effect and reduced ejection fraction. Flecainide's use should be reserved for treatment of documented, life-threatening arrhythmias after failure of conventional therapy.

Pharmacokinetics

Onset: PO, <1 hr
Peak Effect: PO, 2-4 hr
Duration: 12-27 hr (half-life)
Interaction/Toxicity: Additive negative inotropic effects with beta adrenergic blockers, calcium channel blockers; excretion decreased by alkalinization and increased by acidification; altered effects with hypokalemia or hyperkalemia; may cause new or worsened arrhythmias.

Guidelines/Precautions

1. Use with caution in patients with a history of congestive heart failure, myocardial dysfunction, or sick sinus syndrome and those with permanent pacemakers or temporary pacing electrodes.
2. Do not administer to patients with existing poor endocardial pacing thresholds or nonprogrammable pacemakers unless suitable pacing rescue is available.
3. Correct preexisting hypokalemia or hyperkalemia before administration.
4. Increased urinary pH decreases and decreased urinary pH increases flecainide excretion.
5. Potassium status may alter the drug's effect.
6. Initiate therapy in hospital and monitor rhythm. Do not increase dosage more frequently than once every 4 days because optimal effect may not be achieved during the first 2-3 days of therapy.

Principal Adverse Reactions

Cardiovascular: Arrhythmias, new or worsened CHF, AV block, sinus bradycardia, sinus arrest, palpitations, chest pain
Pulmonary: Dyspnea, bronchospasm

CNS: Dizziness, blurred vision, headache, tremor, somnolence, tinnitus
GI: Nausea, vomiting, constipation, diarrhea, abdominal pain
GU: Polyuria, urinary retention
Hematologic: Leukopenia, thrombocytopenia

FLUMAZENIL (ROMAZICON)

Use(s): Diagnostic and therapeutic reversal of benzodiazepine receptor agonists

Dosing: IV bolus, 0.2-1 mg (4-20 μg/kg) at rate of 0.2 mg/min. Titrate to patient response. May repeat at 20 min intervals. Maximum single dose, 1 mg. Maximum total dose, 3 mg in any 1 hr;
Infusion, 30-60 μg/min (0.5-1 μg/kg/min); maximum total dose of 3 mg in any 1 hr.
Lack of patient response at 5 min after cumulative dose above 5 mg implies that the major cause of sedation is unlikely to be benzodiazepines.
Elimination: Hepatic
How Supplied: Injection, 0.1 mg/ml
Storage: Room temperature (15°-30° C).
Dilution for Infusion: IV, 3 mg in 50 mls D_5W or NS (60 μg/ml)

Pharmacology

Flumazenil is a benzodiazepine receptor antagonist with little or no agonist activity. It competitively inhibits the activity at the benzodiazepine recognition site on the GABA/benzodiazepine receptor complex in the central nervous system. It reverses sedation, respiratory depression, amnesia, and psychomotor effects of benzodiazepines (e.g., midazolam, diazepam, flurazepam, lorazepam). Hypoventilation may not be fully reversed. Doses and plasma levels required to reverse each agonist depend on the particular benzodiazepine and the residual plasma level (e.g., higher doses are required to reverse lorazepam than diazepam [a less potent benzodiazepine]). The administration of flumazenil to patients given agonists is remarkably free of cardiovascular effects, unlike opioid reversal with naloxone. Resedation may occur and is more common with larger doses of benzodiazepine (>20 mg of midazolam), long procedures (>60 minutes), and use of neuromuscular blocking agents. Flumazenil does not affect the central nervous system effects of drugs affecting GABA-ergic neurons by means other than the benzodiazepine receptor (including ethanol, barbiturates, or general anesthetics) and does not reverse the effects of opioids. Flumazenil has no direct effects on cerebral blood flow but may reverse the lowering effects on cerebral blood flow (CBF), cerebral metabolic rate (CMR_{O_2}), and intracranial pressure (ICP) of midazolam. Flumazenil produces withdrawal symptoms (seizures, emergent confusion, and agitation) in the presence of physical dependence.

Pharmacokinetics

Onset: 1-2 min
Peak Effect: 2-10 min
Duration: 45-90 min (variable; depends on benzodiazepine plasma concentration)
Interaction/Toxicity: Reversal of sedation; precipitation of benzodiazepine withdrawal (agitation, seizures, cardiac arrhythmias); increased risk of seizures in patients with concurrent tricyclic antidepressant poisoning; may provoke panic attacks in patients with a history of panic disorders.

Guidelines/Precautions

1. The reversal of benzodiazepine effects may be associated with the onset of seizures in certain high-risk populations. Possible risk factors include: concurrent major
   sedative-hypnotic drug withdrawal, recent therapy with
   repeated doses of parenteral benzodiazepines,
   myoclonic jerking or seizure activity before flumazenil
   administration in overdose cases, or concurrent tricyclic
   antidepressant poisoning.
2. Flumazenil is not recommended in cases of serious tricyclic antidepressant poisoning. Such patients should be
   allowed to remain sedated (with ventilatory and circulatory support as needed) until the signs of antidepressant
   toxicity have subsided.
3. Treat convulsions associated with flumazenil administration with benzodiazepines, phenytoin, or barbiturates.
   Because of the presence of flumazenil, higher-than-
   usual doses of benzodiazepines may be required.
4. Patients who have responded to flumazenil should be
   carefully monitored (up to 120 min) for resedation, respiratory depression, or other residual benzodiazepine
   effects because the duration of action of the benzodiazepine may exceed that of flumazenil. Overdose cases
   always should be monitored until the patients are stable
   and resedation is unlikely. The availability of flumazenil
   does not decrease the need for prompt detection of
   hypoventilation and the ability to effectively intervene
   by establishing an airway or assisting ventilation.
5. Necessary measures should be instituted to secure airway, ventilation, and intravenous access before administering flumazenil. Upon arousal, patients may attempt to
   withdraw endotracheal tubes and/or intravenous lines as
   the result of confusion and agitation.

6. Do not use flumazenil until the effects of neuromuscular blockade have been fully reversed.
7. To minimize pain and inflammation at the injection site, administer flumazenil in a large vein. Local irritation may occur after extravasation.

Principal Adverse Reactions

Cardiovascular: Arrhythmias (atrial, nodal, ventricular extrasystoles), tachycardia, bradycardia, hypertension, angina, flushing
CNS: Reversal of sedation, seizures, agitation, emotional lability
GI: Nausea, vomiting
Other: Pain at injection site, thrombophlebitis, rash, shivering

FLURAZEPAM HCL (DALMANE)

Use(s): Premedication, sedative/hypnotic

Dosing: PO, 15-30 mg
Elimination: Hepatic
How Supplied: Capsules, 15 mg, 30 mg
Storage: Room temperature (15°-30° C). Protect from light.

Pharmacology

This benzodiazepine acts on the limbic system, thalamus, and hypothalamus. It exerts antianxiety and skeletal-muscle-relaxing effects by increasing the availability of the glycine inhibitory neurotransmitter, whereas the sedative action reflects the ability of benzodiazepines to facilitate actions of the inhibitory neurotransmitter gamma amino butyric acid (GABA). The site of action for production of anterograde amnesia has not been confirmed. It has no peripheral autonomic blocking action and minimal depressant effects on ventilation and circulation in the absence of other CNS depressant drugs. An active metabolite, desalkylflurazepam has a half-life of 50 to 100 hr.

Pharmacokinetics

Onset: 15 min
Peak Effect: 30-60 min
Duration: 7-8 hr
Interaction/Toxicity: CNS and circulatory depressant effects potentiated by alcohol, sedatives, narcotics, volatile anesthetics; elimination reduced by cimetidine.

Guidelines/Precautions

1. Reduce dose or use a shorter-acting benzodiazepine in elderly, hypovolemic, or high-risk patients and with concomitant use of narcotics or other sedatives.
2. Not for use in children less than 15 yr of age.

Principal Adverse Reactions

Cardiovascular: Palpitations, chest pain, hypotension
Pulmonary: Shortness of breath, respiratory depression
CNS: Drowsiness, dizziness, ataxia, dissociation
GI: Abdominal pain, constipation, nausea, vomiting

FUROSEMIDE (LASIX)

Use(s): Diuretic; treatment of hypertension, increased intracranial pressure, edema associated with congestive heart failure, hepatic cirrhosis, and nephrotic syndrome; differential diagnosis of acute oliguria

Dosing: Adults:

> Slow IV/IM, 5-40 mg (give IV dose slowly over 1-2 min); administer high-dose parenteral therapy as a controlled infusion (dilute in D5W or NS) at a rate not exceeding 4 mg/minute;
>
> PO, 20-160 mg daily (up to 600 mg daily with severe edema)

Children:

> Slow IV/IM, 0.1-1.0 mg/kg;
>
> PO, 1-2 mg/kg daily

Elimination: Renal

How Supplied:

Injection, 10 mg/ml

Tablets, 20 mg, 40 mg, 80 mg.

Oral solution, 10 mg/ml, 40 mg/5 ml

Storage: Injection/tablets/solution: Room temperature (15°-30° C). Protect from light. Do not use discolored solutions or tablets.

Pharmacology

An anthranilic acid derivative, this loop diuretic inhibits reabsorption of sodium and chloride ions primarily in the medullary portion of the loop of Henle. It is the diuretic of choice in acute fluid overload, such as in congestive heart failure. Furosemide may reduce pulmonary wedge pressure even before a diuresis has occurred. It is useful in patients with resistant fluid retention or with chronic renal insufficiency who require diuretic therapy, and as an adjunct in the management of hypertension. The drug decreases intracranial pressure by mobilizing edema fluid and interfering with sodium transport in glial tissue. Its CNS effects are not influenced by alterations in the blood-brain barrier, in contrast to mannitol.

Pharmacokinetics

Onset: IV, 5-15 min; PO, 30 min-1 hr
Peak Effect: IV, 20-60 min; PO, 1-2 hr
Duration: IV, 2 hr; PO, 6-8 hr
Interaction/Toxicity: Ototoxicity associated with rapid injection of large doses; severe renal impairment in concomitant therapy with aminoglycoside antibiotics, ethacrynic acid; reduces clearance of salicylates and lithium; potentiates antihypertensive ganglionic or peripheral adrenergic blocking drugs; induced hypokalemia predisposes to digitalis toxicity and potentiates action of nondepolarizing muscle relaxants; decreased effects with coadministration of indomethacin or other NSAID.

Guidelines/Precautions

1. Do not use to treat acute oliguria because of decreased intravascular volume.
2. Practice periodic monitoring of fluid and electrolytes.
3. Use with caution in patients with liver disease. It may precipitate hepatic encephalopathy.
4. May produce a phototoxicity allergic reaction 1-2 wk after sun exposure.

Principal Adverse Reactions

Cardiovascular: Orthostatic hypotension
CNS: Tinnitus, hearing loss, vertigo, paresthesia
GU: Urinary bladder spasm
GI: Pancreatitis, nausea, vomiting, diarrhea, oral and gastric irritation
Hematologic: Thrombocytopenia, neutropenia, aplastic anemia

Metabolic: Hyperglycemia, hyperuricemia, hypokalemia, hypochloremic alkalosis
Allergic Photosensitivity, pruritus

GALLAMINE TRIETHIODIDE (FLAXEDIL)

Use(s): Skeletal muscle relaxation

Dosing: Intubating: IV, 1-1.5 mg/kg
     Maintenance: IV, 0.1-0.75 mg/kg (10%-50% of
      intubating dose)
     Pretreatment/priming: IV, 10% of intubating dose
      given 3-5 min before depolarizer/nondepolar-
      izer relaxant dose
Elimination: Renal (unchanged)
How Supplied: Injection, 20 mg/ml (for IV use only)
Storage: Room temperature (15°-30° C). Do not permit to freeze.

Pharmacology

A long-acting, nondepolarizing neuromuscular blocking agent that acts by competing for cholinergic receptors at the motor end plate, gallamine triethiodide increases heart rate, mean arterial pressure, and cardiac output by a selective cardiac vagal blockade, activation of the sympathetic nervous system, and inhibition of catecholamine reuptake. Gallamine does not release histamine or block autonomic ganglia.

Pharmacokinetics

Onset: 1-2 min
Peak Effect: 3-5 min
Duration: 25-90 min

Interaction/Toxicity: Effects are potentiated by prior administration of succinylcholine, volatile anesthetics, aminoglycoside, antibiotics, local anesthetics, loop diuretics, magnesium, lithium, ganglionic blocking drugs, hypothermia, hypokalemia, and respiratory acidosis; enhanced neuromuscular blockade will occur in patients with myasthenia gravis or inadequate adrenocortical function; effects are antagonized by anticholinesterases such as neostigmine, edrophonium, pyridostigmine; pretreatment doses of gallamine decrease fasciculations but reduce intensity and shorten duration of succinylcholine neuromuscular blockade; priming doses decrease the time to onset of maximal blockade by about 30-60 sec; there is increased resistance or reversal of effects with use of theophylline, and in patients with burn injury and paresis.

Guidelines/Precautions

1. Monitor response with peripheral nerve stimulator to minimize risk of overdosage.
2. Use is contraindicated in patients with myasthenia gravis and impaired renal function.
3. Reverse effects with anticholinesterases such as neostigmine, edrophonium, or pyridostigmine bromide in conjunction with atropine or glycopyrrolate.
4. Pretreatment doses may produce a degree of neuromuscular blockade sufficient to cause hypoventilation in some patients.

Principal Adverse Reactions

Cardiovascular: Tachycardia, arrhythmias, hypotension
Pulmonary: Hypoventilation, apnea
Musculoskeletal: Inadequate block, prolonged block

GLUCAGON (GLUCAGON)

Use(s): Treatment of hypoglycemia, biliary tract spasm, beta blocker overdose; inotropic agent

Dosing: Hypoglycemia: IV, IM, or SC, 0.5-1 mg
Relaxation of biliary tract: IV/IM, 0.25-2 mg
Inotrope:
IV bolus, 1-5 mg
Infusion, 20 mg/hr

Elimination: Renal, hepatic

How Supplied: Vials containing 1 mg (1 unit), 10 mg (10 units) dry powder for reconstitution

Storage: Room temperature (15°-30° C). Do not permit to freeze. When reconstituted with supplied diluent, solution is stable for 48 hr at 5° C. When reconstituted with sterile water, use immediately.

Dilution for Infusion: Dilute to 1 mg/ml with supplied diluent. If dose used is greater than 2 mg, dilute with sterile water.

Pharmacology

Glucagon is a single-chain polypeptide hormone produced by alpha cells of the pancreas. It acts to convert liver glycogen to glucose. It produces relaxation of the smooth muscle of the common bile duct, stomach, duodenum, small intestine, and colon. In the heart, it enhances the formation of cyclic AMP, but unlike catecholamines does not act via beta receptors. It increases myocardial contractility and heart rate even in the presence of beta adrenergic blockade.

Pharmacokinetics

Onset: Hyperglycemic activity/biliary tract relaxation: IV, <1 min; IM, <5 min

Peak Effect: Hyperglycemic activity/biliary tract relaxation: IV/IM, 5-20 min

Duration:

Hyperglycemic activity: IV/IM, 1-2 hr

Biliary tract relaxation: IV/IM, 10-30 min

Interaction/Toxicity: Paradoxic hypoglycemia, hypokalemia; potentiates hypoprothrombinemic effects of anticoagulants.

Guidelines/Precautions

1. In treatment of hypoglycemic shock, liver glycogen must be available. Parenteral glucose must be given because release of insulin may subsequently cause hypoglycemia.
2. Use cautiously in patients with history of insulinoma or pheochromocytoma.
3. Rapid IV administration may cause a decrease in blood pressure.

Principal Adverse Reactions

Cardiovascular: Hypertension, hypotension

Pulmonary: Respiratory distress

CNS: Dizziness, lightheadedness

GI: Nausea and vomiting

Dermatologic: Urticaria

Metabolic: Hypoglycemia, hyperglycemia

GLYCOPYRROLATE (ROBINUL)

Use(s): Premedication (vagolysis), reversal of neuromuscular blockade (blockade of muscarinic effects of anticholinesterases), adjunctive therapy in treatment of bronchospasm and peptic ulcer

Dosing: Premedication/vagolysis:

IV/IM/SC, 0.1-0.2 mg (4-6 μg/kg)

PO, 50 μg/kg (1 μg/kg). For oral administration, use injectate solution and dilute in 3-5 ml apple juice or carbonated cola beverage.

Reversal of neuromuscular blockade: IV, 0.01 mg/kg with anticholinesterase neostigmine 0.05 mg/kg IV or pyridostigmine 0.25 mg/kg IV (0.2 mg for each 1 mg of neostigmine or 5 mg of pyridostigmine).

Bronchospasm: inhalation: 0.4-0.8 mg q8hr. Dilute injectate solution in 2-3 ml NS and deliver by compressed air nebulizer.

Peptic ulcer/GI disorders: PO, 1 to 2 mg 3 or 4 times daily.

Elimination: Renal, hepatic

How Supplied:

Injection, 0.2 mg/ml

Tablets, 1 mg and 2 mg

Storage: Room temperature (15°-30° C).

Pharmacology

Glycopyrrolate is a semisynthetic, quaternary ammonium anticholinergic. Because of its highly polar nature, it resists passage across the blood-brain barrier and thus unlike atropine, it will not reverse the central effects of physostigmine. Glycopyrrolate inhibits action of acetylcholine by reversibly combining with muscarinic cholinergic receptors. Thus it diminishes volume and free acidity of gastric secretions and controls excessive pharyngeal, tracheal, and bronchial secretions. Glycopyrrolate also relaxes bronchial smooth muscle, inhibits gastrointestinal tone and motility, reduces tone of lower esophageal sphincter, and raises intraocular pressure (IOP) by pupillary dilation. At doses used for premedication, this increase in IOP is not clinically significant. Glycopyrrolate antagonizes muscarinic symptoms (e.g., bronchorrhea, bronchospasm, bradycardia, intestinal hypermotility) induced by cholinergic drugs such as anticholinesterases. It is devoid of sedative effects. Compared with atropine, glycopyrrolate has 2 times more potent antisialagog activity and produces less tachycardia. Like atropine, small doses of glycopyrrolate may produce paradoxic bradycardia because of a weak peripheral muscarinic cholinergic agonist effect.

Pharmacokinetics

Onset: IV, <1 min; IM/SC, 15-30 min; inhalation, 3-5 min; PO, 1 hr
Peak Effect: IV, 5 min; IM/SC, 30-45 min;
Inhalation 1-2 hours
Duration:
IV, vagal blockade 2-3 hr; antisialogog effect, 7 hr
PO, vagal blockade 8-12 hr
Inhalation, vagal blockade 3-6 hr
Interaction/Toxicity: Mental confusion, especially in elderly persons; poorly absorbed orally

Guidelines/Precautions

1. Use with great caution in patients with glaucoma, asthma, coronary artery disease, urinary bladder neck, pyloric or intestinal obstruction.
2. May accumulate and produce systemic effects with multiple dosing by inhalation.

Principal Adverse Reactions

Cardiovascular: Tachycardia (high doses), bradycardia (low doses), palpitation
CNS: Headache, confusion, dizziness
GU: Urinary hesitancy and retention
GI: Nausea, vomiting
Dermal: Urticaria
Eye: Increased intraocular tension

HALOPERIDOL (HALDOL, HALPERON)

Use(s): Tranquilizer; antipsychotic

Dosing: IM haloperidol lactate, 2-5 mg (do not administer IV);

IM haloperidol decanoate (for chronic psychotic patients), give 10-15 times the daily oral dose. Interval between doses is 4 weeks. (Do not administer IV.)

PO, 0.5 to 5 mg bid or tid (children 0.05-0.15 mg/kg/day)

Elimination: Hepatic
How Supplied:
Injection haloperidol lactate, 5 mg/ml (for IM use only)
Injection haloperidol decanoate, 50 mg/ml, 100 mg/ml (for IM use only)

Tablets haloperidol, 0.5 mg, 1 mg, 2 mg, 5 mg, 10 mg, and 20 mg

Oral concentrate haloperidol lactate, 2 mg/ml

Storage: Injection/tablets: Room temperature (15°-30° C). Protect from light.

Pharmacology

This butyrophenone derivative reduces dopaminergic neurotransmission in the CNS. It reduces the anxiety accompanying psychosis. Haloperidol is less effective against acute situational anxiety, such as that present in the preoperative period. It has slight anticholinergic, alpha adrenergic, and ganglionic blocking effects.

Pharmacokinetics

Onset: IM, 10-30 min; PO, 1-2 hr
Peak Effect: IM, 30-45 min; PO, 2-4 hr
Duration: 12-38 hr (half-life)
Interaction/Toxicity: Neuroleptic malignant syndrome; encephalopathic syndrome with coadministration of lithium; extrapyramidal reactions; may lower the seizure threshold; blocks vasopressor activity of epinephrine; potentiates anesthetics, opiates, alcohol.

Guidelines/Precautions

1. Extrapyramidal reactions may consist of dystonic reactions, feelings of motor restlessness (akathisia), and parkinsonian signs and symptoms. Dystonic reactions occur more frequently in children, whereas parkinsonian symptoms predominate in geriatric patients. Therapy should include discontinuation of haloperidol or reduction in dosage, and treatment with an anticholinergic antiparkinsonian agent (e.g., benztropine, trihexyphenidyl) or

with diphenhydramine (IV/PO 25 mg). Maintenance of an adequate airway should be instituted if necessary.

2. Phenylephrine or norepinephrine should be used to treat haloperidol-induced hypotension. Epinephrine may paradoxically further lower the blood pressure.

3. Use cautiously in geriatric patients; patients with glaucoma, prostatic hypertrophy, seizure disorders; and children with acute illnesses (e.g., chickenpox, measles).

4. Neuroleptic malignant syndrome, a rare but potentially fatal side effect, may manifest with hyperpyrexia, muscle rigidity, altered mental status, and evidence of autonomic instability (irregular pulse or blood pressure, tachycardia, diaphoresis, arrhythmias). Discontinue haloperidol, treat symptomatically and with dantrolene or bromocriptine (PO 2.5-10 mg tid).

5. Contraindicated in Parkinson's disease.

Principal Adverse Reactions

Cardiovascular: Tachycardia, hypotension, hypertension
Pulmonary: Laryngospasm, bronchospasm
CNS: Extrapyramidal reaction, tardive dyskinesia
GI: Hypersalivation, diarrhea, nausea and vomiting
Metabolic: Hyperglycemia, hypoglycemia, hyponatremia
Eyes: Retinopathy, visual disturbance

HEPARIN SODIUM (HEPARIN SODIUM)

Use(s): In vitro anticoagulant for blood samples drawn for laboratory purposes; anticoagulation during cardiopulmonary bypass; prophylaxis and treatment of venous, arterial, and intracardiac thrombosis, pulmonary embolism, and atrial fibrillation with embolization; diagnosis and treatment of disseminated intravascular coagulation

Dosing: IV flush, 10 to 100 units

Cardiopulmonary bypass: IV, 350-450 units/kg; maintain activated coagulation time (ACT) of 400-480 sec

Low-dose thrombosis prophylaxis: 5000 units SC 2 hr before surgery then q12hr

Full-dose continuous IV therapy: loading IV, 5000 units (children 50 units/kg IV drip), then infusion 20,000-40,000 units over 24 hr (children 100 units/kg IV every 4 hr or 20,000 units/sq m/24 hr)

Full-dose intermittent IV therapy: loading IV, 10,000 units then IV, 5,000-10,000 units q4-6hr

Full-dose subcutaneous therapy: loading IV, 5,000 units and SQ 10,000-20,000 units then SQ 8,000-10,000 units q8h or 15,000-20,000 units q12hr

Do not administer heparin IM.

Elimination: Hepatic

How Supplied:

Injection, 1000 units/ml, 2500 units/ml, 5000 units/ml, 7500 units/ml, 10,000 units/ml, 20,000 units/ml, 40,000 units/ml

Lock flush solution, 10 units/ml, 100 units/ml

Premixed infusion, in dextrose 40 units/ml, 50 units/ml, 100 units/ml; in sodium chloride, 2 units/ml, 50 units/ml, 100 units/ml

Storage: Injection/solutions: Room temperature (15°-30° C). Avoid excess heat.

Dilution for Infusion: 25,000 units in 250 ml D_5W or NS (100 units/ml)

Pharmacology

This mucopolysaccharide organic acid is present endogenously in the liver and granules of mast cells and basophils. Heparin is obtained from beef lung and porcine intestinal mucosa. It combines with antithrombin III (heparin cofactor), inhibits thrombosis by inactivating activated factors IX, X, XI, XII, inhibiting the conversion of prothrombin to thrombin. It also forms complexes with thrombin resulting in thrombin inactivation and prevents the formation of a stable fibrin clot by inhibiting the activation of fibrin stabilizing factor. Heparin is not teratogenic and does not cross the placenta.

Pharmacokinetics

Onset: IV, immediate; SC, 20-30 min
Peak Effect: SC, 2-4 hr
Duration: 1-3 hr (half-life) dose-dependent
Interaction/Toxicity: Increased risk of bleeding with coadministration of platelet aggregation inhibitors such as aspirin, indomethacin, ibuprofen, dipyridamole, hydroxychloroquine; anticoagulant effects antagonized by protamine; reduced effect with digitalis, propranolol, tetracyclines, nicotine, or antihistamines; increased resistance to therapy in fever, thrombosis, thrombophlebitis, myocardial infarction, cancer, and postsurgical patients.

Guidelines/Precautions

1. Monitor activated partial thromboplastin time (APTT) or activated clotting time (ACT) for therapeutic effects. Usually APTT is 1.5-2 times control when fully anticoagulated. Perform periodic platelet counts, hematocrits, and tests for occult blood in stool and urine during the entire course of heparin therapy.

2. Contraindicated in patients with severe thrombocytopenia, thrombocytopenia induced with acute heparin therapy, or uncontrollable active bleeding not caused by DIC.
3. IV route avoids erratic absorption of IM or SC dosing.
4. Treat bleeding or hyperheparinemia with protamine sulfate (slow IV: 1 mg protamine neutralizes 90 USP units heparin [lung] or 115 USP units heparin [intestinal mucosa]; see Protamine p. 305).

Principal Adverse Reactions

Hematologic: Hemorrhage, thrombocytopenia
GI: Elevated liver enzymes
Dermatologic: Erythema, necrosis at site of SC injection
Other: Osteoporosis, priapism, hypersensitivity

HETASTARCH (HESPAN)

Use(s): Plasma volume expander

Dosing: IV, 250-1000 ml; maximum dose 1500 ml (20 ml/kg)/day
Elimination: Renal (molecules smaller than 40,000 daltons)
How Supplied: 500 ml intravenous infusion bottles of 6% hetastarch in 0.9% sodium chloride.
Storage: Temperature below 40° C. Do not permit to freeze.

Pharmacology

This artificial colloid consists of polysaccharides with an average molecular weight of 450,000. It is composed almost entirely of amylopectin. The colloidal properties approximate those of human albumin. Intravenous infusion results in expansion of plasma volume slightly in excess of the volume infused, which decreases from this maximum over the succeeding 24-36 hr. The expansion of plasma volume may improve the hemodynamic status for 24 hr and longer. Hetastarch has antigenic properties. It does not generally interfere with blood-typing or crossmatching.

Pharmacokinetics

Onset: Immediate
Peak Effect: Few min (after end of infusion)
Duration: 24-36 hr (expansion of plasma volume in excess of volume infused)
Interaction/Toxicity: Large volumes may alter the coagulation mechanism and prolong the bleeding time.

Guidelines/Precautions

1. Contraindicated in patients with severe bleeding disorders or with severe congestive cardiac and renal failure with oliguria or anuria.
2. Use with caution in patients with thrombocytopenia, increased risk of pulmonary edema, or congestive heart failure.
3. It is not a substitute for whole blood or plasma because it does not have oxygen-carrying capacity or contain plasma proteins such as coagulation factors.

Principal Adverse Reactions

Cardiovascular: Circulatory overload
Pulmonary: Pulmonary edema, wheezing
CNS: Headache
GI: Vomiting
Allergic: Urticaria, anaphylactoid reactions
Other: Mild temperature elevation, muscle pain

HYDRALAZINE HCL (APRESOLINE)

Use(s): Antihypertensive; reduction of afterload in the treatment of congestive heart failure

Dosing: IV/IM, 2.5-40 mg (0.1-0.2 mg/kg)
PO, 10-100 mg qid
Higher doses are required in rapid acetylators
Elimination: Hepatic (acetylation)
How Supplied:
Injection, 20 mg/ml
Tablets: 10 mg, 25 mg, 50 mg, and 100 mg
Storage: Injection/tablets: Room temperature (15°-40° C). Do not permit injection to freeze. Protect from light.

Pharmacology

This phthalazine derivative lowers blood pressure almost exclusively by a direct relaxant effect on arteriolar smooth muscle. The vasodilation probably reflects hydralazine- related interference with calcium ion transport in vascular smooth muscle. Decrease in blood pressure is frequently accompanied by an increase in heart rate, only partially explained by a reflex increase, and by increases in cardiac output and stroke volume. The drug maintains or increases renal, uterine, and cerebral blood flow. It also increases plasma renin activity.

Pharmacokinetics

Onset: IV, 5-20 min; IM, 10-30 min; PO, 30-120 min
Peak Effect: IV, 10-80 min; IM, 20-80 min
Duration: IV, 2-4 hr; IM/PO, 2-8 hr
Interaction/Toxicity: Reduced pressor responses to epinephrine; enhanced hypotensive effects in patients on diuretics, monoamine oxidase inhibitors, diazoxide, and other antihypertensives; enhances defluorination of enflu-

rane; lower bioavailability in rapid acetylators (30%) compared with slow acetylators (50%).

Guidelines/Precautions

1. Use cautiously in patients with coronary artery disease, with mitral valvular rheumatic heart disease, and receiving MAO inhibitors.
2. The SLE syndrome is dose-related and occurs more frequently in patients receiving doses greater than 200 mg/kg for extended periods. Genetically slow acetylators are especially predisposed.

Principal Adverse Reactions

Cardiovascular: Hypotension, paradoxic pressor response, tachycardia, palpitations, angina
Pulmonary: Dyspnea, nasal congestion
CNS: Peripheral neuritis, depression, anxiety, headache, dizziness
GI: Nausea, vomiting, diarrhea
Dermatologic: Systemic lupus erythematosus–like syndrome
Allergic: Rash, urticaria, eosinophilia, hypersensitivity
Hematologic: Leukopenia, splenomegaly, agranulocytosis

HYDROCORTISONE (HYDROCORTISONE SODIUM SUCCINATE, SOLU-CORTEF, HYDROCORTISONE SODIUM PHOSPHATE, HYDROCORTISONE ACETATE)

Use(s): Antiinflammatory, treatment of allergic reactions, steroid replacement, organ transplantation

Dosing: Antiinflammatory:
 IV/IM, 20-300 mg (1-2 mg/kg) q2-10hr prn
 Intraarticular/intratissue: 10-50 mg; may repeat
 at 1-3 weeks

Life-threatening shock: IV, 0.5-2 g (50 mg/kg) q2-6hr

Steroid replacement:

IV, 50-100 mg preoperatively, intraoperatively and postoperatively;

PO, 5-30 mg 2-4 times daily for severe inflammation and adrenal insufficiency

Hydrocortisone acetate is for intraarticular or intratissue use only, not for IV use.

Elimination: Hepatic

How Supplied:

Hydrocortisone sodium phosphate: Injection, 50 mg/ml

Hydrocortisone sodium succinate: powder for injection: 100 mg, 250 mg, 500 mg and 1000 mg per vial

Hydrocortisone acetate: powder for injection: 25 mg/ml, 50 mg/ml

Hydrocortisone tablets: 5 mg, 10 mg, 20 mg

Oral suspension, 10 mg/5 ml

Storage:

Injection/tablets: Room temperature (15°-30° C). Do not permit to freeze.

Powder for injection: Room temperature (15°-30° C). Use solution only if clear. Discard reconstituted solution after 3 days. Protect from light.

Pharmacology

A corticosteroid secreted by the adrenal cortex, hydrocortisone has weak antiinflammatory and potent mineralocorticoid activity. Hydrocortisone is the corticosteroid of choice for replacement therapy in patients with adrenocortical insufficiency. For antiinflammatory or immunosuppressive uses, synthetic glucocorticoids (e.g., prednisone) that have minimal mineralocorticoid activity are preferred. Hydrocortisone has a rapid onset but short duration of action. Like other glucocorticoids, hydrocortisone promotes protein catabolism, gluconeogenesis, renal excretion of calcium, and redistribution of fat from peripheral to central areas of the body. Hydrocortisone suppresses the hypothalamic-pituitary-adrenal (HPA) axis.

Pharmacokinetics

Onset of Action: Antiinflammatory effects, IV/IM, few minutes
Peak Effect: Antiinflammatory effects, IV/IM, <1 hr
Duration: Antiinflammatory effects/HPA suppression, 30-36 hr
Interaction/Toxicity: Clearance enhanced by phenytoin, phenobarbital, ephedrine, and rifampin; altered response to coumarin anticoagulants; enhanced effect in patients with hypothyroidism and cirrhosis; interacts with anticholinesterase agents (e.g., neostigmine) to produce severe weakness in patients with myasthenia gravis; potassium-wasting effects enhanced with potassium-depleting diuretics (e.g., thiazides, furosemide); diminished response to toxoids and live or inactivated vaccines.

Guidelines/Precautions

1. Contraindicated in systemic fungal infections.
2. Use cautiously in patients with ocular herpes simplex for fear of corneal perforation.
3. In patients on corticosteroid therapy subjected to any unusual stress, increased dosage of rapidly acting corticosteroid before, during, and after the stressful situation is indicated. Supplemental steroids should be empirical-

ly administered to all patients who have recieved daily steroid replacement for at least 1 week in the year before surgery.
4. Hydrocortisone acetate is not for IV use.

Principal Adverse Reactions

Cardiovascular: Arrhythmias, hypertension, congestive heart failure in susceptible patients

CNS: Seizures, increased intracranial pressure, psychic disturbance

Fluid & Electrolyte: Sodium retention, fluid retention, hypokalemia

Musculoskeletal: Weakness, myopathy, osteoporosis

Endocrine: Growth suppression, secondary adrenocortical and pituitary unresponsiveness to stress, increased requirement for insulin

GI: Increased appetite, nausea

Other: Thromboembolism, weight gain, protein catabolism, glaucoma, increased intraocular tension, erythema, impaired wound healing, diminished response to toxoids and live or inactivated vaccines, increased susceptibility to and masked symptoms of infection

HYDROMORPHONE HCL (DILAUDID, DILAUDID HP)

Use(s): Premedication, analgesia, anesthesia, control of persistent nonproductive cough

Dosing: Analgesia:
       Slow IV, 0.5-2 mg (0.01-0.04 mg/kg)
       IM/SC, 2-4 mg (0.04-0.08 mg/kg)
       PO, 2-4 mg q4-6h prn pain
       Rectal, 3 mg q6-8h

Spinal, 0.1-0.2 mg (2-4 μg/kg)

Epidural, bolus 1-2 mg (20-40 μg/kg), infusion, 0.15-0.3 mg/hr (2-3.5 μg/kg/hr)

Patient controlled analgesia

IV:

Bolus, 0.1-0.5 mg (2-10 μg/kg)

Infusion, 0.1-0.5 mg/hr (2-10 μg/kg/hr)

Lockout interval, 5-15 min

Epidural:

Bolus, 0.15-0.3 mg (3-6 μg/kg)

Infusion, 0.15-0.3 mg/hr (3-6 μg/kg/hr)

Lockout interval, 15-30 min

Antitussive: PO, 0.5-1 mg q3-4hr

Elimination: Hepatic

How Supplied:

Injection, 1 mg/ml, 2 mg/ml, 3 mg/ml, 4 mg/ml,

Injection, Dilaudid HP: 10 mg/ml

Tablets, 1 mg, 2 mg, 3 mg, 4 mg.

Rectal suppositories: 3 mg

Storage:

Injection/tablets: Room temperature (15°-30° C). Protect from light. Do not permit injection to freeze.

Suppositories: Refrigerate (2°-8° C).

Dilution for Infusion:

IV, 5 mg in 100 ml NS (50 μg/ml)

Epidural bolus, 1-2 mg in 10 ml local anesthetic or (preservative-free) NS.

Epidural infusion, 5 mg in 100 ml local anesthetic or (preservative-free) NS (50 μg/ml)

Pharmacology

Hydromorphone is an opiate agonist that is a hydrogenated ketone of morphine. As an analgesic, hydromorphone is 7 times more potent than morphine. Primary effects are on the central nervous system and organs containing smooth muscle. The drug produces analgesia, drowsiness, euphoria, dose-related depression of respiration, interference with adrenocortical response to stress (at high doses), and reduction in peripheral resistance (arteriolar and venous dilation) with little or no effect on cardiac index. Hydromorphone releases histamine, which can cause pruritus. It may induce nausea and vomiting by activating the chemoreceptor trigger zone. It depresses the cough reflex by a direct effect on the cough centers in the medulla.

Pharmacokinetics

Onset: IV, almost immediate; IM/PO/SC, 15-30 min; rectal, 10-15 min; epidural, 5 min
Peak Effect: IV, 5-20 min; IM/PO/SC, 30-60 min; epidural 30 min
Duration: IV, 2-4 hr; IM/PO/SC, 4-6 hr; rectal, 6-8 hr; epidural, 10-16 hr
Interaction/Toxicity: CNS and circulatory depressant effects are potentiated by alcohol, sedatives, narcotics, antihistamines, phenothiazines, butyrophenones, MAO inhibitors, and tricyclic antidepressants; analgesia is enhanced and prolonged by alpha-2 agonists (e.g., clonidine); addition of epinephrine to intrathecal/epidural hydromorphone results in increased side effects (e.g., nausea) and prolonged motor block. Hydromorphone may decrease the effect of diuretics in patients with congestive heart failure.

Guidelines/Precautions

1. Reduce dose in elderly, hypovolemic, and high-risk surgical patients, and with concomitant use of sedatives and other narcotics.

2. The narcotic antagonist naloxone is a specific antidote (IV 0.2-0.4 mg or higher). Reversal of narcotic effect may lead to onset of pain and release of catecholamines.

3. Hydromorphone crosses the placental barrier, and usage in labor may produce depression of respiration in the neonate. Resuscitation may be required; have naloxone available.

4. Do not confuse the highly concentrated Dilaudid HP (10 mg/ml) with other standard parenteral formulations. It is intended for use in narcotic-tolerant patients.

5. Undesirable side effects of epidural, caudal, or intrathecal hydromorphone include delayed respiratory depression, pruritus, nausea and vomiting, and urinary retention. Naloxone (IV 0.2-0.4 mg prn or infusion 5 -10 μg/kg/hr) is effective for prophylaxis and/or treatment of these side effects. Ventilatory support for respiratory depression must be readily available. Antihistamines (e.g., diphenhydramine 12.5-25 mg IV/IM q6hr prn) may be used in treating pruritus. Metoclopramide (10 mg IV q6hr prn) may be used in treating nausea and vomiting. Urinary retention that does not respond to naloxone may require an "in and out" bladder catheter.

6. Epidural, caudal, or intrathecal injections should be avoided when the patient has septicemia, infection at the injection site, or coagulopathy.

Principal Adverse Reactions

Cardovascular: Hypotension, hypertension, bradycardia, arrhythmias
Pulmonary: Bronchospasm, laryngospasm
CNS: Blurred vision, syncope, euphoria, dysphoria
GU: Urinary retention, antidiuretic effect, ureteral spasm
GI: Biliary tract spasm, constipation, anorexia, nausea, vomiting

Eye: Miosis
Allergic: Pruritus, urticaria
Musculoskeletal: Chest wall rigidity

INSULIN REGULAR (REGULAR INSULIN, ILETIN REGULAR, HUMULIN R, NOVOLIN R)

Use(s): Treatment of diabetes mellitus, diabetic ketoacidosis/coma, and hyperkalemia

Dosing: Initiation of therapy: insulin regular: adults SC, 5-10 units 15-30 min before meals and at bedtime; children SC, 2-4 units 15-30 min before meals and at bedtime. Dose and frequency of administration must be carefully individualized. Changes in purity, strength, brand, type, and/or species source may necessitate a change in dosage.

Day of Surgery, patients on insulin and NPO

Blood glucose 150-200 mg/dl: administer half the morning insulin dose. Infuse IV D_5W, D_5LR or D_5NS at 100-200 ml/hr (2-4 ml/kg/hr)

Blood glucose <150 mg/dl: administer one-third the morning insulin dose. Infuse IV D_5W, D_5LR or D_5NS at 100-200 ml/hr (2-4 ml/kg/hr)

Alternative protocol (brief procedures): no glucose, no insulin

Perioperative/postoperative: sliding scale every 4-6 hr;

Glucose level <200, no insulin.

Glucose level 200-250, insulin regular SC 5 units

Glucose level 250-300, insulin regular SC 10 units

Glucose level 300-350, insulin regular SC 15 units

Glucose level >350, insulin regular SC 15 units plus IV 1-2 units/hr. Monitor blood glucose hourly. Correct electrolyte imbalances.

Patients taking oral hypoglycemics should not take the hypoglycemic medications on the day of surgery. Surgery preferably should be scheduled in the morning.

Insulin requirements may increase dramatically with stress associated with sepsis, trauma, or pregnancy.

Diabetic ketoacidosis/coma: insulin regular IV, 10-20 units (0.1-0.2 units/kg) then continuous IV infusion 5-10 units/hr (0.1 units/kg/hr). Infusion rate may be determined by dividing the last serum blood glucose by 150 (or 100 if the patient is receiving steroids, has an infection, or is overweight). Decrease infusion to 1-5 units/hr when blood glucose reaches 250 mg/dl and add dextrose to the infusion. Correct acidosis, dehydration, and electrolyte imbalances.

During the first 2-3 hr of insulin therapy, or after renal function is established, potassium replacement therapy may be needed. Add 20-30 mEq of KCl to 1 L of peripheral IV solution. If serum potassium is <3.5 mEq/L, administer 20 mEq of KCl by controlled infusion. If serum potassium is <2.5 mEq/L and patient is symptomatic, use a higher rate and monitor BP and ECG closely. Decrease potassium replacement with oliguria or renal insufficiency. 100-200 mEq of potassium is usually required during the first 12-24 hr of therapy.

Hyperkalemia: Infusion of combined glucose (0.5 g/kg) and insulin (0.15 unit/kg) in a ratio of 3 g glucose to 1 unit regular insulin to shift potassium into cells. Monitor ECG. Sodium bicarbonate IV 50 to 100 mEq may be administered to reverse acidosis and also produce an intracellular shift. Give 10-20 ml IV calcium gluconate or calcium chloride 10% to reverse ECG changes.

Elimination: Hepatic, renal

How Supplied:

Injection, 100 units/ml, 500 units/ml

Parenteral suspension, 30 units/ml with isophane insulin 70 units/ml

Storage: Refrigerate (2°-8° C) unopened vials. Do not permit to freeze. Vial in use may be stored at room temperature (15°-30° C). Protect from light.

Dilution for Infusion: 25 units in 250 ml NS or D_5W (0.1 unit/ml)

Pharmacology

Insulin, a hormone secreted by the beta cells of the pancreatic islets of Langerhans, is composed of two chains of amino acids connected by disulfide linkages. Insulin facilitates transport of glucose across cell membranes. In the liver, insulin enhances the phosphorylation of glucose to glucose-6-phosphate. which is converted to glycogen or further metabolized. Insulin stimulates protein synthesis and lipogenesis and inhibits lipolysis and release of free fatty acids from adipose cells. Insulin promotes the intracellular shift of pottasium and magnesium and may temporarily decrease elevated serum levels of these ions. Insulin preparations are commonly extracted from pork or beef pancreas. Human insulin is prepared by recombinant DNA technology utilizing special laboratory strains of nonpathogenic *E. coli*. It is less antigenic than either pork or beef insulins. Insulin preparations are classified as rapid (regular, semilente), intermediate (lente, NPH), or long-acting (PZI, ultralente) according to the promptness, duration, and intensity of action after subcutaneous administration. Regular insulin has a rapid onset of action and is the only preparation that may be administered intravenously. It is the preparation of choice for the treatment of abrupt-onset of hyperglycemia or the appearance of ketoacidosis. Insulin is not excreted in breast milk.

Pharmacokinetics

Onset:
Insulin regular SC, 30 min-1 hr
Semilente SC, 30 min-1 hr
Lente SC, 1-2 1/2 hr
NPH SC, 1-2 hr
Ultra lente SC, 4-8 hr
Peak Effect:
Insulin regular SC, 2-3 hr
Semilente SC, 4-7 hr
Lente SC, 7-15 hr
NPH SC, 4-12 hr
Ultra lente SC, 16-18 hr
Duration:
Insulin regular SC, 5-7 hr
Semilente SC, 12-16 hr

Lente SC, 18-24 hr
NPH SC, 18-24 hr
Ultra lente SC, 36 hr
Interaction/Toxicity: Hypoglycemic action increased by concomitant administration of alcohol, anabolic steroids, beta adrenergic blockers, fenfluramine, monoamine oxidase inhibitors, guanethidine, salicylates, phenylbutazone, sulfin-pyrazone, sulfonylureas, tetracycline; hypoglycemic action decreased by dextrothyroxine sodium, thyroid hormones, corticosteroids, dobutamine, epinephrine, diazoxide, pheny-toin, oral contraceptives, thiazide diuretics, furosemide, ethacrynic acid, smoking.

Guidelines/Precautions

1. Hyperinsulinism, resulting in hypoglycemia, may occur in patients with brittle diabetes or in patients who have received an overdose of insulin, a decreased or delayed food intake, or an excess amount of excercise in relation to the insulin dose. Insulin requirements may decrease in diabetic patients who develop Addison's disease or secondary adrenocortical insufficiency.

2. Diabetic ketoacisosis is a life-threatening condition requiring prompt diagnosis and treatment. Hyper-glycemia, ketoacidosis, and hyperglucagonemia may result. Diabetic ketoacidosis may result from stress, illness, insulin omission, or poor insulin control. Treatment involves fluids, continuous infusion of regular insulin, and correction of acidosis, electrolyte imbalances (e.g. hypokalemia, hyponatremia), and hypotension.

3. Pregnancy may make the management of diabetes more difficult. Insulin requirements may increase from the second trimester, decrease for 24-72 hr after delivery, and rise toward the normal prepregnancy dose

during the next 6 wk. Insulin requirements may be decreased by breastfeeding.

4. When mixing two types of insulin, always draw the clear regular insulin into the syringe first. Patients stabilized on such mixtures should have a consistent response if the mixing is standardized. An unexpected response is most likely to occur when switching from separate injections to use of a mixture or vice versa. To avoid dosage errors, do not alter the order of mixing insulins or change the model or brand of syringe or needle. Each different type of insulin used to prepare insulin mixtures must be of the same concentration (units/ml).

5. Insulin adsorption onto plastic IV infusion containers and tubing may result in loss of 20%-30% (or more) of the dose. The lesser the concentration of insulin in solution or the slower the rate of flow of solution, the greater the percentage of adsorption. To saturate insulin binding sites, flush the IV tubing with 60 ml of the infusion mixture and discard the flushing solution.

6. Subcutaneous injections may be administered in the thighs, upper arms, buttocks, and abdomen. Consistent response is obtained from administering insulin in the same area.

7. Treat severe hypoglycemia with 10-30 ml (0.2-0.6 ml/kg) of IV 50% dextrose solution. Administration of glucagon (IV/IM/SC 0.5-1 mg) may be temporarily effective in treating hypoglycemia in patients with adequate liver glycogen. However, parenteral glucose must be given because release of insulin may subsequently cause hypoglycemia.

8. Insulin resistance occurs rarely. It may result in patients with high levels of IgG antibodies to insulin, obesity, acanthosis nigrans, and insulin receptor defects.

9. Excessive insulin action may occur during the night or early morning hours. Hypoglycemia-induced release of epinephrine and other counterregulatory hormones (cortisol, growth hormone, glucagon) may cause rebound hyperglycemia, glucosuria, and ketonuria (Somogyl phenomenon). Prescription of more insulin may result in further hypoglycemia. A good history and frequent blood glucose monitoring are essential in preventing complications.

10. In diabetic ketoacidosis, depletion of total body potassium may occur with deficits of 3-10 mEq/kg. With insulin therapy, further decline in serum potassium may occur (with a nadir at 2-4 hr after start of IV insulin), necessitating parenteral potassium replacement.

11. Facetious hyponatremia may be caused by hyperglycemia or hypertriglyceridemia. Plasma sodium concentration decreases by 1.6 mEq/L for every 100 mg/dl increase in plasma glucose above normal. Normal saline may be infused at rates of 250-1000 ml/hr depending on the degree of volume depletion and on the cardiac status.

Principal Adverse Reactions

Cardiovascular: Hypotension, tachycardia, palpitation
Pulmonary: Shallow breathing
CNS: Headache, tremors, confusion, irreversible brain damage, coma, personality changes
GI: Hunger
Allergic: Itching, redness, swelling, urticaria, angioedema, anaphylaxis
Other: Muscle weakness, blurred vision, atrophy or hypertrophy of subcutaneous fat tissue

ISOPROTERENOL HCL (ISUPREL, MEDIHALER-ISO)

Use(s): Chronotrope, inotrope, bronchodilator; treatment of bradyarrhythmias, bradycardia-dependent long-QT syndrome, carotid sinus hypersensitivity, heart block; management of shock (hypoperfusion) syndromes; resuscitation in cardiac arrest.

Dosing: Arrhythmias/resuscitation:

IM/SC, 0.2 mg

IV push, 0.02-0.06 mg

Infusion, 2-20 μg/min (0.02-0.15 μg/kg/min). Rates greater than 30 μg/min have been used in advanced stages of shock.

Sublingual, 10 mg then 5-50 mg prn.

Bronchospasm:

Metered dose inhaler, 120-262 μg(1 or 2 inhalations of a 0.25% solution) q3-4h. Do not take more than 2 inhalations at any one time. Maximum 6 inhalations/ hour

Nebulizer, adults 1:200 solution. Dilute 0.5 ml in 2.5 ml NS. Deliver solution over 10-20 min. Give treatment q4h (Children 1:200 solution. Dilute 0.25 ml in 2.5 ml NS.)

Elimination: Hepatic

How Supplied:

Injection, 1:50,000 solution (0.02 mg/ml), 1:5000 solution (0.2 mg/ml)

Glossets, sublingual/rectal 10 mg, 15 mg

Aerosol, 80 μg, 120 μg, 131 μg, 160 μg/metered spray

Solution for nebulization, 0.031%, 0.062%, 0.25%, 0.5%, 1%

Dilution for Infusion: 3 mg in 250 ml NS or D_5W (12 μg/ml)

Storage: Injection/glossets/solution: Cool place (8°-15° C). Do not use if solution is brown or discolored or contains a precipitate. Protect from light.

Pharmacology

Isoproterenol is a synthetic sympathomimetic amine that is structurally related to epinephrine but acts almost exclusively on beta-1 and beta-2 adrenergic receptors such as those in heart, bronchiolar smooth muscle, skeletal muscle vasculature, and alimentary tract. It produces a positive inotropic and chronotropic effect and increases the rate of discharge of cardiac pacemakers. Isoproterenol decreases systemic and pulmonary vascular resistance and increases coronary and renal blood flow. It has potent relaxing effects on bronchiolar smooth muscle.

Pharmacokinetics

Onset: IV, immediate; inhalation, 2-5 min; sublingual/subcutaneous, 15-30 min

Peak Effect: IV, 1 min

Duration: IV, 1-5 min; inhalation, 30 min-2 hr; sublingual/subcutaneous, 1-2 hr

Interaction/Toxicity: Arrhythmias with concomitant use of volatile anesthetics and other sympathomimetics such as epinephrine; effects antagonized by beta adrenergic blocking drugs such as propranolol.

Guidelines/Precautions

1. Contraindicated in patients with tachyarrhythmias, tachycardia, and heart block caused by digitalis intoxication.

2. When used for chronotropic support, isoproterenol may exacerbate ischemia and/or hypotension. Electronic pacing provides better control than isoproterenol without increasing myocardial oxygen consumption.
3. Use is not a substitute for the replacement of blood, plasma, fluids, and electrolytes, which should be restored promptly when loss has occurred.
4. Paradoxic bronchoconstriction has occasionally occurred with repeated excessive use of inhalation preparations.

Principal Adverse Reactions

Cardiovascular: Tachyarrhythmias, palpitation, angina, paradoxic precipitation of Adams-Stokes attacks
Pulmonary: Pulmonary edema
CNS: Headache, dizziness, tremors
GI: Nausea and vomiting, anorexia

KETAMINE HCL (KETALAR)

Use(s): Dissociative anesthetic; induction and maintenance of anesthesia, especially in hypovolemic or high-risk patients; sole anesthetic for short surgical procedures

Dosing: Sedation/analgesia:
IV, 0.5-1 mg/kg
IM/rectal, 2.5-5 mg/kg
PO, 5-6 mg/kg. Dilute injectate solution in 5-10 ml (0.2 ml/kg) cola-flavored drink.
Induction: IV, 1-2.5 mg/kg; IM/rectal, 5-10 mg/kg
Infusion: 15-80 μg/kg/min (augment with 2-5 mg IV diazepam or 1-2 mg IV midazolam as needed)

Epidural/caudal: 0.5 mg/kg; dilute in (preservative-free) NS or local anesthetic (1 ml/kg)

Elimination: Hepatic

How Supplied: Injection: 10 mg/ml, 50 mg/ml, 100 mg/ml

Storage: Room temperature (15°-30° C). Protect from light and heat.

Dilution for Infusion: 250 mg in 250 ml D_5W or NS (1 mg/ml)

Pharmacology

This phencyclidine derivative produces rapid-acting dissociative anesthesia characterized by normal or slightly enhanced pharyngeal-laryngeal reflexes, normal or slightly enhanced skeletal muscle tone, respiratory stimulation, and occasionally a transient and minimal respiratory depression. Anesthetic effects of ketamine may be partly due to an antagonist effect on excitatory N-methyl aspartate receptors, a subgroup of opioid receptors. Ketamine also may act on norepinephrine, serotonin, and muscarinic cholinergic receptors in the CNS. The central sympathetic stimulation, neuronal release of catecholamines, and inhibition of neuronal uptake of catecholamines usually override the direct myocardial depressant effects of ketamine. Hemodynamic effects (which depend on intact sympathetic responses) include increases in systemic and pulmonary arterial pressure, heart rate, and cardiac output. Ketamine is a useful anesthetic agent in patients with hemodynamic compromise based on either hypovolemia or intrinsic cardiac (but not coronary artery) disease (e.g., cardiac tamponade, cyanotic heart disease). It is a bronchial smooth muscle relaxant and is as effective as the inhalational anesthetics in preventing experimentally induced bronchospasm. Ketamine effects on the EEG include an increase in the alpha, delta, and theta activity with no change in the beta waves. The seizure threshold in epileptic patients is not altered. Cerebral metabolism, cerebral blood flow, and intracranial pressure are increased in the presence of normocapnia. Ketamine produces dose-related increases in uterine tone without adverse effects on uterine blood flow (at dosages <1 mg/kg). Salivary and tracheobronchial secretions are increased. Ketamine does not release histamine.

Pharmacokinetics

Onset: IV, <30 sec; IM/rectal, 3-4 min
Peak Effect: IV, 1 min; IM/rectal, 5-20 min; PO, 30 min
Duration: IV, 5-15 min; IM/rectal, 12-25 min; epidural, 4 hr
Interaction/Toxicity: Emergence delirium; decreased requirements for volatile anesthetics; hypertension, arrhythmias, myocardial ischemia with concomitant use of sympathomimetics (e.g., epinephrine); hemodynamic depression may occur in presence of alpha blockers, beta blockers, calcium channel blockers, benzodiazepines, opioids, volatile anesthetics, ganglionic blockade, cervical epidural anesthesia, and spinal cord transection; concomitant use with benzodiazepines, barbiturates, volatile anesthetics may prolong recovery; enhancement of depolarizing and nondepolarizing neuromuscular blockers; reduction of seizure threshold when administered with aminophylline.

Guidelines/Precautions

1. Critically ill patients with catecholamine depletion may respond to ketamine with unexpected reductions in blood pressure and cardiac output.
2. Emergence reactions (dreaming, hallucinations, confusion) are more common with adults (15-65 years of age), high doses, and rapid administration, and are

reduced by premedication with benzodiazepines and droperidol.

3. Ketamine-induced increase in intracranial pressure may be attenuated by hyperventilation and benzodiazepine pretreatment.

4. Do not mix with barbiturates in same syringe. Precipitate formation occurs.

5. Use with caution in patients with severe hypertension, ischemic heart disease, or aneurysms, those with increased intracranial pressure, chronic alcoholics, and the acutely alcohol-intoxicated patient.

6. Avoid use of ketamine after topical nasal cocaine, in acute cocaine intoxication, or with concomitant administration of sympathomimetics. Hypertension, arrhythmias, and myocardial ischemia may be the end result.

7. Increased salivary secretions may cause upper airway obstruction and laryngospasm, especially in children. Administer an antisialagog (e.g., glycopyrrolate) preoperatively.

8. Avoid intramuscular ketamine sedation (1-2 mg/kg) in preterm infants. It may cause prolonged apnea with bradycardia.

Principal Adverse Reactions

Cardiovascular: Hypertension, tachycardia, hypotension, arrhythmias, bradycardia

Pulmonary: Respiratory depression, apnea, laryngospasm

CNS: Tonic, clonic movements, emergence delirium

GI: Hypersalivation, nausea, vomiting

Eye: Diplopia, nystagmus, slight elevation in intraocular tension

KETOROLAC (TORADOL)

Use(s): Analgesia

Dosing: Loading: IM/slow IV, 30-60 mg (0.5-1 mg/kg)

Maintenance: IM/slow IV, 15-30 mg (0.25-0.5 mg/kg) q6 hr prn and/or 10 mg PO q4-6hr prn

Maximum total dose (combined oral and parenteral): 150 mg (2-3 mg/kg/day) for the first day and 120 mg/day (1.5-2.5 mg/kg/day) thereafter. Maximum PO dose 40 mg daily.

IV doses should be infused slowly (> 15 sec) to reduce risk of phlebitis. Combined duration of use for parenteral and oral ketorolac in all patients should not exceed 5 days. (Note: The intravenous route is approved for general clinical use in the United States.)

Elimination: Hepatic, renal

How Supplied:

Injection, 15 mg/ml, 30 mg/ml

Tablets, 10 mg

Storage: Injection/tablets: Room temperature (15°-30° C). Protect from light.

Pharmacology

This nonsteroidal antiinflammatory drug (NSAID) exhibits analgesic, antiinflammatory, and antipyretic activity. It inhibits synthesis of prostaglandins and may be considered a peripherally acting analgesic. Analgesic potency of ketorolac 30 mg IM is equivalent to morphine 9 mg with less drowsiness, nausea, and vomiting, and no significant change in ventilatory function. Analgesic potency of

ketorolac 10 or 20 mg PO is equivalent to aspirin 650 mg
or acetaminophen 600 mg with codeine 60 mg. Unlike opioids, ketorolac does not decrease the MAC for volatile
anesthetics. At clinical doses, there are no significant
changes in cardiac or hemodynamic parameters. Ketorolac
inhibits platelet aggregation and prolongs bleeding time.
Inhibition of platelet function disappears within 24-48
hours after the the drug is discontinued. It does not affect
platelet count, prothrombin time (PT), or partial thromboplastin time (PTT).

Pharmacokinetics

Onset: IV, <1 min; IM, <10 min; PO, <1 hr
Peak Effect: IV/IM/PO, 1-3 hr
Duration: IV/IM/PO, 3-7 hr
Interaction/Toxicity: Effects are potentiated by concomitant use of salicylates; enhances toxicity of lithium,
methotrexate; risk of bleeding is increased with concomitant NSAIDs, anticoagulant, or low-dose heparin therapy;
may precipitate renal failure in patients with impaired renal
function, heart failure, or liver dysfunction, patients on
diuretic therapy, and the elderly.

Guidelines/Precautions

1. Use with caution in patients with impaired renal or
   hepatic function. Ketorolac may cause fluid retention
   and edema in patients with cardiac decompensation or
   hypertension.
2. Observe carefully patients with coagulation disorders
   and those receiving drug therapy that interferes with
   hemostasis.
3. Ketorolac is contraindicated in patients with previously
   demonstrated hypersensitivity to ketorolac, or with the

complete or partial syndrome of nasal polyps, angioedema, or bronchospastic reactivity to aspirin or other nonsteroidal antiinflammatory drugs (NSAIDs).
4. Do not use for obstetric analgesia.
5. Not recommended for premedication because it prolongs bleeding time.
6. Ketorolac is incompatible and should not be mixed with solutions of morphine sulfate, meperidine, promethazine, or hydroxyzine.

Principal Adverse Reactions

Cardiovascular: Vasodilation, pallor, angina
Pulmonary: Dyspnea, asthma
CNS: Drowsiness, dizziness, headache, sweating, depression, euphoria
GI: Ulceration, bleeding, dyspepsia, nausea, vomiting, diarrhea, gastrointestinal pain
Dermatologic: Pruritus, urticaria

LABETALOL HCL (NORMODYNE, TRANDATE)

Use(s): Antihypertensive

Dosing: IV bolus, 2.5-20 mg (0.25 mg/kg) slowly over 2 min (titrate to blood pressure response)
Infusion, 0.5-2 mg/min; maximum cumulative dose of 1-4 mg/kg
PO, 100-400 mg twice daily
Elimination: Hepatic; urine and feces
How Supplied:
Injection, 5 mg/ml
Tablets, 100 mg, 200 mg, and 300 mg
Storage: Injection/tablets: Temperature (2°-30° C). Protect injection from light and freezing.

Dilution for Infusion: 200 mg in 200 ml D_5W or NS (1 mg/ml)

Pharmacology

Labetalol is an adrenergic-receptor blocking agent with mild alpha-1 and predominant beta-adrenergic-receptor blocking actions (alpha:beta blockade ratio of 1:7 for IV and 1:3 for PO administration). Labetalol produces dose-related decrease in blood pressure without reflex tachycardia and without profound reduction in heart rate. Beta-2 adrenergic blockade may result in bronchoconstriction in patients subject to bronchospasm. Cerebral blood flow and intracranial pressure are unchanged.

Pharmacokinetics

Onset: IV, 2-5 min; PO, 20 min-2 hr
Peak Effect: IV, 5-15 min; PO, 1-4 hr
Duration: IV, 2-4 hr; PO, 8-24 hr
Interaction/Toxicity: Bioavailability increased by cimetidine; increases resistance to beta agonist bronchodilators; blunts reflex tachycardia produced by nitroglycerin; hypotensive effect potentiated by volatile anesthetics.

Guidelines/Precautions

1. Contraindicated in bronchial asthma, overt cardiac failure, greater than first-degree heart block, cardiogenic shock, and severe bradycardia.
2. Manifestations of excessive vagal tone and myocardial depression (profound bradycardia, hypotension) may be corrected with IV atropine (1-2 mg), IV isoproterenol (0.02-0.15 μg/kg/min), IV glucagon (1-5 mg), transvenous cardiac pacemaker, or a vasopressor (e.g., epinephrine, dopamine, dobutamine).

3. Risk of ischemia or infarction is increased in patients with coronary artery disease if drug is withdrawn abruptly.
4. Labetalol may block signs of acute hypoglycemia.

Principal Adverse Reactions

Cardiovascular: Hypotension, bradycardia, ventricular arrhythmias, congestive heart failure, chest pain
Pulmonary: Dyspnea, bronchospasm
CNS: Headache, drowsiness, paresthesia, vertigo, tremor, mental depression, fatigue, numbness
GI: Diarrhea, cholestasis, elevated liver enzymes
Dermatologic: Rashes
Other: Systemic lupus erythematosus, positive antinuclear antibody (ANA) titer

LIDOCAINE HCL (XYLOCAINE)

Use(s): Regional anesthesia; treatment of ventricular arrhythmias, especially when associated with acute myocardial infarction or cardiac surgery; attenuation of pressor response (blood pressure/intracranial pressure) to intubation; attenuation of succinylcholine-induced fasciculations

Dosing: Antiarrhythmic:
Slow IV bolus, 1 mg/kg (1%-2% solution) followed by 0.5 mg/kg every 2-5 min (to maximum of 3 mg/kg/hr)
Infusion, (0.1%-0.4% solution) 1-4 mg/min (20-50 μg/kg/min);
IM, 4-5 mg/kg; may be repeated 60-90 min later

Reduce doses in the elderly and patients with heart failure, liver disease, or who are receiving beta blockers or cimetidine.

Attenuation of pressor response:

IV, 1.5-2 mg/kg (1%-2% solution), give 3-4 min before laryngoscopy.

Laryngotracheal, 2 mg/kg (4% solution); instill translaryngeally (with cannula) just before intubation. Reduction of pressor responses to intubation is indicated only in patients who are hemodynamically stable.

Attenuation of fasciculations: IV, 1.5 mg/kg (1%-2% solution), give 3 min before succinylcholine dose. May be combined with pretreatment doses of nondepolarizing muscle relaxants.

Local anesthesia:

Topical, 0.6-3 mg/kg (2%-4% solution)

Infiltration/peripheral nerve block, 0.5-5 mg/kg (0.5%-2% solution)

Transtracheal, 80-120 mg (2-3 ml of 4% solution)

Superior laryngeal nerve: 40-60 mg (2-3 ml of 2% solution on each side)

Intravenous regional:

Upper extremities, 200-250 mg (40-50 ml of 0.5% solution)

Lower extremities, 250-300 mg (100-120 ml of 0.25% solution)

Do not add epinephrine for intravenous regional block. If desired, add fentanyl 50 μg to enhance the block and/or muscle relaxant (pretreatment doses only) (e.g., pancuronium 0.5 mg). This combination may enable the use of lower concentrations of the local anesthetic (e.g., lidocaine 50 ml of 0.25% for upper extremity block).

Brachial plexus block: 300-750 mg (30-50 ml of 1%-1.5% solution); children, 0.5-0.75 ml/kg.

With high doses (>4 mg/kg), add epinephrine 1:200,000 to decrease systemic toxicity (in the absence of any contraindications). Regional blockade may be potentiated by addition of tetracaine 0.5-1 mg/kg or fentanyl 1-2 μg/kg or morphine (0.05-0.1 mg/kg).

Stellate ganglion block: 10-20 ml of 1% solution (100-200 mg) with or without epinephrine 1:200,000

Caudal, 150-300 mg (15-20 ml of 1% or 1.5% solution), children, 0.4-0.7-1.0 ml/kg (L2-T10-T7 level of anesthesia);

Epidural bolus, 200-400 mg (1%-2% solution), children, 7-9 mg/kg infusion 6-12 ml/hr (0.5% solution with or without epidural narcotics); Children, 0.2-0.35 ml/kg/hr

Rate of onset and potency of local anesthetic action may be enhanced by carbonation. (Add 1 ml of 8.4% sodium bicarbonate with 10 ml of 0.5%-2% lidocaine. Do not use if there is precipitation.)

Spinal bolus/infusion, 50-100 mg (0.5%-5% solution with or without glucose 7.5%)

Therapeutic level: 1.5-6 μg/ml

Maximum safe dose: 4 mg/kg without epinephrine, 7 mg/kg with epinephrine 1:200,000

IV: Use only lidocaine injection without preservatives and clearly labeled for IV use. Doses for epidural or spinal anesthesia should be reduced in pregnant patients. Solutions containing preservatives should not be used for spinal, epidural, or caudal block. Except where contraindicated, vasoconstrictor drugs may be added to increase effect and prolong local or regional anesthesia. For dosage/route guidelines, see Epinephrine, Dosing or Phenylephrine, Dosing. Do not use vasoconstrictor drugs for IV regional anesthesia or local anesthesia of end organs (digits, penis, nose, ears).

Elimination: Hepatic, pulmonary

How Supplied:

Parenteral administration, injection for IM injection, 10%; injection for direct IV, 1%, 2%; injection for IV admixture, 4%, 10%, 20%; injection for IV infusion, 0.2%, 0.4%, 0.8%

Infiltration/peripheral nerve block, 0.5%, 1%, 1.5%, 2% with or without epinephrine 1:50,000, 1:100,000, 1:200,000

Epidural, 1%, 1.5%, 2% preservative free

Spinal (hyperbaric solution), 1.5%, 5% solution with 7.5% dextrose/glucose

Laryngotracheal, (with laryngotracheal cannula) 4% sterile solution

Storage: Room temperature (15°-30° C). Protect from light.

Dilution for Infusion:

IV, 500 mg-2 gm in 500 ml D5W (0.1%-0.4% or 1-4 mg/ml)

Epidural, 20 ml 1% in 20 ml (preservative-free) NS (0.5% solution)

Pharmacology

This amide-derivative local anesthetic has a rapid onset of action. It stabilizes neuronal membrane by inhibiting the sodium flux required for the initiation and conduction of impulses. The drug is also a Class 1B antidysrhythmic agent that suppresses automaticity and shortens the effective refractory period and action potential duration of the His/Purkinje system. Action potential duration and effective refractory period of ventricular muscle also are decreased. Intravenous and laryngotracheal lidocaine decrease the blood pressure responses evoked by tracheal intubation. Given intravenously, this is partly due to an analgesic effect and the local anesthetic effect (reflecting delivery of the drug to the highly vascular tracheobronchial tree). Dose-dependent decrease in intracranial pressure is secondary to an increase in cerebral vascular resistance and decrease in cerebral blood flow. High plasma levels (as occur in paracervical blocks) produce uterine vasoconstriction and decrease in uterine blood flow. Therapeutic doses do not significantly decrease systemic arterial blood pressure, myocardial contractility, or cardiac output. Repeated doses cause significant increases in blood level because of slow accumulation.

Pharmacokinetics

Onset: IV(antiarrhythmic effects), 45-90 sec; intratracheal (antiarrhythmic effects), 10-15 sec; infiltration, 0.5-1 min; epidural, 5-15 min

Peak Effect: IV (antiarrhythmic effects), 1-2 min; infiltration/epidural, <30 min

Duration: IV (antiarrhythmic effects) 10-20 min; intratracheal (antiarrhythmic effects), 30-50 min; infiltration, 0.5-1 hr, w/epinephrine 2-6 hr; epidural, 1-3 hr

Interaction/Toxicity: Cardiac effects with other antiar-rhythmics, such as phenytoin, procainamide, propranolol, or quinidine, may be additive or antagonistic; may potenti-ate the neuromuscular blocking effect of succinylcholine, tubocurarine; clearance is reduced with concomitant use of beta blocking agents, cimetidine; seizures, respiratory and circulatory depression occur at high plasma levels; benzodi-azepines, barbiturates, and volatile anesthetics increase seizure threshold; duration of regional anesthesia is pro-longed by vasoconstrictor agents (e.g., epinephrine), alpha-2 agonists (e.g., clonidine), and narcotics (e.g., fentanyl); alkalinization increases rate of onset and potency of local or regional anesthesia.

Guidelines/Precautions

1. Use with caution in patients with hypovolemia, severe congestive heart failure, shock, and all forms of heart block.
2. Contraindicated in patients with hypersensitivity to amide-type local anesthetics.
3. Benzodiazepines increase seizure threshold.
4. Use for paracervical block associated with fetal brady-cardia and acidosis.
5. If intravenous access is not available, the drug may be diluted 1:1 in sterile NS and injected via an endotra-cheal tube. The absorption rate, duration, and pharma-cologic effects of intratracheal drug administration compare favorably with the IV route.
6. In intravenous regional blocks, deflate the cuff after 40 min and not less than 20 min. Between 20- 40 min, the cuff can be deflated, reinflated immediately, and finally deflated after a minute to reduce the sudden absorption of anesthetic into the systemic circulation.

7. Cauda equina syndrome with permanent neurologic deficit has occured in patients receiving greater than 100 mg of a 5% lidocaine solution with a continuous spinal technique. Transient neurologic deficits have occurred with bolus injections of hyperbaric 5% lidocaine (in 7.5% dextrose), especially for surgery performed in the lithotomy position when perfusion of the cauda equina may be compromised and the nerves may be more vulnerable. Consistent neurologic damage is produced more commonly by hyperbaric 5% lidocaine than bupivacaine.

8. The recommended volumes for brachial plexus block are consistent with available data on plasma levels (subtoxic) after brachial plexus block. The risks of systemic toxicity may be decreased by adding epinephrine to the local anesthetic and avoiding IV injection, which may result in an immediate toxic reaction.

9. Toxic plasma levels (e.g., from accidental intravascular injection) may cause cardiopulmonary collapse and seizures. Premonitory signs and symptoms manifest as numbness of the tongue and circumoral tissues, metallic taste, restlessness, tinnitus, and tremors. Support of circulation (IV fluids, vasopressors, IV sodium bicarbonate 1-2 mEq/kg to treat cardiac toxicity [sodium channel blockade], IV bretylium 5 mg/kg, DC cardioversion/defibrillation for ventricular arrhythmias) and securing a patent airway (ventilate with 100% oxygen) are paramount. Thiopental (1-2 mg/kg IV), midazolam (0.02-0.04 mg/kg IV), or diazepam (0.1 mg/kg IV) may be used for prophylaxis and/or treatment of seizures.

10. The level of sympathetic blockade (bradycardia with block above T5) determines the degree of hypotension (often heralded by nausea and vomiting) after epidural

or intrathecal lidocaine. Fluid hydration (10-20 ml/kg NS or lactated Ringer's solution), vasopressor agents (e.g., ephedrine), and left uterine displacement in pregnant patients may be used for prophylaxis and/or treatment. Administer atropine to treat bradycardia.

11. Epidural, caudal, or intrathecal injections should be avoided when the patient has hypovolemic shock, septicemia, infection at the injection site, or coagulopathy.

12. Monitor for hypoventilation with release of the cuff when a muscle relaxant is added to the local anesthetic solution for intravenous regional blockade.

Principal Adverse Reactions

Cardiovascular: Hypotension, bradycardia, arrhythmias, heart block
Pulmonary: Respiratory depression, arrest
CNS: Tinnitus, seizures, loss of hearing, euphoria, anxiety, diplopia, postspinal headache, arachnoiditis, palsies
Allergic: Urticaria, pruritus, angioneurotic edema
Epidural/caudal/spinal: High spinal, loss of bladder and bowel control, permanent motor, sensory, autonomic (sphincter control) deficit of lower segments

LORAZEPAM (ATIVAN)

Use(s): Premedication, amnesia, induction agent, treatment of acute alcohol withdrawal and chemotherapy-induced/postoperative nausea and vomiting

Dosing: Sedation:

IV/IM, 1-4 mg (0.02-0.08 mg/kg). Before IV administration dilute with equal volume of D_5W or NS. For IM administration use undiluted injectate solution.

> PO, 2-3 mg bid or tid (elderly 1-2 mg/day in
> divided doses).
Antiemetic:
> IV, 0.5-1 mg (0.01-0.02 mg/kg);
> PO, 1-2 mg bid or tid
> Induction: IV, 0.5-1 mg/kg

Elimination: Hepatic, renal

How Supplied:

Injection, 2 mg/ml, 4 mg/ml

Tablets, 0.5 mg, 1 mg, 2 mg

Oral solution, 2 mg/ml

Storage: Injection: Refrigerate (2°-8° C). Protect from light and freezing. Tablets: Room temperature (15°-30° C).

Pharmacology

This benzodiazepine produces a dose-related sedation, relief of preoperative anxiety, and lack of recall of events relating to the day of surgery in a majority of patients. Like other benzodiazepines, the drug is thought to influence the effect of gamma amino butyric acid, an inhibitory neurotransmitter, in the brain. It produces minimal depressant effects on ventilation and circulation in the absence of other CNS depressant drugs. Lorazepam has an unpredictable blood level–CNS response relationship. It is intermediate in speed of onset compared with other benzodiazepines.

Pharmacokinetics

Onset: IV, 1-5 min; IM, 15-30 min; PO, 20-30 min

Peak Effect: IV, 15-20 min; PO, 2 hr

Duration: IV/IM/PO, 6-10 hr

Interaction/Toxicity: CNS and circulatory depressant effects potentiated by alcohol, narcotics, sedatives, barbiturates, phenothiazines, MAO inhibitors, and volatile anesthetics; decreased requirements for volatile anesthetics; effects antagonized by flumazenil.

Guidelines/Precautions

1. Intraarterial injection may produce arteriospasm resulting in gangrene. Treat with local infiltration of phentolamine (5-10 mg in 10 ml NS) and if necessary sympathetic block.
2. For optimal amnesic effects, administer IV 15-20 min or PO 2 hr before anticipated operative procedure.
3. Unexpected hypotension and respiratory depression may occur when combined with opioids.
4. Use with caution in elderly patients because excessive sedation and hypoventilation may occur.
5. Not for use in children less than 12 years of age.
6. Treat overdose with supportive measures and flumazenil (slow IV 0.2-1 mg).
7. Contraindicated in patients with known hypersensitivity to benzodiazepines or any ingredients in the parenteral formulation (i.e., polyethylene glycol, propylene glycol, or benzyl alcohol) and in patients with acute-angle closure glaucoma.

Principal Adverse Reactions

Cardiovascular: Hypotension, hypertension, bradycardia, tachycardia
Pulmonary: Respiratory depression
CNS: Sedation, dizziness, weakness, depression, agitation, amnesia
Psychologic: Hysteria, psychosis
GI: Change in appetite
Other: Visual disturbances, urticaria, pruritus

MAGNESIUM SULFATE (MAGNESIUM SULFATE)

Use(s): Prevention and control of seizures in toxemia/eclampsia of pregnancy, epilepsy, nephritis and hypomagnesemia; treatment of acute magnesium deficiency; tocolytic therapy; adjunctive therapy of acute MI, *torsades de pointes* ventricular tachycardia, and hypokalemia-related arrhythmias

Dosing: Toxemia/eclampsia/tocolysis:
      Slow IV, 1-4 g of 10%-20% solution then, infusion, 1-2 g/hr
      IM, 1-5 g of a 25%-50% solution q4h prn
      Therapeutic plasma level 4-6 mEq/L
    Hypomagnesemia:
      IV, 10-15 mg/kg of 10%-20% solution over 15-20 min, then infusion, 1 g/hr;
      IM, 10-15 mg/kg q6h for 4 doses;
      PO, 3 g q6h for 4 doses
      Normal plasma level, 1.5-2.2 mEq/L

Elimination: Renal

How Supplied: Injection: 10% (0.8 mEq/100 mg/ml), 12.5% (1 mEq/125 mg/ml), 50% (4 mEq/500 mg/ml)

Storage: Room temperature (15°-40° C). Protect from freezing.

Dilution for Infusion: 10 g in 1000 ml D_5W (10 mg/ml)

Pharmacology

This mineral is present in the body and distributed principally in intracellular space. It regulates presynaptic release of acetylcholine from nerve endings, activates enzyme systems such as alkaline phosphatase, and is an essential cofactor in oxidative phosphorylation. At the neuromuscular junction, it decreases acetylcholine, release, reduces the sensitivity of the motor end plate to acetylcholine, and decreases the amplitude of the motor end plate potential. These effects are opposed by calcium. Hypocalcemia and hypokalemia often follow low serum levels of magnesium. Magnesium exerts CNS and respiratory depressant effects. It slows the rate of sinoatrial node impulse formation and prolongs conduction time. The drug produces vasodilation and at high doses may decrease systemic arterial pressure. Effects of magnesium in pregnancy include transient decrease in uterine vascular resistance and increase in uteroplacental blood flow.

Pharmacokinetics

Onset: IV, immediate; IM, <1 hr
Peak Effect: IV, few min; IM, 1-3 hr
Duration: IV, 30 min; IM, 3-4 hr
Interaction/Toxicity: Potentiates both depolarizing and nondepolarizing muscle relaxants; cardiac depression, respiratory paralysis, loss of deep tendon reflexes occur at serum levels exceeding 10-12 mEq/L; potentiates CNS depressant effects of sedatives, narcotics, volatile anesthetics; CNS depression and peripheral neuromuscular blockade produced by hypermagnesemia are antagonized by calcium.

Guidelines/Precautions

1. Treat life-threatening hypermagnesemia with intravenous administration of calcium 5-10 mEq (10-20 ml of 10% calcium gluconate) followed by fluid loading and drug-induced diuresis.

2. Periodic monitoring of plasma magnesium concentrations is essential during magnesium therapy. Disappearance of the patellar reflex is a useful clinical sign to detect the onset of magnesium intoxication. Knee-jerk reflex should be tested before repeat doses, and if it is absent, no additional magnesium should be given until it returns.
3. Use is contraindicated in heart block or in patients with extensive myocardial damage.
4. Maintain urine output at a minimum of 100 ml every 4 hr.

Principal Adverse Reactions

Cardiovascular: Hypotension, circulatory collapse, heart block
Pulmonary: Respiratory paralysis
CNS: Flaccid paralysis, depressed reflexes
Metabolic: Hypocalcemia
Other: Flushing, sweating, hypothermia

MANNITOL (OSMITROL)

Use(s): Diuretic, differential diagnosis of acute oliguria, "renal protection" in presence of myoglobin, hemoglobinuria, and for aortic aneurysmectomy; treatment of increased intracranial and intraocular pressure

Dosing: Acute oliguria: Infusion: 12.5-50 g (0.25-1 g/kg or 2-4 ml/kg of a 5%-25% solution)
Reduction of intracranial/intraocular pressure: Slow IV/infusion: 12.5-100 g (0.25-2 g/kg or 2-8 ml/kg of a 20%-25% solution)
Elimination: Renal
How Supplied: 5%, 10%, 15%, 20%, 25% solution

Storage: Room temperature (15°-30° C). Do not permit to freeze.

Pharmacology

Mannitol is a six-carbon sugar that is pharmacologically inert and resists metabolism. Because it is freely filtered at the glomerulus, mannitol raises the osmolarity of the renal tubular fluid and inhibits tubular reabsorption of water and electrolyte. Urinary excretion of water, sodium, chloride, and bicarbonate ions are increased. Urinary pH is not altered. Plasma osmolarity is also increased, with an acute expansion of intravascular fluid volume. Shift of fluid from extracellular to intracellular sites decreases brain size and may increase renal blood flow.

Pharmacokinetics

Onset: Diuresis, 15-60 min; reduction of: IOP, 30-60 min; ICP, <15 min
Peak Effect: Diuresis, 1 hr; reduction of IOP, 1-2 hr
Duration: Diuresis, 3-8 hr; reduction of: IOP, 4-6 hr; ICP, 3-8 hr
Interaction/Toxicity: Increases urinary excretion of lithium.

Guidelines/Precautions

1. If urine output continues to decline during infusion, review the patient's clinical status and suspend infusion, if necessary. Accumulation of mannitol may result in overexpansion of the extracellular fluid, which may intensify existing or latent congestive heart failure and pulmonary edema.
2. Conduct periodic monitoring of fluids and electrolytes.
3. If blood-brain barrier is not intact, mannitol may enter the brain, producing rebound cerebral edema.

4. Use is contraindicated in severe pulmonary congestion, frank pulmonary edema, or anuria caused by severe renal disease. May be contraindicated with intracerebral bleeding, aneurysm, or arteriovenous malformation, because by shrinking healthy brain tissue, hematoma may expand and fragile bridging veins may rupture, producing subdural hematoma.
5. Do not give electrolyte-free mannitol solutions with blood. If blood is given simultaneously, add at least 20 mEq of sodium chloride to each liter of mannitol solution to avoid pseudoagglutination.
6. Obligatory response after rapid infusion may further aggravate preexisting hemoconcentration.

Principal Adverse Reactions

Cardiovascular: Edema, hypertension, hypotension, tachycardia, chest pain
Pulmonary: Pulmonary edema
CNS: Seizures, headaches, blurred vision, dizziness
GI: Nausea, vomiting, diarrhea
Dermatologic: Skin necrosis, urticaria
Metabolic: Hypernatremia, hyponatremia, hyperkalemia, acidosis, dehydration
Other: Chills, fever, thirst, dry mouth, rhinitis

MEPERIDINE HCL (DEMEROL)

Use(s): Premedication, analgesia, prevention and treatment of postoperative shivering

Dosing: Analgesia:
PO/IM/SC, 50-150 mg (1-3 mg/kg)
Slow IV, 25-100 mg (0.5-2 mg/kg)

Epidural:

Bolus, 50-100 mg (1-2 mg/kg). Dilute in 10 ml (preservative-free) NS or local anesthetic.

Infusion, 10-20 mg/hr (0.2-0.4 mg/kg/hr)

Spinal:

Bolus, 10-50 mg (0.2-1 mg/kg). Use preservative-free 5% solution (50 mg/ml).

Infusion, 5-10 mg/hour (0.1-0.2 mg/kg/hr)

Patient-controlled analgesia:

IV:

Bolus, 5-30 mg (0.1-0.6 mg/kg)

Infusion, 5-40 mg/hr (0.1-0.8 mg/kg/hr)

Lockout interval 5-15 min

Epidural:

Bolus, 5-30 mg (0.1-0.6 mg/kg/hr);

Infusion, 5-10 mg/hr (0.1-0.2 mg/kg/hr)

Lockout interval, 5-15 min

Prevention/treatment of shivering: IV/IM, 25-75 mg (0.5-2 mg/kg)

Maximum recommended dose: 1 g/day (20 mg/kg/day). Meperidine serum levels (normal, <0.55 μg/ml) and normeperidine serum levels (normal, <0.5 μg/ml) should be monitored at higher doses.

Elimination: Hepatic

How Supplied:

Injection, 10 mg/ml, 25 mg/ml, 50 mg/ml, 75 mg/ml, 100 mg/ml

Tablets, 50 mg, 100 mg.

Oral solution, 50 mg/5 ml

Storage: Injection: Room temperature (15°-25°C). Protect from light.

Tablets: Room temperature (15°-30° C).
Solutions: Temperature below 40° C). Protect from freezing.
Dilution for Infusion: IV, 100 mg in 50 ml D_5W or NS
(2 mg/ml); epidural infusion, 100-500 mg in 50 ml local
anesthetic or (preservative-free) NS (2-10 mg/ml)

Pharmacology

This synthetic opioid agonist is approximately one tenth as
potent as morphine with a slightly more rapid onset and
shorter duration of action. Compared with morphine,
meperidine may be more effective in neuropathic pain.
Meperidine has mild vagolytic and antispasmodic effects. It
may produce orthostatic hypotension at therapeutic doses
and has a direct myocardial depressant effect at high doses.
Normeperidine, the active metabolite, is a cerebral stimulant and excreted primarily in the urine. It may accumulate
with prolonged administration of meperidine (>3 days).
Meperidine decreases cerebral blood flow, cerebral metabolic rate, and intracranial pressure. Meperidine crosses the
placental barrier and may produce depression in the
neonate. Maximum placental transfer and neonatal depression occur 2-3 hr after parenteral administration. Spinal and
epidural administration of meperidine produces analgesia
by specific binding and activation of opioid receptors in the
substantia gelatinosa. Once activated, the opioid receptors
inhibit the release of substance P from nociceptive afferent
C fibers. Unlike other opiates, meperidine has potent local
anesthetic activity and epidural/spinal analgesia is accompanied by sensory, motor, and autonomic blockade.
Meperidine is not used as a topical anesthetic because of
local irritation.

Pharmacokinetics

Onset: PO, 10-45 min; IV, <1 min; IM, 1-5 min; epidural/spinal, 2-12 min
Peak Effect: PO, <1 hr; IV, 5-20 min; IM, 30-50 min; epidural/spinal, 30 min
Duration: PO/IV/IM, 2-4 hr; epidural/spinal, 0.5-3 hr
Interaction/Toxicity: Seizures, myoclonus, delirium with repeated high doses and in patients with renal/hepatic impairment; potentiates CNS and circulatory depression of narcotics, sedative-hypnotics, volatile anesthetics, tricyclic antidepressants; severe, sometimes fatal reaction (hyperthermia, hypertension, seizures) with MAO inhibitors; aggravates adverse effects of isoniazid; chemically incompatible mixture with barbiturates; analgesia enhanced and prolonged by alpha-2 agonists (e.g., clonidine); addition of epinephrine to intrathecal/epidural meperidine results in increased side effects (e.g., nausea) and prolonged motor block.

Guidelines/Precautions

1. Causes severe and occasionally fatal reactions in patients who are receiving or have just received MAO inhibitors. Treat with hydrocortisone IV. Use chlorpromazine IV to treat the associated hypertension.
2. Do not use in high doses for anesthesia.
3. Use with caution in patients with asthma, chronic obstructive pulmonary disease, increased intracranial pressure, and supraventricular tachycardia.
4. Reduce doses in elderly, hypovolemic, and high-risk surgical patients and with concomitant use of sedatives and other narcotics.
5. The narcotic antagonist naloxone is a specific antidote (IV 0.2-0.4 mg or higher). Reversal of narcotic effect may lead to onset of pain and release of catecholamines.

The duration of reversal may be shorter than duration of narcotic effect. Naloxone may precipitate seizures, especially in patients receiving meperidine.

6. Meperidine crosses the placental barrier, and usage in labor may produce depression of respiration in the neonate. Resuscitation may be required; have naloxone available.

7. Undesirable side effects of epidural, caudal, or intrathecal meperidine include delayed respiratory depression (up to 8 hr after single dose), pruritus, nausea and vomiting, and urinary retention. Naloxone (IV 0.2-0.4 mg prn or infusion 5-10 μg/kg/hr) is effective for prophylaxis and/or treatment of these side effects. Ventilatory support for respiratory depression must be readily available. Antihistamines (e.g., diphenhydramine 12.5-25 mg IV/IM q6h prn) may be used in treating pruritus. Metoclopramide (10 mg IV q6h) may be used in treating nausea and vomiting. Urinary retention that does not respond to naloxone may require an "in and out" bladder catheter.

8. Epidural, caudal, or intrathecal meperidine should be avoided when the patient has septicemia, infection at the injection site, or coagulopathy.

Principal Adverse Reactions

Cardiovascular: Hypotension, cardiac arrest
Pulmonary: Respiratory depression, arrest, laryngospasm
CNS: Euphoria, dysphoria, sedation, seizures, psychic dependence
GI: Constipation, biliary tract spasm
Musculoskeletal: Chest wall rigidity
Allergic: Urticaria, pruritus

MEPHENTERMINE SULFATE (WYAMINE)

Use(s): Inotropic agent, vasoconstrictor

Dosing: IV/IM, 15-45 mg (0.4 mg/kg)
        Infusion: 0.2-5 mg/min (4-100 μg/kg/min)
Elimination: Hepatic
How Supplied: Injection, 15 mg/ml, 30 mg/ml
Storage: Room temperature (15°-30° C).
Dilution for Infusion: 250 mg in 250 ml D_5W (1 mg/ml)

Pharmacology

A synthetic noncatecholamine sympathomimetic that stimulates alpha and beta receptors, mephentermine acts directly and indirectly by releasing norepinephrine from neuronal storage sites. Mephentermine increases blood pressure, heart rate, and cardiac output primarily by an increase in myocardial contractility and to a lesser degree by an increase in peripheral vascular resistance. It increases cerebral blood flow and produces CNS stimulation.

Pharmacokinetics

Onset: IV, 1-5 min; IM, 5-15 min
Peak Effect: IV, 5 min; IM, 15-60 min
Duration: IV, 15-30 min; IM, 1-2 hr
Interaction/Toxicity: Increased risk of arrhythmias with use of volatile anesthetics, especially halothane; pressor effect potentiated in patients treated with MAO inhibitors, tricyclic antidepressants, oxytocics; ineffective in patients treated with reserpine or guanethidine; potentiates rather than corrects hypotension secondary to the adrenolytic effects of chlorpromazine.

Guidelines/Precautions

1. Use is not a substitute for the replacement of blood, plasma, fluids, and electrolytes, which should be restored promptly when loss has occurred.
2. Use with caution in patients with severe hypertension or hyperthyroidism.
3. May increase uterine contractions, especially during the third trimester of pregnancy. It is not recommended for use in pregnant women.

Principal Adverse Reactions

Cardiovascular: Hypertension, arrhythmias
CNS: Anxiety, seizures, euphoria, paranoid psychosis

MEPIVACAINE HCL (CARBOCAINE, POLOCAINE)

Use(s): Regional anesthesia

Dosing: Infiltration, 50-400 mg (0.5-1.5% solution)
Brachial plexus block: 300-750 mg (30-50 ml of 1%-1.5% solution); children 0.5-0.75 ml/kg.
High doses (>4 mg/kg) are not recommended without addition of epinephrine 1:200,000 to decrease systemic toxicity (in the absence of any contraindications). Regional blockade may be potentiated by addition of tetracaine 0.5-1 mg/kg or fentanyl 1-2 μg/kg or morphine (0.05-0.1 mg/kg);
Epidural:
Bolus, 150-400 mg (15-20 ml of 1%-2% solution);
Infusion, 6-12 ml/hr (0.25%-0.5% solution with or without epidural narcotics)

Rate of onset and potency of local anesthetic action may be enhanced by carbonation. (Add 1 ml of 8.4% sodium bicarbonate with 10 ml of 1%-3% mepivacaine. Do not use if there is precipitation.)

Caudal: 150-400 mg (15-20 ml of 1%-2% solution); children, 0.4-0.7-1.0 ml/kg (L2-T10-T7 level of anesthesia);

Maximum safe dose: 4 mg/kg without epinephrine; 7 mg/kg with epinephrine 1:200,000.

Solutions containing preservatives should not be used for epidural or caudal block. Except where contraindicated, vasoconstrictor drugs may be added to increase effect and prolong local or regional anesthesia For dosage/route guidelines, see Epinephrine, Dosing or Phenylephrine, Dosing. Do not use vasoconstrictor drugs for local anesthesia of end organs (digits, penis, nose, ears).

Elimination: Hepatic

How Supplied: Injection, 1%, 1.5%, 2%, 3%

Storage: Room temperature (15°-30° C). Protect from light.

Pharmacology

This tertiary amine local anesthetic stabilizes the neuronal membrane and prevents the initiation and transmission of impulses. The amide structure is not detoxified by plasma esterases, and metabolism occurs primarily by hepatic microsomal enzymes. Similar to lidocaine in potency and speed of onset, mepivacaine has a slightly longer duration of action and lacks vasodilator activity. High plasma levels (as occur in paracervical blocks) produce uterine vasoconstriction and decrease in uterine blood flow.

Pharmacokinetics

Onset: Infiltration, 3-5 min; epidural, 5-15 min
Peak Effect: Infiltration/epidural, 15-45 min
Duration: Infiltration, 0.75-1.5 hr; with epinephrine, 2-6 hr; epidural, 3-5 hr/prolonged with epinephrine
Interaction/Toxicity: Reduced clearance with coadministration of beta blockers, cimetidine; seizures, respiratory and circulatory depression at high plasma levels; benzodiazepines, barbiturates, and volatile anesthetics increase seizure threshold; duration of local or regional anesthesia prolonged by vasoconstrictor agents (e.g., epinephrine) and alpha-2 agonists (e.g., clonidine); alkalinization increases rate of onset and potency of local or regional anesthesia.

Guidelines/Precaution

1. Do not use for spinal anesthesia.
2. Not recommended for obstetric anesthesia. High neonatal blood levels are due to placental transfer and impaired elimination.
3. Use for paracervical block may be associated with fetal bradycardia and acidosis.
4. Use with caution in patients with severe disturbance of cardiac rhythm and heart block.
5. Contraindicated in patients with hypersensitivity to amide-type local anesthetics.
6. The recommended volumes for brachial plexus block are consistent with available data on (subtoxic) plasma levels after brachial plexus block. The risks of systemic toxicity may be decreased by adding epinephrine to the local anesthetic and avoiding IV injection, which may result in an immediate toxic reaction.
7. Toxic plasma levels (e.g., from accidental intravascular

injection) may cause cardiopulmonary collapse and
seizures. Premonitory signs and symptoms manifest as
numbness of the tongue and circumoral tissues, metallic
taste, restlessness, tinnitus, and tremors. Support of circulation (IV fluids, vasopressors, IV sodium bicarbonate
1-2 mEq/kg to treat cardiac toxicity [sodium channel
blockade], IV bretylium 5 mg/kg, and DC cardiover-
sion/defibrillation for ventricular arrhythmias) and
securing a patent airway (ventilate with 100% oxygen)
are paramount. Thiopental (0.5-2 mg/kg IV), midazolam
(0.02-0.04 mg/kg IV), or diazepam (0.1 mg /kg IV) may
be used for prophylaxis and/or treatment of seizures.

8. The level of sympathetic blockade (bradycardia with
   block above T5) determines the degree of hypotension
   (often heralded by nausea and vomiting) after epidural
   or intrathecal mepivacaine. Fluid hydration (10-20
   ml/kg NS or lactated Ringer's solution), vasopressor
   agents (e.g., ephedrine), and left uterine displacement in
   pregnant patients may be used for prophylaxis and/or
   treatment. Administer atropine to treat bradycardia.

9. Epidural or caudal injections should be avoided when
   the patient has hypovolemic shock, septicemia, infection
   at the injection site, or coagulopathy.

Principal Adverse Reactions

Cardiovascular: Hypotension, bradycardia, cardiac arrest
Pulmonary: Respiratory depression, arrest
CNS: Tinnitus, seizures, loss of hearing, euphoria, dysphoria
Allergic: Urticaria, pruritus, angioneurotic edema
Epidural/Caudal: High spinal, loss of bladder and bowel
control, and permanent motor, sensory, autonomic (sphinc-
ter control) deficit of lower segments

METARAMINOL BITARTRATE (ARAMINE)

Use(s): Vasoconstrictor; treatment of hypotension and shock

Dosing: Hypotension during spinal or inhalation anesthesia:
>> SC or IM, 2-10 mg
>> Infusion, titrate to effect
> Shock:
>> Direct IV, 0.5-5 mg (0.01 mg/kg)
>> Intratracheal (if IV access not available), 5 mg diluted in 10 ml NS, inject via the endotracheal tube and continue ventilation

Elimination: Tissue uptake, renal

How Supplied: Injection: 10 mg/ml

Storage: Room temperature (15°-40° C). Do not permit to freeze. Infusion solutions should be used within 24 hr. Protect from light.

Dilution for Infusion: 50 mg in 500 ml D_5W or NS (0.1 mg/ml)

Pharmacology

A potent sympathomimetic, metaraminol directly activates alpha adrenergic receptors. It may act indirectly by release of norepinephrine from storage sites, and prolonged infusions may deplete norepinephrine from sympathetic nerve endings. Metaraminol also directly stimulates beta-1 receptors of the heart but has no effect on beta-2 receptors of the bronchi or peripheral blood vessels. The drug produces intense peripheral vasoconstriction, increased systolic and diastolic blood pressures, and a reflex bradycardia, which can result in decreased cardiac output. Pulmonary artery pressure is elevated. Renal, splanchnic, and cutaneous blood flows are reduced, but coronary blood flow is

increased because of increased work. At clinical doses and
with an intact blood-brain barrier, metaraminol does not
have any significant effects on cerebral vascular resistance,
cerebral blood flow, or intracranial pressure. In patients
with hypotension, cerebral perfusion pressure is increased
because of the increase in systemic arterial pressure (CPP =
MAP−ICP).

Pharmacokinetics

Onset: IV, 1-2 min; IM/SC, 10-20 min
Peak Effect: IV, >2 min
Duration: IV/IM/SC, 20-90 min
Interaction/Toxicity: Pressor effects potentiated with oxytocics, MAO inhibitors, guanethidine, bretylium, and other
sympathomimetics; decreased pressor effects with use of
tricyclic antidepressants, alpha adrenergic blockers (e.g.,
phentolamine); sensitization of myocardium by volatile
anesthetics may increase risk of arrhythmias with use of
metaraminol; extravasation may cause sloughing and
necrosis.

Guidelines/Precautions

1. Use with extreme caution in elderly patients and patients
   with hyperthyroidism, bradycardia, partial heart block,
   or severe arteriosclerosis. In pregnant patients, metaraminol is not recommended for treatment of spinal
   hypotension, because the drug-induced decrease in
   uterine blood flow may lead to fetal asphyxia.
2. Use is not a substitute for the replacement of blood,
   plasma, fluids, and electrolytes, which should be
   restored promptly when loss has occurred.
3. Infuse into large veins to prevent extravasation. Treat
   any extravasation with local infiltration of phentolamine
   (5 to 10 mg in 10 ml NS) or sympathetic block.

4. Hypotension may occur after prolonged metaraminol therapy because of depletion of norepinephrine tissue stores. In some patients, it may be necessary to administer norepinephrine to replace tissue stores before metaraminol may be discontinued.
5. Metaraminol (and other sympathomimetic amines) may provoke a relapse in patients with a history of malaria.

Principal Adverse Reactions

Cardiovascular: Reflex bradycardia, palpitations, precordial pain, arrhythmias, hypertension, hypotension
Pulmonary: Acute pulmonary edema, respiratory distress
CNS: Headache, anxiety, cerebral hemorrhage, dizziness
GU: Decreased renal perfusion, renal necrosis, oliguria
GI: Hepatic necrosis, nausea
Dermatologic: Tissue necrosis, sloughing at site of injection

METHADONE HCL (DOLOPHINE)

Use(s): Premedication, analgesia, detoxification treatment of narcotic addiction

Dosing: Analgesia:
Initial: IM/SC/PO, 2.5-10 mg (0.05-0.1 mg/kg) every 3-4 hr
Maintenance:
PO, 5-20 mg (0.1-0.4 mg/kg) every 6-8 hr. Once stable blood levels are achieved (2-3 wk), dosing intervals may be increased to 12-24 hr.
Epidural (bolus), 1-5 mg (0.02-0.1 mg/kg)
Maintenance methadone therapy (more than 3 weeks) may be provided only at approved methadone programs.

       Narcotic abstinence syndrome: PO, 15 to 120 mg
         daily (highly individualized);
       Patient Controlled Analgesia
         IV: bolus, 0.5-3.0 mg (0.01-0.06 mg/kg)
         Lockout interval 10-20 min

Elimination: Hepatic

How Supplied:

Injection, 10 mg/ml;

Tablets, 5 mg, 10 mg, 40 mg

Oral solution, 1 mg/ml, 2 mg/ml

Solution concentrate, 10 mg/ml

Storage: Injection/tablets/oral solution: Room temperature (15°-30° C).

Solution, concentrate: Cool place (15°-20° C.)

Dilution for Infusion: Epidural bolus, 1-5 mg in 10 ml local anesthetic or (preservative-free) NS

Pharmacology

Methadone is a synthetic opioid agonist with multiple actions quantitatively similar to those of morphine, mainly involving the central nervous system and organs composed of smooth muscle. As an analgesic, methadone is 3 times more potent than morphine. The methadone abstinence syndrome, although qualitatively similar to that of morphine, differs in that the onset is slower, the course is more prolonged, and the symptoms are less severe. Cumulative effect occurs with repeated use, resulting in a prolonged duration of action. Oral methadone is approximately one half as potent as parenteral.

Pharmacokinetics

Onset: IV, <1 min; IM, 1-5 min; PO, 30-60 min; epidural, 5-10 min

Peak Effect: IV, 5-20 min; IM, 30-60 min
Duration: IV/IM, 4-6 hr; PO, 22-48 hr (patients on methadone maintenance); epidural, 6-10 hr
Interaction/Toxicity: Blood concentration may be reduced by rifampin with production of withdrawal symptoms; severe reaction with MAO inhibitors; withdrawal symptoms precipitated by pentazocine in heroin addicts on methadone therapy; potentiates CNS and circulatory depressant effects of other narcotic analgesics, volatile anesthetics, phenothiazines, sedative-hypnotics, alcohol, tricyclic antidepressants; analgesia enhanced and prolonged by alpha-2 agonists (e.g., clonidine); addition of epinephrine to epidural methadone results in increased side effects (e.g., nausea) and prolonged motor block.

Guidelines/Precautions

1. Do not give pentazocine to heroin addicts on methadone.
2. Methadone is ineffective for relief of general anxiety.
3. Use with caution in patients with asthma, chronic obstructive pulmonary disease, or increased intracranial pressure.
4. Reduce dosage in elderly, hypovolemic, or high-risk surgical patients and with concomitant use of narcotics and sedative hypnotics.
5. Methadone can produce drug dependence of the morphine type and therefore has the potential for being abused.
6. Use of doses greater than 120 mg requires special federal approval.
7. Methadone is not recommended for obstetric analgesia because of its long duration of action.

8. Undesirable side effects of epidural methadone include delayed respiratory depression, pruritus, nausea and vomiting, and urinary retention. Naloxone (IV 0.2-0.4 mg prn or infusion 5-10 μg/kg/hr) is effective for pro- phylaxis and/or treatment of these side effects. Ventila- tory support for respiratory depression must be readily available. Antihistamines (e.g., diphenhydramine 12.5- 25 mg IV/IM q6h prn) may be used in treating pruritus. Metoclopramide (10 mg IV q6h) may be used in treating nausea and vomiting. Urinary retention that does not respond to naloxone may require straight bladder catheterization.

9. Epidural injections should be avoided when the patient has septicemia, infection at the injection site, or coagu- lopathy.

Principal Adverse Reactions

Cardiovascular: Hypotension, circulatory depression, bra- dycardia, syncope
Pulmonary: Respiratory depression
CNS: Euphoria, dysphoria, disorientation
GU: Urinary retention
GI: Biliary tract spasm, constipation, anorexia
Eye: Miosis
Allergic: Rash, pruritus, urticaria

METHOHEXITAL SODIUM (BREVITAL)

Use(s): Induction agent, supplementation of anesthesia, sole anesthetic for pain-free procedures (e.g., cardioversion)

Dosing: Sedation: IV, 0.25-1 mg/kg

    Induction:
        IV, 1.5-2.5 mg/kg
        IM, 7-10 mg/kg
        Rectal, 20-30 mg/kg; 5% aqueous solution for
            children (500 mg injectate powder in 10 ml
            sterile water; give through a well-lubricated
            catheter)
    Infusion: 50-150 μg/kg/min (0.2% solution)
    Do not administer intravenously in a concentra-
        tion greater than 1% (10 mg/ml).

Elimination: Hepatic

How Supplied: Powder for injection, 500 mg, 2.5 g, 5.0 g with 50 ml, 250 ml, 500 ml diluent respectively.

Storage: Room temperature (15°-30° C). When reconstituted in sterile water, solution is stable at room temperature (<25° C) for at least 6 weeks. When reconstituted in D_5W or normal saline, solutions are stable for 24 hr.

Dilution for Infusion: 500 mg in 250 ml D_5W or NS (2 mg/ml)

Pharmacology

A methylated oxybarbiturate that produces a rapid ultrashort-acting anesthesia, methohexital depresses the sensory cortex, decreases motor activity, alters cerebellar function, and produces dose-dependent drowsiness, sedation, and hypnosis. These effects are thought to be mediated by enhanced gamma-aminobutyric acid (GABA) actions in the CNS. GABA is thought to be a major inhibitory transmitter in the CNS. Methohexital causes an initial increase in the alpha amplitude, followed by a progressive decrease in activity of the EEG. Burst suppression and a flat EEG occur at high doses. It does not produce analgesia and has no muscle-relaxant properties. Methohexital may induce paradoxic excitement in elderly persons and children and in the presence of acute or chronic pain. It has a more rapid recovery of consciousness compared with thiopental. Induction may be accompanied by excitatory phenomenon (e.g., involuntary muscle movements). Cardiovascular effects are secondary to a decrease in myocardial contractility and peripheral vasodilation.

Pharmacokinetics

Onset: IV, 20-40 sec; rectal, <5 min
Peak Effect: IV, 45 sec; rectal, 5-10 min
Duration: IV, 5-10 min; rectal, 30-90 min
Interaction/Toxicity: Potentiates CNS and circulatory depressant effects of narcotics, sedative hypnotics, alcohol, and volatile anesthetics; decreases effects of oral anticoagulants, digoxin, beta blockers, corticosteroids, quinidine, theophylline; actions are prolonged by MAO inhibitors, chloramphenicol.

Guidelines/Precautions

1. Premedication with opioids reduces incidences of excitatory phenomenon.
2. Extravascular injection may cause necrosis, and intraarterial injection may lead to gangrene. Treat the latter by injection in the artery (use subclavian artery if in spasm) of 10 ml of 1% procaine, 40-80 mg dilute solution of papaverine, or local infiltration of phentolamine (2.5-5 mg in 10 ml) to produce vasodilation. Sympathectomy may be achieved by stellate ganglion or brachial plexus block.
3. Contraindicated in patients with latent or manifest porphyria.
4. Use with caution in patients in status asthmaticus.
5. Reduce dosage in elderly, hypovolemic, and high-risk

surgical patients and with concomitant use of narcotics and other sedative hypnotics.

6. Incompatible with lactated Ringer's solution and other acid solutions such as atropine sulfate, metocurine iodide, and succinylcholine chloride.

Principal Adverse Reactions

Cardiovascular: Myocardial depression, arrhythmias
Pulmonary: Respiratory depression, laryngospasm, bronchospasm
CNS: Emergence delirium, prolonged somnolence, headache
GI: Nausea, emesis, hiccups
Other: Rash, skeletal muscle hyperactivity, shivering

METHOXAMINE HCL (VASOXYL)

Use(s): Vasoconstrictor; treatment of paroxysmal atrial tachycardia

Dosing: IV, 1-5 mg (Give slowly. May repeat dose after 15 min)
IM, 5-15 mg (0.25 mg/kg) (for prolonged effect)
Elimination: Hepatic
How Supplied: Injection, 20 mg/ml
Storage: Room temperature (15°-30° C). Protect from light.

Pharmacology

Methoxamine is a selective alpha-1 receptor agonist that produces a prompt and prolonged rise in blood pressure by increasing peripheral resistance. It is already O-methylated and cannot be inactivated by COMT or metabolized by MAO and thus has a long duration of action. It has no direct effect on the heart and may produce reflex bradycardia secondary to increased systolic and diastolic blood pressures. Increased afterload decreases cardiac output in patients with heart failure. Methoxamine produces uterine hypertonus and decrease in uterine blood flow. Fetal acid-base status may be adversely affected.

Pharmacokinetics

Onset: IV, almost immediate; IM, 15-20 min
Peak Effect: IV, 0.5-2 min; IM, 15-20 min
Duration: IV, 15-60 min; IM, 60-90 min
Interaction/Toxicity: Pressor effects are potentiated with oxytocics, with other sympathomimetic amines, and in patients receiving MAO inhibitors or tricyclic antidepressants; severe hypertensive response occurs with concomitant administration of beta-adrenergic blocking agents, guanethidine, and reserpine; increases risk of cardiac arrhythmias during halothane anesthesia; extravasation may cause sloughing and necrosis.

Guidelines/Precautions

1. Use with extreme caution in elderly patients and patients with hyperthyroidism, bradycardia, partial heart block, myocardial disease, or severe arteriosclerosis.
2. Use is not a substitute for the replacement of blood, plasma, fluids, and electrolytes, which should be restored promptly when loss has occurred.
3. Infuse into large veins to prevent extravasation. Treat any extravasation with local infiltration of phentolamine (5 to 10 mg in 10 ml NS) or sympathetic block.
4. The drug formulation contains sulfites and may cause allergic-type reactions (wheezing, anaphylaxis) in susceptible populations.

Principal Adverse Reactions

Cardiovascular: Reflex bradycardia, hypertension, hypotension

Pulmonary: Respiratory distress

CNS: Anxiety, tremors, dizziness, seizures, cerebral hemorrhage, headache

GI: Projectile vomiting

GU: Desire to void

METHYLDOPA (ALDOMET, METHYLDOPATE)

Use(s): Antihypertensive

Dosing: IV/PO, 250-500 mg bid or tid (20-40 mg/kg/day)

Elimination: Hepatic, renal

How Supplied:

Injection, 250 mg/5 ml

Tablets, 125 mg, 250 mg, 500 mg

Oral solution, 250 mg/5 ml

Storage:

Injection: Temperature below 26° C. Do not permit to freeze.

Tablets: Room temperature (15°-30° C).

Pharmacology

Methyldopa acts in the central nervous system to lower blood pressure. After it is in brain, the drug is converted to alpha-methylnorepinephrine by the enzyme dopa decarboxylase. Alpha-methylnorepinephrine lowers arterial pressure through activation of alpha-2 adrenergic receptors and lowered sympathetic outflow.

Pharmacokinetics

Onset: IV, 1-2 hr; PO, 3-6 hr
Peak Effect: IV/PO, 4-6 hr
Duration: IV, 10-16 hr; PO, 12-24 hr
Interaction/Toxicity: Reduces MAC for volatile anesthetics; produces false-positive test for pheochromocytoma; produces paradoxic hypertensive response with coadministration of propranolol (which blocks beta-2 vasodilating component of alpha methyl norepinephrine); produces dementia in patients who subsequently receive haloperidol; Coombs positive hemolytic anemia and liver dysfunction occur with prolonged therapy.

Guidelines/Precautions

1. Contraindicated in patients with active hepatic disease, such as acute hepatitis or cirrhosis.
2. Paradoxic pressor response has been reported with IV methyldopa.

Principal Adverse Reactions

Cardiovascular: Bradycardia, paradoxic pressor response, hypotension, pericarditis
CNS: Sedation, vertigo, headache, paresthesias, cerebrovascular insufficiency, Bell's palsy, choreoathetotic movements
GI: Nausea, vomiting
Hepatic: Jaundice, hepatitis, abnormal liver function tests
Endocrine: Gynecomastia, lactation, amenorrhea
Hematologic: Thrombocytopenia, hemolytic anemia, positive Coomb's test

METHYLENE BLUE (UROLENE BLUE)

Use(s): Treatment of drug-induced methemoglobinemia; dye effect to delineate body structures and fistulas and to confirm rupture of amniotic membranes; urinary antiseptic (oral route)

Dosing: IV, 1-2 mg/kg (inject over several minutes)
PO, 65-130 mg tid after meals with a full glass of water

Elimination: Renal

How Supplied:
Injection, 10 mg/ml
Tablets, 55 mg, 65 mg

Storage: Tablets: Room temperature (15°-30° C).

Pharmacology

This compound has an oxidation-reduction action and a tissue-staining property. It has opposite actions on hemoglobin, depending on the concentration. In high concentrations, methylene blue converts the ferrous iron of reduced hemoglobin to the ferric form, and as a result methemoglobin is produced. In contrast, low concentrations (recommended doses) are capable of hastening the conversion of methemoglobin to hemoglobin.

Pharmacokinetics

Onset: IV, almost immediate
Peak Effect: IV, <1 hr
Duration: IV/PO, varies
Interaction/Toxicity: Discoloration of urine and feces; high concentrations in blood interfere with pulse oximetry,

producing artifactual decrease in measured oxygen saturation (Sao_2); methemoglobinemia produced may alter measured oxygen saturation (falsely low at Sao_2 >85% and falsely high at Sao_2 <85%); releases free cyanide from cyanomethemoglobin.

Guidelines/Precautions

1. Contraindicated in patients allergic to methylene blue, with renal insufficiency, with G-6-PD deficiency (hemolysis), in intraspinal injection, and in treatment of methemoglobinemia in cyanide poisoning.
2. Requires periodic monitoring of hemoglobin. Continued administration may cause marked anemia.
3. Administer with slow IV injection to prevent local high concentration from producing additional methemoglobin.
4. Methylene blue stains skin blue. The staining may be removed by hypochlorite solution.
5. Intraamniotic injection may result in fetal tachycardia, neonatal hemolytic anemia, hyperbilirubinemia, methemoglobinemia, and blue skin.

Principal Adverse Reactions

Cardiovascular: Tachycardia, hypertension, precordial pain
Pulmonary: Cyanosis
CNS: Confusion, headache, dizziness
GU: Bladder irritation
GI: Nausea, vomiting, diarrhea, abdominal pain
Dermatologic: Stains skin blue (may be removed by hypochlorite solution), necrotic abscesses
Other: Methemoglobinemia, hemolytic anemia, hyperbilirubinemia

METHYLERGONOVINE MALEATE (METHERGINE)

Use(s): Treatment of postpartum uterine atony and bleeding

Dosing: IV or IM, 0.2 mg (give IV over 60 sec); repeat as required every 2-4 hr; then PO, 0.2-0.4 mg every 4-6 hr for 2-7 days

Elimination: Hepatic

How Supplied:

Injection, 0.2 mg/ml

Tablets: 0.2 mg

Storage: Injection/tablets: Temperature below 25°C. Protect from light.

Pharmacology

Methylergonovine is a semisynthetic ergot alkaloid that acts directly on the smooth muscle of the uterus and increases the tone, rate, and amplitude of rhythmic uterine contractions. Thus it induces a rapid and sustained tetanic uterotonic effect that shortens the third stage of labor and reduces blood loss. The drug also constricts peripheral, mainly venous capacitance, vessels, and raises central venous pressure and blood pressure. Compared with ergonovine, methylergonovine is associated with a lower incidence of hypertension.

Pharmacokinetics

Onset: IV, immediate; IM, 2-5 min; PO, 5-15 min

Peak Effect: IV, <5 min; IM/PO, <30 min

Duration: IV, 45 min; IM/PO, 4-6 hr

Interaction/Toxicity: Vasoconstriction potentiated by sympathomimetics such as ephedrine, phenylephrine, and nicotine.

Guidelines/Precautions

1. Use cautiously in patients with preeclampsia, hypertension, or cardiac disease. The drug may produce severe maternal hypertension, cerebrovascular accidents, and retinal detachment.
2. Avoid in patients with peripheral vascular disease.
3. Discontinue if patients complain of tingling sensations in the extremities.
4. Inhibits lactation and is excreted in breast milk.

Principal Adverse Reactions

Cardiovascular: Hypertension, hypotension, chest pain
Pulmonary: Dyspnea, increased pulmonary artery pressure
CNS: Dizziness, tinnitus, seizures, headache
GI: Diarrhea, nausea, vomiting
Other: Hematuria, thrombophlebitis, diaphoresis, gangrene of the fingers and toes

METHYLPREDNISOLONE SODIUM SUCCINATE (SOLU-MEDROL)

METHYLPREDNISOLONE ACETATE (DEPO-MEDROL)

METHYLPREDNISOLONE (MEDROL)

Use(s): Antiinflammatory, treatment of nerve root irritation and myofascial pain with trigger points, treatment of allergic reactions, short-term management of bronchodilator-unresponsive asthma and chronic obstructive pulmonary disease, steroid replacement, organ transplantation, adjunct treatment of sympathetic mediated pain

Dosing: Inflammatory diseases/asthma/steroid replacement:

Methylprednisolone (Medrol): PO, 2-60 mg (0.1-1.6 mg/kg) daily in 4 divided doses. May be given as alternate doses to minimize side effects.

Methylprednisolone sodium succinate (Solu-Medrol): IV/IM, 10 mg-1.5 g (0.03-30 mg/kg) daily. Usual dose, 10-250 mg up to 6 times daily.

Acute spinal cord injury/life-threatening shock: Methylprednisolone sodium succinate (Solu-Medrol): IV, 30 mg/kg infused over 10-20 min every 4-6 hr if needed.

Inflammatory diseases/myofascial pain: Methylprednisolone acetate (Depo-Medrol): intraarticular/intratissue, 4-80 mg. May repeat at 1-5 weeks.

Sympathetic mediated pain: IV regional block: Methylprednisolone sodium succinate (Solu-Medrol): 80 mg. Dilute in 50 ml of NS or 0.5% lidocaine. May be combined with guanethidine 20-40 mg or bretylium (1-2 mg/kg)

Herniated disk/back pain: Epidural methylprednisolone acetate (Depo-Medrol): 40-80 mg in 5-10 ml (preservative-free) NS or local anesthetic. (Dilute in 20-25 ml for the caudal route.) May repeat at 2-3 weeks if response is partial. Additional relief does not occur with more than 3 injections. Do not administer intrathecally.

Elimination: Hepatic

How Supplied:

Methylprednisolone sodium succinate: powder for injection, 40 mg, 125 mg, 500 mg, 1000 mg, and 2000 mg per vial

Methylprednisolone acetate injection, 20 mg/ml, 40 mg/ml, 80 mg/ml

Methylprednisolone tablets, 2 mg, 4 mg, 8 mg, 16 mg, 24 mg, 32 mg

Storage:

Injection/tablets: Room temperature (15°-30° C). Do not permit to freeze.

Powder for injection: Room temperature (15°-30°C). Use solution only if clear. Discard reconstituted solution after 2 days. Protect from light.

Pharmacology

This methyl derivative of prednisolone is a potent antiinflammatory steroid. Antiinflammatory potency of 4 mg of methylprednisolone is equivalent to that of 0.75 mg of dexamethasone, 5 mg of prednisolone, and 20 mg of cortisol. Methylprednisolone may decrease the number and activity of inflammatory cells, enhance the effects of beta adrenergic drugs on cyclic-AMP production, and inhibit bronchoconstrictor mechanisms. It has less tendency to cause salt and water retention than prednisolone, hydrocortisone, or cortisone, and a rapid onset but short duration of action. It may suppress the hypothalamic-pituitary-adrenal (HPA) axis.

Pharmacokinetics

Onset: Antiinflammatory effects: IV, almost immediate
Peak Effect: Antiinflammatory effects: IV,<1 hr
Duration: Antiinflammatory effects/HPA suppression: IV, 12-36 hr
Interaction/Toxicity: Clearance enhanced by phenytoin, phenobarbital, ephedrine, and rifampin; altered response to coumarin anticoagulants; enhanced effect in patients with hypothyroidism and cirrhosis; interacts with anticholinesterase agents (e.g., neostigmine) to produce severe

weakness in patients with myasthenia gravis; potassium-wasting effects enhanced with potassium-depleting diuretics (e.g., thiazides, furosemide); diminished response to toxoids and live or inactivated vaccines; increased risk of GI bleeding with concomitant NSAIA.

Guidelines/Precautions

1. Contraindicated in systemic fungal infections.
2. Use cautiously in patients with ocular herpes simplex for fear of corneal perforation.
3. After prolonged therapy, abrupt discontinuation may result in a withdrawal syndrome without evidence of adrenal insufficiency. To minimize morbidity associated with adrenal insufficiency, discontinue exogenous corticosteroid therapy gradually.
4. In patients receiving corticosteroid therapy who are subjected to any unusual stress, increased doses of rapidly acting corticosteroid should be administered before, during, and after the stressful situation. Supplemental steroids should be empirically administered to all patients who have received daily steroid replacement for at least 1 week in the year before surgery.
5. Methylprednisolone may mask signs of infection. There may be decreased resistance and inability of the host defense mechanisms to prevent dissemination of infection.
6. Epidural injections should be avoided when the patient has septicemia, infection at the injection site, or coagulopathy.

Principal Adverse Reactions

Cardiovascular: Arrhythmias, hypertension, congestive heart failure in susceptible patients
CNS: Seizures, psychosis, increased intracranial pressure
GI: Pancreatitis, peptic ulcer with perforation and hemorrhage

Dermatologic: Impaired wound healing, petechiae, lupus erythematosus-like syndrome
Musculoskeletal: Weakness, myopathy, osteoporosis, aseptic necrosis
Endocrine: Amenorrhea, growth suppression, hyperglycemia, negative nitrogen balance
Fluid and Electrolyte Imbalances: Sodium and water retention, hypokalemia, metabolic alkalosis, hypocalcemia
Intraspinal: Meningitis, arachnoiditis
Other: Thromboembolism, diminished response to toxoids and live or inactivated vaccines, increased susceptibility to and masked symptoms of infection

METOCLOPRAMIDE (REGLAN)

Use(s): Stimulate gastric emptying, antiemetic, treatment of symptomatic gastroesophageal reflux and diabetic gastroparesis

Dosing: IV/IM, 10 mg (give IV injection over 1 to 2 min)
PO, 10 mg 30 min before meals and at bedtime
Elimination: Renal
How Supplied:
Injection: 5 mg/ml, 10 mg/ml
Tablets, 5 mg, 10 mg
Oral solution: 5 mg/5 ml
Storage: Injection/tablets/oral solution: Room temperature (15°-30° C). Do not permit to freeze.

Pharmacology

Metoclopramide is a derivative of procainamide. It stimulates motility of the upper gastrointestinal tract and increases lower esophageal sphincter tone by 10-20 cm H_2O. Gastric acid secretion is not altered. Net effect is accelerated gastric emptying and intestinal transit. The drug sensitizes gastrointestinal smooth muscle to the effects of acetylcholine and may cause release of acetylcholine from cholinergic nerve endings. Antiemetic effects may result from its antagonism of central and peripheral dopamine receptors and inhibition of chemoreceptor-trigger-zone–mediated vomiting. Metoclopramide produces minimal sedation and rarely may produce extrapyramidal reactions.

Pharmacokinetics

Onset: IV, 1-3 min; IM, 10-15 min; PO, 30-60 min
Peak Effect: IV/IM, <1 hr; PO, 1-2 hr
Duration: IV/IM/PO, 1-2 hr
Interaction/Toxicity: Effects on gastrointestinal motility are antagonized by anticholinergic drugs (e.g., atropine) and narcotic analgesics; sedative effects are potentiated by alcohol, sedative hypnotics, tranquilizers, narcotics; hastens the onset of action of tetracycline, acetaminophen, levodopa, and ethanol, which are mainly absorbed in the small bowel; prolongs the duration of action of succinylcholine (by release of acetylcholine and inhibition of plasma cholinesterase); releases catecholamines in patients with essential hypertension and pheochromocytoma; may produce intense feelings of anxiety and restlessness after rapid intravenous injection; may produce extrapyramidal reactions.

Guidelines/Precautions

1. Use cautiously in patients with hypertension or those receiving MAO inhibitors. Metoclopramide-induced hypertensive crisis in patients with pheochromocytoma may be controlled with phentolamine.

2. Metoclopramide is not recommended in pediatric patients because of its increased incidence of extrapyramidal reactions.
3. Metoclopramide is contraindicated in patients with pheochromocytoma, epilepsy, or gastrointestinal hemorrhage, obstruction, or perforation; or those receiving other drugs likely to cause extrapyramidal reactions.
4. Extrapyramidal reactions may consist of dystonic reactions, feelings of motor restlessness (akathisia), and parkinsonian signs and symptoms. Therapy should include discontinuation of metoclopramide or reduction in dosage and treatment with an anticholinergic antiparkinsonian agent (e.g., benztropine, trihexyphenidyl) or with diphenhydramine (IV/PO 25 mg). Maintenance of an adequate airway should be instituted if necessary.

Principal Adverse Reactions

Cardiovascular: Hypertension, hypotension, arrhythmia
CNS: Drowsiness, extrapyramidal reactions, akathisia, insomnia, anxiety
GI: Nausea, diarrhea
Other: Galactorrhea, gynecomastia, hypoglycemia

METOCURINE IODIDE (METUBINE IODIDE)

Use(s): Skeletal muscle relaxation

Dosing: Intubation: IV, 0.2-0.4 mg/kg
Maintenance: IV, 0.04-0.2 mg/kg (10%-50% of intubating dose)
Pretreatment/priming: IV, 10% of intubating dose given 3-5 min before depolarizer/ nondepolarizer relaxant dose

Elimination: Renal
How Supplied: Injection, 2 mg/ml
Storage: Refrigerate (2°-8° C). Do not permit to freeze.
Protect from light.

Pharmacology

Metocurine is a methyl analog of tubocurarine that produces a nondepolarizing neuromuscular blockade at the myoneural junction. It does not produce autonomic ganglion blockade. Histamine release occurs less frequently than with d-tubocurarine and is related to dosage and rapidity of administration. Repeated doses may be accompanied by a cumulative effect. Effects on the cardiovascular system (e.g., changes in pulse rate, hypotension) are less than those reported with equipotent doses of tubocurarine and gallamine.

Pharmacokinetics

Onset: <3 min
Peak Effect: 3-5 min
Duration: 35-60 min
Interaction/Toxicity: Effects are potentiated by volatile anesthetics, aminoglycoside antibiotics, local anesthetics, quinidine, diuretics, magnesium, lithium, respiratory acidosis, hypokalemia; enhanced neuromuscular blockade will occur in patients with myasthenia gravis or inadequate adrenocortical function; effects are antagonized by anticholinesterases such as neostigmine, edrophonium, and pyridostigmine; pretreatment doses of metocurine decrease fasciculations but reduce intensity and shorten duration of succinylcholine neuromuscular blockade; priming doses decrease the time to onset of maximal blockade by about

30-60 sec; resistance occurs with concomitant use of phenytoin and in patients with burn injury and paresis; metocurine is chemically incompatible with alkaline solutions, including solutions of barbiturate, meperidine, and morphine sulfate.

Guidelines/Precautions

1. Monitor response with peripheral nerve stimulator to minimize risk of overdosage.
2. Reverse effects with anticholinesterases such as neostigmine, edrophonium, or pyridostigmine bromide in conjunction with atropine or glycopyrrolate.
3. Rapid intravenous injection may produce hypotension, tachycardia, and signs of histamine release.
4. Pretreatment doses may induce a degree of neuromuscular blockade sufficient to cause hypoventilation in some patients.
5. Use is contraindicated in patients sensitive to iodide.

Principal Adverse Reactions

Cardiovascular: Hypotension
Pulmonary: Hypoventilation, apnea, bronchospasm
Musculoskeletal: Inadequate block, prolonged block
Dermatologic: Erythema, flushing, anaphylactoid reactions

METOPROLOL TARTRATE (LOPRESSOR)

Use(s): Antihypertensive, treatment of supraventricular and ventricular arrhythmias and acute myocardial infarction; antianginal; symptomatic relief in thyrotoxic patients; adjunct treatment of alcohol withdrawal; prophylaxis of migraine headaches

Dosing: Hypertension/angina: PO, 100-450 mg daily in single or divided doses. Begin with 100 mg/day and increase at weekly intervals.

Acute myocardial infarction:

Early: IV, 15 mg (5 mg q2min for 3 doses) then PO, 50 mg q6h for 48 hr, then PO, 100 mg twice daily.

Patients intolerant of full IV dose: PO, 25-50 mg q6h

Late treatment: PO, 100 mg twice daily.

Migraine prophylaxis: PO, 50-100 mg twice daily

Elimination: Hepatic

How Supplied:

Tablets, 50 mg and 100 mg

Injection, 1 mg/ml

Storage: Injection/Tablets: Room temperature (15°-30° C). Do not permit injection to freeze.

Pharmacology

Metoprolol is a cardioselective beta blocker but can inhibit beta-2 receptors in high doses. The mechanism for the anti-hypertensive effects of the drug is unknown. Reduced cardiac output, decreased renin release, or a central action may play a role. The antiarrhythmic effect is secondary to the reduction in sympathetic nervous system activity, and the antianginal effect reflects the decrease in myocardial oxygen consumption secondary to a reduction in heart rate and cardiac output. Metoprolol may prevent common migraine and reduce the number of attacks in some patients. It is not effective for a migraine attack that has already start-ed. The antimigraine effect may be partly due to inhibition of vasodilation. The drug also may inhibit arteriolar spasm of the pial vessels in the brain. Metoprolol increases uterine activity more in the nonpregnant than in the pregnant uterus.

Pharmacokinetics

Onset: Antihypertensive effects: IV, almost immediate; PO, <15 min

Peak Effect: Antihypertensive effects: IV, 20 min; antimigraine effects: PO, 4-6 weeks

Duration: Antihypertensive effects: IV/PO, 5-8 hr

Interaction/Toxicity: Hypotensive effect potentiated by volatile anesthetics, catecholamine-depleting drugs (e.g., reserpine); may unmask negative inotropic effects of ketamine; prolongs elevation of plasma potassium after the administration of succinylcholine; potentiates depolarizing and nondepolarizing muscle relaxants (e.g., succinylcholine, tubocurarine); may mask symptoms of hypoglycemia (e.g., tachycardia); increases serum levels of digoxin and morphine; rebound hypertension may occur with abrupt withdrawal; may produce bradycardia, AV block, bronchospasm, and cardiac failure.

Guidelines/Precautions

1. Excessive myocardial depression may be treated with IV atropine (1-2 mg), IV isoproterenol (0.02- 0.15 μg/kg/min), IV glucagon (1-5 mg), or a transvenous cardiac pacemaker.
2. Use is contraindicated in sinus bradycardia, heart block greater than first degree, cardiogenic shock, and overt failure.
3. Use with extreme caution if at all in patients with bronchospastic disease.
4. Risk of ischemia or infarction is increased in patients with coronary artery disease if drug is withdrawn abruptly.

Principal Adverse Reactions

Cardiovascular: Hypotension, arrhythmias, rebound angina
Pulmonary: Bronchospasm, dyspnea, cough
CNS: Fatigue, depression, disorientation
GI: Nausea, vomiting, pancreatitis
Hematologic: Thrombocytopenic purpura
Musculoskeletal: Arthralgia

MIDAZOLAM HCL (VERSED)

Use(s): Premedication, conscious sedation, induction agent, supplementation of anesthesia

Dosing: Premedication:

IM, 2.5-10 mg (0.05-0.2 mg/kg)

PO, 20-40 mg (0.5-0.75 mg/kg). Use high-potency injectate solution (5 mg/ml). Dilute in 3-5 ml apple juice or carbonated cola beverage. Atropine 0.03 mg/kg PO may be added to reduce secretions.

Intranasal, 0.2-0.3 mg/kg. Use high-potency injectate solution (5 mg/ml).

Rectal, 15-20 mg (0.3-0.35 mg/kg). Dilute in 5 ml NS.

Conscious sedation: IV, 0.5-5 mg (0.025-0.1 mg/kg). Titrate slowly to the desired effect (e.g., onset of slurred speech). Monitor respiratory and cardiac function continuously.

Sedation: Infusion 1-15 mg/hr (20-300 µg/kg/hr). Respiratory support and continuous monitoring are required.

Induction:

IV, 50-350 µg/kg

Infusion, 0.25-5 µg/kg/min

       Anticonvulsant: IV/IM, 2-5 mg (0.025-0.1
       mg/kg) q10-15min as needed

Elimination: Renal

How Supplied: Injection, 1 mg/ml, 5 mg/ml

Storage: Room temperature (15°-30° C). Protect from light.

Dilution for Infusion: 50 mg in 250 ml D_5W or NS (200 μg/ml)

Pharmacology

This short-acting benzodiazepine possesses antianxiety, sedative, amnesic, anticonvulsant, and skeletal muscle relaxant properties. Neuromuscular transmission is not affected, and the action of nondepolarizing drugs is not altered. Because of the imidazole ring in its structure, midazolam is highly water-soluble at a low pH (<4) with the ring opened and lipophilic at physiologic pH (>4) with the ring closed. The water solubility facilitates intravenous admixtures, and the lipophilic properties minimize venous irritation. The mechanism of action is unknown, but midazolam is thought to act by facilitating the effects of gamma aminobutyric acid, like other benzodiazepine drugs. With a midazolam induction, the awake alpha rhythm changes to a beta rhythm on the EEG. Alpha activity returns after 30 min. Cerebral blood flow, cerebral metabolic rate, and intracranial pressure are decreased. Midazolam depresses ventilation and decreases peripheral vascular resistance and blood pressure, especially in presence of narcotic premedication and/or hypovolemia. Uterine blood flow depends on systemic arterial pressure. Compared with diazepam, midazolam has a more rapid onset with fewer local reactions, a shorter duration of action, greater amnesic effect, and 3-4 times the sedative potency. Recovery is slightly slower compared with patients who received thiopental for induction. The blood level–CNS response relationship is predictable.

Pharmacokinetics

Onset: IV, 30 sec-1 min; IM, 15 min; PO/rectal, <10 min; intranasal, <5 min
Peak Effect: IV, 3-5 min; IM, 15-30 min; PO, 30 min; intranasal, 10 min; rectal, 20-30 min
Duration: IV/IM, 15-80 min; PO/rectal, 2-6 hr
Interaction/Toxicity: CNS and circulatory depressant effects potentiated by alcohol, narcotics, sedatives, volatile anesthetics; decreases MAC for volatile anesthetics; effects antagonized by flumazenil.

Guidelines/Precautions

1. Reduce doses in elderly, hypovolemic, high-risk patients and with concomitant use of other sedatives or narcotics.
2. Patients with COPD are unusually sensitive to the respiratory depressant effect.
3. Use is contraindicated in acute narrow-angle or open-angle glaucoma unless patients are receiving appropriate therapy.
4. Unexpected hypotension and respiratory depression may occur when given with opioids; consider smaller doses.
5. Respiratory depression and arrest may occur when used for conscious sedation. When used for conscious sedation, do not administer as a bolus. Treat overdose with supportive measures and flumazenil (slow IV 0.2-1 mg)

Principal Adverse Reactions

Cardiovascular: Tachycardia, vasovagal episode, premature ventricular complexes, hypotension
Pulmonary: Bronchospasm, laryngospasm, apnea, hypoventilation
CNS: Euphoria, emergence delirium, prolonged emergence, tonic-clonic movements, agitation, hyperactivity
GI: Salivation, retching, acid taste
Dermatologic: Rash, pruritus, warmth or coldness at injection site

MIVACURIUM CHLORIDE (MIVACRON)

Use(s): Skeletal muscle relaxation

Dosing: Intubation:
  Single dose: IV, 0.15-0.2 mg/kg (adults) or 0.2 mg/kg (children); administer over 15-30 sec.
  Divided dose: IV, 0.25 mg/kg (adults and children) in 2 divided doses separated by 30 sec.
 Maintenance:
  IV, 0.01-0.1 mg/kg (10%-50% of intubating dose).
  Infusion: 1-15 μg/kg/min.
 Pretreatment/priming: IV, 10% of intubating dose given 3-5 min before depolarizer/nondepolarizer relaxant dose
Elimination: Plasma cholinesterase
How Supplied:
Injection, 2 mg/ml
Premixed infusion: 0.5 mg/ml in 5% dextrose
Storage: Room temperature (15°-30° C).
Dilution for Infusion: Injectate solution, 25 mg in 50 ml

D_5W or NS (0.5 mg/ml); undiluted injectate solution (2 mg/ml) may be used for infusion.

Pharmacology

This bis-benzylisoquinolinium diester compound is a short-acting nondepolarizing neuromuscular blocking agent. Mivacurium competes for cholinergic receptors at the motor end plate. It is metabolized by plasma cholinesterase, and the duration of neuromuscular activity is one third that of atracurium, one half that of vecuronium, and 2 to 2.5 times that of succinylcholine. The time to onset of maximum effect is similar for recommended doses of mivacurium and intermediate-acting neuromuscular blockers (e.g., atracurium, vecuronium), but longer than that for succinylcholine. Unlike these intermediate-acting agents, increasing the dosage of mivacurium does not markedly increase the duration of action. Repeated doses are not associated with tachyphylaxis and have minimal cumulative effect on duration of blockade. Doses higher than($>$0.3 mg/kg)may be associated with transient decreases in mean arterial pressure, transient increases in heart rate, and elevation of plasma histamine concentrations.

Pharmacokinetics

Onset: <2 min
Peak Effect: 1-3 min
Duration: 6-16 min
Interaction/Toxicity: Neuromuscular blockade potentiated by aminoglycoside, antibiotics, local anesthetics, loop diuretics, magnesium, lithium, ganglionic blocking drugs, hypothermia, hypokalemia, respiratory acidosis, and prior administration of succinylcholine; dosage requirements decreased (about 30%-45%) and duration of neuromuscular

blockade prolonged (up to 25%) by volatile anesthetics; recurrent paralysis with quinidine; enhanced neuromuscular blockade in patients with low plasma cholinesterase, myasthenia gravis, or inadequate adrenocortical function; pretreatment doses of mivacurium decrease fasciculations but reduce intensity and shorten duration of succinylcholine neuromuscular blockade; priming doses decrease the time to onset of maximal blockade by about 30-60 sec; sensitivity to mivacurium is increased during pregnancy secondary to decreased pseudocholinesterase; effects are antagonized by anticholinesterases such as neostigmine, edrophonium, and pyridostigmine; resistance is increased or effects are reversed with use of theophylline and in patients with burn injury and paresis; mivacurium is incompatible with alkaline solutions having a pH greater than 8.5 (e.g., barbiturate solutions).

Guidelines/Precautions

1. Monitor response with peripheral nerve stimulator to minimize risk of overdosage.
2. Reverse effects with anticholinesterases such as neostigmine, edrophonium, or pyridostigmine bromide in conjunction with atropine or glycopyrrolate.
3. Pretreatment doses may induce a degree of neuromuscular blockade sufficient to cause hypoventilation in some patients.
4. Prolonged neuromuscular blockade may occur in patients with low plasma pseudocholinesterase, as in severe liver disease or cirrhosis, burns, malignant tumors, infections, decompensated heart disease, myxedema, peptic ulcer, pregnancy, dehydration, collagen disease, and abnormal body temperatures, in patients receiving MAO inhibitors, oral contraceptives, or glucocorticoids, or in those with a

recessive hereditary trait. Administer test doses of not more than 0.015-0.020 mg/kg mivacurium.

5. Use with caution in patients with any history suggesting a greater sensitivity to the release of histamine or related mediators (e.g., asthma). Initial dose of mivacurium should be 0.15 mg/kg or less administered over 60 sec with adequate hydration and careful monitoring of hemodynamic status.

6. Initial dose requirements are higher in children, and maintenance doses are generally required more frequently.

7. Use is contraindicated in patients known to have allergic hypersensitivity to mivacurium chloride or other benzylisoquinolinium agents. Use of mivacurium from multidose vials is contraindicated in patients with a known allergy to benzyl alcohol.

Principal Adverse Reactions

Cardiovascular: Hypotension, vasodilation, tachycardia, bradycardia
Pulmonary: Hypoventilation, apnea, bronchospasm, laryngospasm, dyspnea
Dermatologic: Rash, urticaria, erythema, injection-site reaction
Musculoskeletal: Inadequate block, prolonged block

MORPHINE SULFATE (MORPHINE, MS Contin, ASTRAMORPH, DURAMORPH, INFUMORPH)

Use(s): Premedication, analgesia, anesthesia, treatment of pain associated with myocardial ischemia, and for dyspnea associated with acute left-ventricular failure and pulmonary edema

Dosing: Analgesia:

   IV, 2.5-15 mg (Children 0.05-0.2 mg/kg; maximum 15 mg);

   IM/SC, 2.5-20 mg (Children 0.05-0.2 mg/kg; maximum 15 mg)

   PO, 10 - 30 mg q4h prn pain

   PO extended release, 15-60 mg q8-12hr

   Rectal 10-20 mg q4h

   Intraarticular, 0.5-1 mg (dilute in 40 ml normal saline or 0.0625%-0.25% bupivacaine)

   Induction: IV, 1 mg/kg

   Epidural:

    Bolus, 2-5 mg (40-100 μg/kg), dilute in 10 ml (preservative-free) NS or local anesthetic.

    Infusion, 0.1-1 μg/hr (2-20 μg/kg/hr) (use preservative-free solution).

   Spinal: 0.1-1 mg (4-20 μg/kg) (use preservative-free solution).

  Patient controlled analgesia:

   IV:

    Bolus, 0.5-3.0 mg (10-60 μg/kg)

    Infusion, 0.5-10 mg/hr (15-200 μg/kg/hr)

    Lockout interval, 5-20 min

   Epidural:

    Bolus, 0.1 mg (2 μg/kg)

    Infusion, 0.4 mg/hr (8 μg/kg)

    Lockout interval, 10 min

  Pulmonary edema: IV, 0.05-0.1 mg/kg; add a diuretic if required

Elimination: Hepatic
How Supplied:
Injection, 0.5 mg/ml, 1 mg/ml, 2 mg/ml, 3 mg/ml 4 mg/ml, 5 mg/ml, 8 mg/ml, 10 mg/ml, 15 mg/ml

Preservative-free injection, 0.5 mg/ml, 1 mg/ml
Tablets, 10 mg, 15 mg, 30 mg
Tablets, extended release, 30 mg, 60 mg
Oral solution, 10 mg/5 ml, 20 mg/ml, 20 mg/5 ml, 100 mg/5 ml
Rectal suppositories, 5 mg, 10 mg, 20 mg, 30 mg
Storage: Injection/tablets/oral solution: Room temperature (15°-30° C). Protect from light. Do not permit injection/oral solution to freeze.
Dilution for Infusion:
IV, 20 mg in 100 ml NS (0.2 mg/ml)
Epidural infusion, 10 mg in 100 ml local anesthetic or (preservative-free) NS (0.1 mg/ml)

Pharmacology

This alkaloid of opium exerts its primary effects on the central nervous system and organs containing smooth muscle. It produces analgesia, drowsiness, euphoria, dose-related depression of respiration, interference with adrenocortical response to stress (at high doses), and reduction in peripheral resistance (arteriolar and venous dilation) with little or no effect on cardiac index. The therapeutic effect of the drug in pulmonary edema is secondary to the increase in the capacitance bed. Constipating effects of morphine result from induction of nonpropulsive contractions through the GI tract. Morphine (and other opioids) may cause biliary tract spasm and increase common bile duct pressure (15%, pentazocine; 53%, morphine; 61%, meperidine; 99%, fentanyl) above predrug levels. Depression of the cough reflex is by a direct effect on the cough centers in the medulla. Morphine decreases cerebral blood flow, cerebral metabolic rate, and intracranial pressure. It may induce nausea and vomiting by activating the chemoreceptor trigger zone. Morphine releases histamine and can cause pruritus after oral or systemic administration. Altered sensory modulation secondary to direct binding of morphine (and other opioids) to opiate receptors in the medulla oblongata may be the mechanism for pruritus after epidural/intrathecal administration. Intraarticular analgesia occurs secondary to binding of morphine to opiate receptors in the synovium.

Pharmacokinetics

Onset: IV, <1 min; IM, 1-5 min; SC, 15-30 min; PO, 15-60 min; PO slow release, 60-90 min; epidural/ spinal, 15-60 min

Peak Effect: IV, 5-20 min; IM, 30-60 min; SC, 50-90 min; PO, 30-60 min; PO slow release, 1-4 hr; rectal, 20-60 min; epidural/spinal, 90 min

Duration: IV/IM/SC, 2-7 hr; PO slow release, 6-12 hr; epidural/spinal, 6-24 hr

Interaction/Toxicity: CNS and circulatory depressant effects are potentiated by alcohol, sedatives, narcotics, antihistamines, phenothiazines, butyrophenones, MAO inhibitors, and tricyclic antidepressants; may decrease the effect of diuretics in patients with congestive heart failure; analgesia is enhanced and prolonged by alpha-2 agonists (e.g., clonidine, epinephrine); addition of epinephrine to intrathecal/epidural morphine results in increased side effects (e.g., nausea) and prolonged motor block.

Guidelines/Precautions

1. Reduce dose in elderly, hypovolemic, and high-risk surgical patients and with concomitant use of sedatives and other narcotics.
2. The narcotic antagonist naloxone is a specific antidote (IV 0.2-0.4 mg or higher). Reversal of narcotic effect may lead to onset of pain and release of catecholamines.
3. Opioid-induced biliary tract spasm may be reversed with

naloxone (IV/IM 0.2-0.4 mg) or glucagon (IV/IM 0.25-0.2 mg). Reversal of analgesia may occur with naloxone but not glucagon.

4. Morphine crosses the placental barrier, and usage in labor may produce depression of respiration in the neonate. Resuscitation may be required; have naloxone available.

5. Incidences of reactivation of herpes simplex have occurred after administration of epidural or spinal morphine. The herpes virus may be reactivated directly by mechanical irritation of the sensory nerves when patients scratch (in response to itching) or by opioid activity in the medulla.

6. Undesirable side effects of epidural, caudal, or intrathecal morphine include delayed respiratory depression (up to 24 hr after single dose), pruritus, nausea and vomiting, and urinary retention. Naloxone (IV 0.2-0.4 mg prn or infusion 5-10 μg/kg/hr) is effective for prophylaxis and/or treatment of these side effects. Ventilatory support for respiratory depression must be readily available. Antihistamines (e.g., diphenhydramine 12.5-25 mg IV/IM q6h prn) may be used in treating pruritus. Metoclopramide (10 mg IV q6h prn) may be used in treating nausea and vomiting. Urinary retention that does not respond to naloxone may require straight bladder catheterization.

7. Epidural, caudal, or intrathecal morphine should be avoided when the patient has septicemia, infection at the injection site, or coagulopathy.

Principal Adverse Reactions

Cardiovascular: Hypotension, hypertension, bradycardia, arrhythmias, chest wall rigidity
Pulmonary: Bronchospasm, laryngospasm
CNS: Blurred vision, syncope, euphoria, dysphoria

GU: Urinary retention, antidiuretic effect, ureteral spasm
GI: Biliary tract spasm, constipation, anorexia, nausea, vomiting, delayed gastric emptying
Eye: Miosis
Musculoskeletal: Chest wall rigidity
Allergic: Pruritus, urticaria

NALBUPHINE HCL (NUBAIN)

Use(s): Analgesia; anesthesia

Dosing: Sedation/analgesia: IV/IM/SC, 5-10 mg (0.1-0.3 mg/kg)
Induction: IV, 0.3-3 mg/kg
Patient controlled analgesia IV:
Bolus, 1-5 mg (0.02-0.1 mg/kg)
Infusion, 1-8 mg/hr (0.02-0.15 mg/kg/hr)
Lockout interval, 5-15 min
Elimination: Hepatic
How Supplied: Injection: 10 mg/ml, 20 mg/ml
Storage: Room temperature (15°-30° C). Protect from light.

Pharmacology

Nalbuphine is a synthetic opioid agonist-antagonist and a potent analgesic. It is related chemically to oxymorphone and naloxone. Nalbuphine is equal in potency as an analgesic to morphine and one fourth as potent as nalorphine as an antagonist. It exhibits ceiling effect at high doses (greater than 30 mg) for respiratory depression and analgesia. It is effective in reversing the ventilatory depression of agonist opioids (e.g., fentanyl), while maintaining reasonable analgesia. Cardiovascular stability is good.

Pharmacokinetics

Onset: IV, 2-3 min; IM/SC, <15 min
Peak Effect: IV, 5-15 min
Duration: IV/IM/SC, 3-6 hr
Interaction/Toxicity: In nondependent patients, nalbuphine potentiates depressant effect of other narcotics, volatile anesthetics, sedative hypnotics, phenothiazines; precipitates withdrawal symptoms in narcotic-dependent patients; may produce pruritus, bronchospasm, hypotension, hypertension.

Guidelines/Precautions

1. Reduce dose in elderly, hypovolemic, and high-risk surgical patients and with concomitant use of narcotics and sedatives.
2. Naloxone is a specific antidote (IV 0.2-0.4 mg or higher).
3. Nalbuphine may worsen gallbladder pain.
4. It crosses the placental barrier, and usage in labor may produce depression of respiration in the neonate. Resuscitation may be required; have naloxone available.
5. Use with caution in patients who have been chronically receiving opiate agonists. High doses of nalbuphine may precipitate withdrawal symptoms as a result of opiate antagonist effect.

Principal Adverse Reactions

Cardiovascular: Hypertension, hypotension, bradycardia, tachycardia
Pulmonary: Respiratory depression, dyspnea, asthma
CNS: Euphoria, dysphoria, confusion, sedation
GI: Cramps, dyspepsia, bitter taste
Eye: Miosis
Dermatologic: Itching, burning, urticaria

Other: Speech difficulty, urinary urgency, blurred vision, flushing

NALOXONE HCL (NARCAN)

Use(s): Reversal of narcotic depression and biliary tract spasm, adjunct treatment of captopril, clonidine, codeine, dextromethorphan, diphenoxylate, and propoxyphene overdose; prophylaxis/treatment of narcotic side effects (e.g., pruritus, nausea); adjunct therapy of septic and cardiogenic shock

Dosing: Narcotic depression/drug overdose:

IV/IM/SC, 0.1-2 mg (neonates/children 10-100 μg/kg), titrate to patient response. May repeat at 2-3 min intervals. Response should occur with a maximum dose of 10 mg.

Infusion, 5-15 μg/kg/hr (children 10-150 μg/kg/hr). Titrate to patient response.

Prophylaxis/treatment of narcotic side effects:

IV/IM/SC, 0.1-0.8 mg

Infusion, 50-250 μg/hr (1-5 μg/kg/hr); infusion rate of <125 ml/hr if 1-2 ampules of naloxone are diluted in 1000 ml of patient's maintenance intravenous fluid.

Septic shock:

IV, 30 μg/kg

Infusion, 30-200 μg/kg/hr (for 1-16 hr)

Elimination: Hepatic

How Supplied:

Injection, 0.4 mg/ml, 1 mg/ml

Neonatal injection, 0.02 mg/ml

Storage: Room temperature (15°-30° C). Protect from light.

Dilution for Infusion:

Narcotic depression/drug overdose: IV, 1 mg in 100 ml D_5W or NS (10 μg/ml)

Narcotic side effects: IV, 0.4-0.8 mg (1-2 ampules) in 1000 ml

Pharmacology

Naloxone is a pure opioid antagonist with no agonist activity. It competitively inhibits opiate agonists at mu, delta, and kappa receptor sites and prevents or reverses the effects of opioids, including respiratory depression, sedation, hypotension, analgesia, and biliary tract spasm. Naloxone also can reverse the psychotomimetic and dysphoric effects of agonists-antagonists such as pentazocine. CNS and respiratory depression secondary to captopril, clonidine, codeine, dextromethorphan, diphenoxylate, and propoxyphene overdose may be reversed with naloxone. Naloxone may reverse the hypotension and cardiovascular instability secondary to endogenous endorphins (potent vasodilators) released in patients with septic or cardiogenic shock. Naloxone does not produce respiratory depression, psychotomimetic effects, or pupillary constriction. It shows no pharmacologic activity in the absence of narcotics and produces withdrawal symptoms in the presence of physical dependence.

Pharmacokinetics

Onset: IV, 1-2 min; IM/SC, 2-5 min
Peak Effect: IV/IM/SC, 5-15 min
Duration: IV/IM/SC, 1-4 hr
Interaction/Toxicity: Reversal of analgesia; increased sympathetic nervous system activity, including tachycardia, hypertension, pulmonary edema, and cardiac arrhythmias; nausea and vomiting related to dose and speed of injection.

Guidelines/Precautions

1. Use with caution in patients with preexisting cardiac disease or who have received potentially cardiotoxic drugs.
2. Titrate slowly to desired effect. Excessive dosage of naloxone may result in reversal of analgesia and other significant side effects (hypertension, excitement, acute pulmonary edema, cardiac arrhythmias).
3. Patients who have responded to naloxone should be carefully monitored because the duration of action of some opiates may exceed that of naloxone. Repeated doses of naloxone should be administered to those patients when necessary.
4. If intravenous access is not available, the drug may be diluted 1:1 in sterile NS and injected via an endotracheal tube. The absorption rate, duration, and pharmacologic effects of endotracheal drug administration compare favorably with the IV route.
5. Administer cautiously to persons who are known or suspected to be physically dependent on opioids, including newborns of mothers with narcotic dependence. Reversal of narcotic effects will precipitate acute abstinence syndrome.

Principal Adverse Reactions

Cardiovascular: Tachycardia, hypertension, hypotension, arrhythmias
Pulmonary: Pulmonary edema
CNS: Tremulousness, reversal of analgesia, seizures
GI: Nausea, vomiting
Other: Sweating

NEOSTIGMINE (PROSTIGMINE)

Use(s): Reversal of nondepolarizing muscle relaxants, treatment of myasthenia gravis, postoperative ileus and urinary retention, adjunct treatment of sinus or supraventricular tachycardia

Dosing: Reversal: slow IV, 0.05 mg/kg (maximum dose 5 mg) (with atropine 0.015 mg/kg, or glycopyrrolate 0.01 mg/kg)

Myasthenia gravis:
PO, 15 to 375 mg daily (3 divided doses); or
IM/slow IV, 0.5 to 2 mg (dose must be individualized)

Postoperative ileus/urinary retention: IM/SC, 0.25 to 1 mg q4-6h

Sinus or supraventricular tachycardia: IV, 0.25-0.5 mg; treat precipitating causes of tachycardia (e.g., hypovolemia). Monitor for hypotension or bronchospasm.

Elimination: Hepatic, plasma esterases

How Supplied:

Injection, 0.25 mg/ml (1:4000), 0.5 mg/ml (1:2000), 1 mg/ml (1:1000).

Tablets, 15 mg

Storage: Injection/tablets: Room temperature (15°-40° C). Protect from light. Do not permit (injection) to freeze.

Pharmacology

Neostigmine inhibits the hydrolysis of acetylcholine by competing with acetylcholine for attachment to acetylcholinesterase at the esteratic site. Buildup of acetylcholine facilitates the transmission of impulses across the neuromuscular junction. In myasthenia gravis there is an increased response of skeletal muscle to repetitive impulses caused by increased availability of acetylcholine. Cholinergic stimulation is useful in treating postoperative ileus and sinus or supraventricular tachycardia. When used for reversal of neuromuscular blockade, the muscarinic cholinergic effects (bradycardia, salivation) may be prevented by concurrent use of atropine or glycopyrrolate.

Pharmacokinetics

Onset:
Reversal: IV, <3 min
Myasthenia: IM, <20 min; PO, 45-75 min
Peak Effect:
Reversal: IV, 3-14 min (twitch height >20% control)
Reversal: IV, 8-29 min (twitch height <20% control)
Myasthenia: IM, 20-30 min
Duration:
Reversal: IV, 40-60 min
Myasthenia: IM/PO, 2-4 hr
Interaction/Toxicity: Does not antagonize and may prolong the phase-1 block of depolarizing muscle relaxants, such as succinylcholine; antagonizes the effects of nondepolarizing muscle relaxants, such as tubocurarine, atracurium, vecuronium, and pancuronium; antagonism of neuromuscular blockade is reduced by aminoglycoside antibiotics, hypothermia, hypokalemia, and respiratory and metabolic acidosis.

Guidelines/Precautions

1. Use is contraindicated in patients with peritonitis or mechanical obstruction of the intestines or urinary tract.

2. Neostigmine overdosage may induce a cholinergic crisis characterized by nausea, vomiting, bradycardia or tachycardia, excessive salivation and sweating, bronchospasm, weakness, and paralysis.

3. Treatment of a cholinergic crisis includes discontinuation of neostigmine and administration of atropine (10 μg/kg IV q3-10min until muscarinic symptoms disappear) and if necessary pralidoxime (15 mg/kg IV over 2 min) for reversal of nicotinic symptoms. Give other supportive treatment as indicated (e.g., artificial respiration, tracheostomy, oxygen).

4. Use with caution in patients with bradycardia, bronchial asthma, epilepsy, cardiac arrhythmias, or peptic ulcer.

Principal Adverse Reactions

Cardiovascular: Bradycardia, tachycardia, AV block, nodal rhythm, hypotension
Pulmonary: Increased oral, pharyngeal, and bronchial secretions, bronchospasm, respiratory depression
CNS: Seizures, dysarthria, headaches
GI: Nausea, emesis, flatulence, increased peristalsis
GU: Urinary frequency
Dermatologic: Rash, urticaria
Allergic: Allergic reactions, anaphylaxis

NIFEDIPINE (PROCARDIA, ADALAT)

Use(s): Antianginal, antihypertensive, suppression of preterm labor

Dosing: Angina/hypertension:
        PO, 10-30 mg tid, maximum 180 mg/day
        PO sustained release (PO-SR), 30-60 mg once
           daily

Unlabeled route:

Sublingual: puncture capsule and apply contents sublingually

Intrabuccal: puncture capsule 10 times and chew

Preterm labor: sublingual, 10 mg q20min until cessation of contractions (maximum dose: 40 mg in 1 hr) then PO, 20 mg q8h for 3 days

Elimination: Hepatic, renal

How Supplied:

Capsules, 10 mg, 20 mg

Tablets (SR), 30 mg, 60 mg, 90 mg

Storage:

Capsules: Room temperature (15°-25° C). Protect from light.

Tablets: Temperature below 30° C. Protect from light.

Pharmacology

Nifedipine is a dihydropyridine calcium channel blocker. It inhibits the transmembrane influx of calcium ions into cardiac muscle and smooth muscle. It possesses greater coronary and peripheral arterial vasodilator properties than verapamil and minimal effects on venous capacitance. It has little or no direct depressant effect on SA node or AV node activity and consequently, may be safely used in patients with low heart rates. The antihypertensive effects are probably due to decreased peripheral vascular resistance. A reflex increase in heart rate, cardiac output, and fluid retention from peripheral vasodilation may offset the antihypertensive effect. Nifedipine improves myocardial oxygen supply-and-demand balance, which accounts for its effectiveness in the treatment of angina pectoris. Nifedipine, like other calcium channel blockers, is a cerebral vasodilator. It increases cerebral blood flow and intracranial pressure. Cerebral perfusion pressure is decreased (CPP = MAP − ICP).

Pharmacokinetics

Onset: PO, 20 min; SL, 5 min
Peak Effect: PO, 30 min; PO-SR, 6 hr; SL, 20-45 min
Duration: PO/SL, 4-12 hr; PO-SR, 24 hr
Interaction/Toxicity: Potentiates effects of depolarizing and nondepolarizing muscle relaxants; has additive cardiovascular depressant effects with use of volatile anesthetics, other antihypertensives such as diuretics, angiotensin-converting enzyme inhibitors, and vasodilators; increases toxicity of digoxin, benzodiazepines, carbamazepine, oral hypoglycemics, and possibly quinidine and theophylline; cardiac failure, AV conduction disturbances, and sinus bradycardia may occur with concurrent use of beta blockers; severe hypotension and bradycardia may occur with bupivacaine; concomitant use of IV verapamil and IV dantrolene may result in cardiovascular collapse; decreases lithium effect and neurotoxicity; decreases clearance with cimetidine; is chemically incompatible with solutions of bicarbonate or nafcillin; may be displaced from binding sites by, or may displace from binding sites, other highly protein-bound drugs such as oral anticoagulants, hydantoins, salicylates, sulfonamides, and sulfonylureas.

Guidelines/Precautions

1. Nifedipine requires careful monitoring of blood pressure during initial administration and titration.
2. Use with caution in the elderly, hypovolemic patients, and those with acute MI, aortic stenosis, obstructive cardiomyopathy, unstable angina, severe myocardial depression or increased intracranial pressure.
3. Do not chew or divide sustained-release tablets.

Principal Adverse Reactions

Cardiovascular: Hypotension, palpitations, peripheral edema

Pulmonary: Bronchospasm, shortness of breath, nasal and chest congestion

CNS: Headache, dizziness, nervousness

GI: Nausea, diarrhea, constipation

Musculoskeletal: Inflammation, joint stiffness, peripheral edema

Dermatologic: Pruritus, urticaria

Other: Fever, chills, sweating

NITROGLYCERIN (NITROL, NITROSTAT, TRIDIL, NITROGARD, NITROCINE, NITROLIN, NITROGLYN, NITRONG, NITRO-BID, TRANSDERM-NITRO, NITRODISC and NITRO OINTMENT)

Use(s): Controlled hypotension, antianginal, treatment of pulmonary edema and congestive heart failure associated with acute myocardial infarction, uterine relaxation (for manual extraction of a retained placenta)

Dosing: Controlled hypotension/antianginal/pulmonary edema/CHF:

IV infusion, 5-200 μg/min (0.1-4 μg/kg/min). Absorbed in plastic and polyvinylchloride (PVC) tubings. Use glass bottle and supplied infusion set.

Slow IV bolus, 25-100 μg (0.5-2 μg/kg), dilute 1 mg of parenteral concentrate with 20 ml D_5W or NS (50 μg/ml)

Antianginal/CHF:

Tablets:

Sublingual, 0.15-0.6 mg q5min prn to maximum of 3 doses in a 15 min period;

Sustained-release buccal, 1-2 mg q3-5h. Place tablet between lip and gum above incisors.

Sustained-release oral, 1.3-9 mg q8-12h prn

Capsules: sustained-release oral, 1.3-9 mg q8-12h prn

Ointment: $\frac{1}{2}$-2 inches q8h. Maximum 4-5 inches q4h

Transdermal systems: Apply pad once each day. Titrate to a higher dose strength as needed for optimal effect.

Aerosol: 1 or 2 metered doses on oral mucosa. Maximum of 3 doses in 15 min.

Uterine relaxation: Slow IV bolus, 50-100 μg (1-2 μg/kg) Dilute 1 mg of parenteral concentrate with 20 ml D_5W or NS (50 μg/ml)

Elimination: Hepatic, renal

How Supplied:

Injection: concentrate for infusion, 0.5 mg/ml, 0.8 mg/ml, 5 mg/ml, 10 mg/ml

Tablets:

Sublingual, 0.15 mg (1/400 gr), 0.3 mg (1/200 gr), 0.4 mg (1/150 gr), 0.6 mg (1/100 gr)

Sustained-release, buccal, 1 mg, 2 mg, 3 mg

Sustained-release, oral, 2.5 mg, 2.6 mg, 6.5 mg, 9 mg

Capsules: sustained release, oral, 2.5 mg, 6.5 mg, 9 mg

Aerosol translingual: 0.4 mg per metered dose

Transdermal systems: 2.5 mg/24 hr, 5 mg/24 hr, 7.5 mg/24 hr, 10 mg/24 hr, 15 mg/24 hr

Ointment 2% (1 inch contains 15 mg nitroglycerin)

Storage: Injection/tablets/aerosol/ointment/transdermal systems: Room temperature (15°-30° C). Protect from heat. Do not permit injection to freeze. Aerosol should not be punctured, exposed to heat, or stored at a temperature greater than 49° C.

Dilution for Infusion:

8 mg vial, dilute in 250 ml D_5W or NS (32 $\mu g/ml$)

50 mg vial, dilute in 250 ml D_5W or NS (200 $\mu g/ml$)

100 mg vial, dilute in 250 ml D_5W or NS (400 $\mu g/ml$)

Pharmacology

This organic nitrate produces a vasodilator effect principally on venous capacitance vessels. This produces peripheral pooling of blood, decreasing venous return, and reducing left ventricular end diastolic pressure (preload) and ventricular size. The decreased diameter of the left ventricle reduces wall tension according to the law of Laplace and decreases cardiac work. At higher doses, arteriolar relaxation reduces systemic vascular resistance and arterial pressure (afterload). All of these factors help improve the myocardial oxygen supply-demand ratio. The drug also causes the redistribution of blood to ischemic areas of the subendocardium in angina pectoris and may decrease the area of damage in myocardial infarction. Nitroglycerin may alter pulmonary ventilation:perfusion ratio and increase cerebral blood flow. Nitroglycerin produces a brief relaxation of the smooth muscle present in the cervix, uterus, and vagina. Uterine blood flow is increased.

Pharmacokinetics

Onset: IV, 1-2 min; SL, 1-3 min; PO sustained release, 20-45 min; transdermal, 40-60 min

Peak Effect: IV, 1-5 min

Duration: IV, 3-5 min; SL, 30-60 min; PO sustained release, 3-8 hr; transdermal, 18-24 hr; aerosol translingual, 30-60 min

Interaction/Toxicity: Hypotensive effects are potentiated by alcohol, phenothiazines, calcium channel blockers, beta-adrenergic blockers, other nitrates, nitrites, and antihypertensives; may antagonize the anticoagulant effect of heparin; methemoglobinemia may occur at high doses.

Guidelines/Precautions

1. Use cautiously in patients with hypotension, uncorrected hypovolemia, increased intracranial pressure, constrictive pericarditis and pericardial tamponade, and inadequate cerebral circulation.
2. Infusion pumps may fail to occlude the non-PVC infusion sets completely because the non-PVC tubing is less pliable than standard PVC tubing. The results may be excessive flow at low infusion rate settings, causing alarms or unregulated gravity flow when the infusion pump is stopped. This could lead to overinfusion.
3. Methemoglobinemia may be caused by high doses of nitrites, especially in individuals with methemoglobin reductase deficiency. Treat with high-flow oxygen and administer methylene blue slowly IV at a dose of 0.1-0.2 ml/kg (1-2 mg/kg).
4. Nitroglycerin transdermal systems should be removed from the site(s) of application before attempting defibrillation or cardioversion because altered electrical conductivity and enhanced potential for arcing may occur.
5. Because of alcohol present in IV nitroglycerin solutions, prolonged administration of high doses may result in mild alcoholic intoxication.

6. Prehydration with intravenous crystalloid solution is recommended during obstetric use to minimize hypotension.

Principal Adverse Reactions

Cardiovascular: Tachycardia, palpitations, hypotension, paradoxic bradycardia and increased angina, collapse
CNS: Headache, dizziness, vertigo
GI: Nausea, vomiting, abdominal pain
Dermatologic: Flushing, exfoliative or contact dermatitis
Other: Methemoglobinemia

NOREPINEPHRINE BITARTRATE (LEVOPHED)

Use(s): Vasoconstrictor, inotrope

Dosing: Infusion, 2-20 μg/min (0.04-0.4 μg/kg/min)
Elimination: Enzymatic degradation, pulmonary
How Supplied: Injection, 1 mg/ml
Storage: Room temperature (15°-30° C). Protect from light. Do not use solution if it is discolored (pink, dark yellow, brown) or contains a precipitate.
Dilution for Infusion: 8 mg in 500 ml D_5W (16 μg/ml)

Pharmacology

This catecholamine produces potent peripheral vasoconstrictor actions on both arterial and venous vascular beds (alpha adrenergic action). It is a potent inotropic stimulator of the heart (beta-1 adrenergic action), but to a lesser degree than epinephrine or isoproterenol. Norepinephrine does not stimulate beta-2 adrenergic receptors of the bronchi or peripheral blood vessels. Systolic and diastolic blood pressure and coronary artery blood flow are increased. Cardiac output varies reflexively with systemic hypertension but is usually increased in hypotensive subjects when blood pressure is raised to an optimal level. On other occasions, increased baroreceptor activity reflexively decreases the heart rate. The drug reduces renal, hepatic, cerebral, and muscle blood flow.

Pharmacokinetics

Onset: <1 min
Peak Effect: 1-2 min
Duration: 2-10 min
Interaction/Toxicity: Increased risk of arrhythmias with use of volatile anesthetics or bretylium or in patients with profound hypoxia or hypercarbia; pulmonary extraction decreased and pressor effect increased by halothane, nitrous oxide; pressor effect potentiated in patients receiving MAO inhibitors, tricyclic antidepressants, guanethidine, oxytocics; necrosis or gangrene may occur with extravasation.

Guidelines/Precautions

1. Administer into large vein to minimize extravasation. Treat extravasation immediately with local infiltration of phentolamine (5-10 mg in 10 ml NS) or sympathetic block.
2. Use is not a substitute for the replacement of blood, plasma, fluids, and electrolytes, which should be restored promptly when loss has occurred.
3. Use is contraindicated in patients with mesenteric or peripheral vascular thrombosis.

Principal Adverse Reactions

Cardiovascular: Bradycardia, tachyarrhythmias, hypertension, decreased cardiac output
CNS: Headache
Other: Plasma volume depletion

ONDANSETRON (ZOFRAN)

Use(s): Prevention and treatment of chemotherapy-induced and postoperative nausea and vomiting

Dosing: Chemotherapy-induced nausea:

IV, 32 mg in 1 dose. Dilute in 50 ml D_5W and infuse over 15 min beginning a half hour before the start of chemotherapy; or,

IV, 0.15 mg/kg, 3 doses. Dilute each dose in 50 ml D_5W and infuse over 15 min. Give dose a half hour before the start of chemotherapy and repeat dose 4 hr and 8 hr after.

Dosage should be reduced (maximum daily dose of 8 mg) in patients with hepatic impairment.

Postoperative nausea:

PO, 16 mg (1 hr prior to induction of anesthesia)

Slow IV, 4 mg, give undiluted over 1-5 min. Dose may be repeated if necessary.

Elimination: Hepatic

How Supplied: Injection, 2 mg/ml

Storage: Temperature between 2°-30° C. Protect from light.

Pharmacology

Ondansetron is a selective serotonin 5-HT3 receptor antagonist. 5-HT3 receptors are present both peripherally on vagal nerve terminals and centrally in the chemoreceptor trigger zone of the area postrema. Ondansetron may antagonize the emetic effects of serotonin at either or both receptor sites. Ondansetron does not antagonize dopamine receptors. Transient increases in hepatic transaminase levels may occur after therapy. The drug may cross the placenta and may be excreted in breast milk. It should be used with caution in pregnant and nursing mothers.

Pharmacokinetics

Onset: IV, <30 min
Peak Effect: IV, variable
Duration: IV, 12-24 hr
Interaction/Toxicity: Serum levels may be altered with concomitant administration of phenytoin, phenobarbital, and rifampin.

Guidelines/Precautions

1. Ondansetron does not stimulate gastric or intestinal peristalsis. It should not be used in place of a nasogastric tube. As with other antiemetics, the use of ondansetron in abdominal surgery may mask a progressive ileus and/or gastric distension.

Principal Adverse Reactions

Cardiovascular: Hypotension, bradycardia, tachycardia, angina, second-degree heart block
Pulmonary: Bronchospasm, shortness of breath
CNS: Extrapyramidal reactions, seizures
GI: Constipation, hepatic dysfunction
Other: Blurred vision, hypokalemia, pain and redness at site of injection

OXYTOCIN (SYNTOCINON, PITOCIN)

Use(s): Improvement of uterine contractions, control of postpartum hemorrhage

Dosing: Antepartum: infusion, 1-20 mU/min
        Postpartum:
                Infusion, 20-40 mU/min; titrate to control uterine atony
                IV bolus, 0.6-1.8 units, IM, 3-10 units

Elimination: Hepatic

How Supplied:

Injection, 10 units/ml

Nasal solution, 40 units/ml

Storage: Injection: Refrigerate (2°-8° C). Stable for 3 months at room temperature (15°-25° C). Protect from freezing.

Dilution for Infusion: 10-40 units in 1 L NS (10-40 mU/ml)

Pharmacology

This naturally occurring nonapeptide hormone stimulates uterine smooth muscle contractions. It increases both the force and frequency of existing rhythmic contractions and raises the tone of the uterine musculature. The sensitivity of the uterus to oxytocin increases gradually during gestation and sharply immediately before parturition. The hormone is structurally similar to antidiuretic hormone and may produce water intoxication. High doses produce a marked but transient vasodilation, hypotension, and flushing accompanied by a reflex tachycardia and increased cardiac output.

Pharmacokinetics

Onset: IV, almost immediate; IM, 3-5 min
Peak Effect: IV, <20 min; IM, 40 min
Duration: IV, 20 min-1 hr; IM, 2-3 hr
Interaction/Toxicity: Potentiates pressor effects of sympathomimetics (e.g., ephedrine, phenylephrine)

Guidelines/Precautions

1. When used for induction or stimulation of labor, administer only by the IV route.
2. Monitor uterine activity and fetal heart rate throughout the infusion of oxytocin. Discontinue infusion in event of uterine hyperactivity or fetal distress and administer oxygen to the mother, who should be put in the lateral position.
3. When administering by continuous infusion, monitor fluid intake to minimize risk of water intoxication.
4. Use is contraindicated in significant cephalopelvic disproportion, in fetal distress where delivery is not imminent, and when vaginal delivery is contraindicated.
5. Use cautiously in patients with preeclampsia, essential hypertension, or cardiac disease.

Principal Adverse Reactions

Cardiovascular: Arrhythmia, hypotension, hypertension, tachycardia
CNS: Subarachnoid hemorrhage
GI: Nausea, vomiting
Allergic: Anaphylactic reactions, flushing
Uteral: Hypertonicity, spasm, rupture
Fetal: Bradycardia, arrhythmias, brain damage, low Apgar scores at 5 min
Other: Afibrinogenemia, water retention, hyponatremia

PANCURONIUM (PAVULON)

Use(s): Skeletal muscle relaxation

Dosing: Intubation: IV, 0.04-0.1 mg/kg
Maintenance: IV, 0.01-0.05 mg/kg (10%-50% of
intubating dose)
Infusion: 1-15 μg/kg/min
Pretreatment/priming: IV, 10% of intubating dose
given 3-5 min before depolarizer/nondepolariz-
er relaxant dose

Elimination: Renal, hepatic

How Supplied: Injection, 1 mg/ml, 2 mg/ml

Storage: Stable through the expiration date (e.g., 18
months) when refrigerated (2°-8° C). Stable for 6 months at
room temperature (18°-22° C).

Pharmacology

This synthetic bisquaternary amino steroid is a long-acting
nondepolarizing neuromuscular blocking agent. It acts by
competing for cholinergic receptors at the motor end plate.
Pancuronium is associated with increases in heart rate,
blood pressure, and cardiac output. The increased heart rate
may result from vagolytic actions on the heart. Increased
mean arterial pressure and cardiac output may occur by an
activation of the sympathetic nervous system and inhibition
of catecholamine reuptake. With continuous infusions (>16
hr), recovery may be prolonged because of the accumulation of active metabolites. Histamine release rarely occurs.

Pharmacokinetics

Onset: 1-3 min
Peak Effect: 3-5 min

Duration: 40-65 min

Interaction/Toxicity: Neuromuscular blockade potentiated by aminoglycoside, antibiotics, local anesthetics, loop diuretics, magnesium, lithium, ganglionic blocking drugs, hypothermia, hypokalemia, respiratory acidosis, and prior administration of succinylcholine; dosage requirements are decreased (about 30%-45%) and duration of neuromuscular blockade is prolonged (up to 25%) by volatile anesthetics; inhibits pseudocholinesterase, and pretreatment doses prolong the duration of succinylcholine neuromuscular blockade; priming doses decrease the time to onset of maximal blockade by about 30-60 sec; increases risk of arrhythmia in patients receiving tricyclic antidepressants and volatile anesthetics; recurrent paralysis occurs with quinidine; neuromuscular blockade is enhanced in patients with myasthenia gravis or inadequate adrenocortical function; effects are antagonized by anticholinesterases such as neostigmine, edrophonium, pyridostigmine; resistance is increased or effects are reversed with use of theophylline and in patients with burn injury and paresis.

Guidelines/Precautions

1. Monitor response with peripheral nerve stimulator to minimize risk of overdosage.
2. Reverse effects with anticholinesterases such as neostigmine, edrophonium, or pyridostigmine bromide in conjunction with atropine or glycopyrrolate.
3. Pretreatment doses may induce a degree of neuromuscular blockade sufficient to cause hypoventilation in some patients.
4. Prolonged paralysis (days to months) may occur after termination of long-term infusions in intensive care patients, especially those with renal failure, electrolyte

imbalance (hypokalemia, hypocalcemia, hypermagnesemia), or concomitant corticosteroids and/or aminoglycosides. This is due to development of acute myopathy and persistent neuromuscular blockade secondary to accumulation of active metabolites, particularly 3-desacetyl pancuronium.

Principal Adverse Reactions

Cardiovascular: Tachycardia, hypertension
Pulmonary: Hypoventilation, apnea, bronchospasm
GI: Salivation
Allergic: Flushing, anaphylactoid reactions
Musculoskeletal: Inadequate block, prolonged block

PHENTOLAMINE (REGITINE)

Use(s): Arterial dilator, controlled hypotension, treatment of acute hypertensive crises that may accompany intraoperative manipulation of a pheochromocytoma, treatment of autonomic hyperreflexia, MAO inhibitor/ sympathomimetic amine interactions, treatment of rebound hypertension on withdrawal of antihypertensives, prevention or treatment of dermal necrosis and sloughing after IV administration or extravasation of a barbiturate or sympathomimetic

Dosing: Antihypertensive: IV/IM, 2.5-5 mg (0.05-0.1 mg/kg)
Infusion, 0.1-1 mg/min (10-20 μg/kg/min)
Antisloughing: infiltration, 5-10 mg (0.1-0.2 mg/kg to maximum of 10 mg). Dilute in 10 ml NS.
Elimination: Hepatic
How Supplied: Injection, 5 mg/ml
Storage: Injection: Room temperature (15°-30° C).

Reconstituted solution is stable for 1 week when refrigerated (2°-8° C) and for 48 hr at room temperature (15°-30° C).
Dilution for Infusion: 200 mg in 100 ml D_5W or NS (2 mg/ml)

Pharmacology

Phentolamine is an imidazoline sympathomimetic that blocks both alpha-1 and alpha-2 adrenergic receptors in the periphery. It produces peripheral vasodilation. Blockade of autoregulatory, presynaptic alpha-2 receptors leads to enhanced neuronal release of norepinephrine from catecholaminergic neurons. This action may enhance the positive inotropic and chronotropic effects produced by phentolamine stimulation of beta adrenergic receptors. Blood pressure response to phentolamine depends on the relative contributions of its vasodilating and cardiac-stimulating effects. At usual doses (and IV infusion rates ≥0.3 mg/min) vasodilation predominates, decreasing blood pressure and masking the inotropic effect. Pulmonary vascular resistance and pulmonary arterial pressure are decreased. Cerebral blood flow and intracranial pressure are generally maintained.

Pharmacokinetics

Onset: IV, 1-2 min; IM, 5-20 min
Peak Effect: IV, 2 min; IM, <30 min
Duration: IV, 10-15 min; IM, 30-45 min
Interaction/Toxicity: Use of epinephrine, ephedrine, dobutamine, or isoproterenol after phentolamine may cause paradoxic fall in blood pressure.

Guidelines/Precautions

1. Do not use epinephrine, ephedrine, dobutamine, or isoproterenol to treat phentolamine-induced hypotension.

Phentolamine alpha-receptor blockade will potentiate the $\beta2$ adrenergic vasodilation of epinephrine, ephedrine, dobutamine, or isoproterenol. Treat phentolamine hypotension with norepinephrine.

2. Use with caution in patients with ischemic heart disease.

Principal Adverse Reactions

Cardiovascular: Hypotension, tachycardia, arrhythmias, myocardial infarction
CNS: Dizziness, cerebrovascular spasm and occlusion
GI: Nausea, vomiting, diarrhea
Allergic: Flushing

PHENYLEPHRINE HCL (NEOSYNEPHRINE)

Use(s): Vasoconstrictor; treatment of hypotension, shock, supraventricular tachyarrhythmias; reversal of right-to-left shunting; prolongation of duration of local anesthetics

Dosing: Hypotension during spinal or inhalation anesthesia:
SC or IM, 2-5 mg
IV, 50-100 μg (0.01% solution, dilute 0.1 ml of 1% solution with 10 ml sterile water or NS to give 100 μg/ml); children, 1-2 μg/kg.
Infusion, 10-200 μg/min (0.15-4 μg/kg/min)
Shunt reversal: IV, 50-100 μg (1-2 μg/kg)
Paroxysmal supraventricular tachycardia: IV, 0.5-1 mg, give rapidly within 20-30 sec. If cardiac rhythm fails to convert within 60-90 sec, give an additional 2 mg IV slowly.
Vasoconstrictor for spinal anesthesia: 2-5 mg (40-80 μg/kg) added to anesthetic solution
Vasoconstrictor for infiltration/plexus/epidural/caudal/intra-pleural anesthesia: 1:20,000 dilu-

tion (1 mg diluted in 20 ml local anesthetic
solution or 50 μg/ml)

Nasal/topical: 2 or 3 drops/1 or 2 sprays of
0.25%-0.5% solution. Use 0.125% solution in
children younger than 6 years of age.

Elimination: Hepatic

How Supplied:

Injection, 1% solution (10 mg/ml)

Nasal solution, 0.125%, 0.16%, 0.2%, 0.5%, 0.25%, 1%

Storage: Injection: Room temperature (15°-30° C). Protect from light. Do not use solutions if they are brown or contain a precipitate.

Dilution for Infusion: 30 mg in 500 ml D$_5$W or NS (60 μg/ml)

Pharmacology

Phenylephrine activates alpha adrenergic receptors with minimal beta activation. It produces intense peripheral vasoconstriction, increased systolic and diastolic blood pressures, and a reflex bradycardia that can result in decreased cardiac output. Renal, splanchnic, and cutaneous blood flows are reduced, but coronary blood flow is increased because of increased work. Pulmonary artery pressure is elevated. Reflex vagal effects can be used to slow the heart rate in supraventricular tachyarrhythmias. In acute cyanotic spells in tetralogy of Fallot, phenylephrine-induced increase in systemic vascular resistance may decrease right-to-left shunt and increase pulmonary blood flow. Phenylephrine (and other predominant alpha agonists) increases uterine vascular resistance and decreases uterine blood flow. At therapeutic levels and in the absence of maternal hypertension, there are no adverse fetal effects. At clinical doses and with an intact blood-brain barrier, phenylephrine does not have any significant effects on cerebral vascular resistance, cerebral blood flow, or intracranial pressure. In patients with hypotension, cerebral perfusion pressure is increased because of the increase in systemic arterial pressure (CPP = MAP−ICP) Phenylephrine decreases the rate of absorption of local anesthetics. It prolongs the duration of anesthesia and decreases the risk of systemic toxicity.

Pharmacokinetics

Onset: IV, <1 min; IM/SC, 10-15 min
Peak Effect: IV, 1 min
Duration: IV, 15-20 min; IM/SC, 30 min-2 hr
Interaction/Toxicity: Pressor effects are potentiated with oxytocics, MAO inhibitors, guanethidine, bretylium, and other sympathomimetics; decreased or increased effects may occur with use of tricyclic antidepressants; sensitization of myocardium produced by volatile anesthetics may increase risk of arrhythmias with use of phenylephrine; extravasation may cause sloughing and necrosis.

Guidelines/Precautions

1. Use with extreme caution in elderly patients, patients with hyperthyroidism, bradycardia, partial heart block, or severe arteriosclerosis. In pregnant patients, phenylephrine is not recommended for treatment of spinal hypotension, because the drug-induced decrease in uterine blood flow may lead to fetal asphyxia.
2. Use is not a substitute for the replacement of blood, plasma, fluids, and electrolytes, which should be restored promptly when loss has occurred.
3. Infuse into large veins to prevent extravasation. Treat any extravasation with local infiltration of phentolamine (5 to 10 mg in 10 ml NS) or sympathetic block.
4. Use is contraindicated for IV regional anesthesia or local anesthesia of end organs (digits, penis, ears).

Principal Adverse Reactions

Cardiovascular: Reflex bradycardia, palpitations, precordial pain, arrhythmias, hypertension, hypotension
Pulmonary: Acute pulmonary edema, respiratory distress
CNS: Headache, anxiety, cerebral hemorrhage, dizziness
GU: Decreased renal perfusion, renal necrosis, oliguria
GI: Hepatic necrosis, nausea
Dermatologic: Tissue necrosis, sloughing at site of injection

PHENYTOIN SODIUM (DILANTIN)

Use(s): Anticonvulsant, treatment of trigeminal neuralgia (tic douloureux), digitalis toxic arrhythmias, lidocaine-resistant ventricular arrhythmias, congenital prolonged-QT syndrome and ventricular arrhythmias occurring after congenital heart surgery

Dosing: Anticonvulsant:

Loading IV/PO, 1 g (10-15 mg/kg) in 3 divided doses over 6 hr; do not exceed IV rate of 50 mg/min or 0.5-1.5 mg/kg/min in children. Administer with glucose-free solutions to avoid precipitation.

Maintenance IV/PO, 100 mg q6-8hr (children 5 mg/kg/day)

Therapeutic range, 10-20 μg/ml.

Antiarrhythmic:

IV, 1.5 mg/kg every 5 min until arrhythmia is suppressed or undesirable effects appear (maximum dose 10-15 mg/kg)

PO, 200-400 mg once daily (2-4 mg/kg/day)

Elimination: Hepatic

How Supplied:
Injection, 50 mg/ml
Capsules, 30 mg, 100 mg
Capsules extended release, 30 mg, 100 mg
Tablets, chewable, 50 mg
Oral suspension, 30 mg/5 ml, 125 mg/5 ml

Storage:
Injection: Room temperature (15°-30° C). Protect from freezing. Refrigerated or frozen injections may contain precipitate, which dissolves on warming to room temperature.
Suspension/tablets/capsules: Temperature below 30° C. Do
not permit freezing of oral suspension.

Pharmacology

Also called diphenylhydantoin, phenytoin is an anticonvulsant with primary site of action in the motor cortex. There it
stabilizes the neuronal membranes and prevents the spread
of activity through neuronal nets. Cellular electrical activity
is stabilized by phenytoin, either by preventing influx or
enhancing efflux of sodium ions. It may be used for treatment of all kinds of epilepsy except petit mal epilepsy. It is
also a class 1b antiarrhythmic. It decreases automaticity,
duration of action potential, velocity of conduction, and
effective refractory period of cardiac fibers.

Pharmacokinetics

Onset: IV, few minutes
Peak Effect: IV, 1-2 hr; PO, 4-12 hr
Duration: 10-15 hr (half-life)
Interaction/Toxicity: Serum level increased by diazepam,
chloramphenicol, dicumarol, disulfiram, tolbutamide, salicylates, halothane, cimetidine, acute alcohol intake, sulfonamides, chlordiazepoxide; serum levels are decreased by

chronic alcohol abuse, reserpine, carbamazepine; oral absorption decreased by calcium-containing antacids; seizures may be precipitated with use of tricyclic antidepressants; decreases effects of corticosteroids, coumarin anticoagulants, quinidine, digitoxin, and furosemide; rapid IV administration may cause hypotension; may cause hyperglycemia, confusional states, and systemic lupus erythematosus.

Guidelines/Precautions

1. Monitor serum blood levels to achieve optimal therapeutic effect.
2. Phenytoin may be associated with exfoliative dermatitis and the Stevens-Johnson syndrome as a non–dose-related hypersensitivity reaction. Discontinue the drug if a rash occurs.
3. Because of its effect on ventricular automaticity, do not use IV phenytoin in sinus bradycardia, sinoatrial block, or second- and third-degree AV block, or in patients with Adams-Stokes syndrome.
4. Use with caution in hypotension and severe myocardial insufficiency.
5. Abrupt withdrawal in epileptic patients may precipitate status epilepticus. Reduce dosage, discontinue, or substitute other anticonvulsant medications gradually.
6. Administration of phenytoin during pregnancy may result in the fetal hydantoin syndrome. This may manifest as wide-set eyes, broad mandible, and finger deformities.

Principal Adverse Reactions

Cardiovascular: Hypotension, cardiovascular collapse, atrial and ventricular conduction depression, ventricular fibrillation

CNS: Ataxia, confusion, dizziness, tremors, headaches, peripheral neuropathy
GI: Nausea, vomiting, constipation
Dermatologic: Stevens-Johnson syndrome, lupus erythematosus, rash
Hematologic: Thrombocytopenia, leukopenia, megaloblastic anemia
Other: Hyperglycemia, gingival hyperplasia

PHYSOSTIGMINE SALICYLATE (ANTILIRIUM)

Use(s): Reversal of drug-induced (anticholinergic) CNS effects, topical treatment of glaucoma

Dosing: Anticholinergic reversal: slow IV/IM, 0.5-2 mg (10-30 μg/kg) rate of $\leq$1 mg/min. Repeat at intervals of 10-30 min if desired patient response is not obtained.
Elimination: Plasma esterases
How Supplied: Injection, 1 mg/ml
Storage: Room temperature (15°-30° C). Do not use solution if more than slightly discolored.

Pharmacology

This tertiary amine anticholinesterase agent effectively increases the concentration of acetylcholine at sites of cholinergic transmission and facilitates the transmission of impulses across the neuromuscular junction. Unlike neostigmine, physostigmine penetrates the blood-brain barrier. It reverses the central anticholinergic syndrome (anxiety, confusion, seizures) and peripheral anticholinergia (hyperpyrexia, vasodilation, urinary retention) associated with anticholinergic drugs (e.g., atropine, scopolamine, tricyclic antidepres-

sants). Physostigmine also reverse the sedative effects of
benzodiazepines (e.g., diazepam), phenothiazines, and the
ventilatory depressant effects of opioids. It may reduce postoperative somnolence after use of a volatile anesthetic.

Pharmacokinetics

Onset: IV/IM, 3-8 min
Peak Effect: IV/IM, 5-10 min
Duration: IV/IM, 30 min-5 hr
Interaction/Toxicity: Overdosage may cause cholinergic
crisis (bronchoconstriction, excessive salivation and sweating, bradycardia, skeletal muscle paresis or paralysis, hallucinations, seizures)

Guidelines/Precautions

1. Because of its potential for producing serious adverse
   effects (e.g., seizures), routine use of physostigmine as
   an antidote for overdosage of anticholinergic drugs is
   controversial.
2. High doses may cause tremors, ataxia, muscle fasciculations, and ultimately a depolarization block.
3. Rapid IV administration can cause bradycardia, hypersalivation leading to respiratory problems, or possibly
   seizures.
4. Treatment of cholinergic crisis includes mechanical ventilation with repeated bronchial aspiration and IV
   atropine 2-4 mg every 3-10 min until control of muscarinic symptoms is achieved or signs of atropine overdosage appear. IV pralidoxime (15 mg/kg over 2 min)
   may be useful in counteracting the ganglionic and skeletal muscle effects of physostigmine.
5. Use with caution in patients with epilepsy, parkinsonian
   syndrome, or bradycardia.

6. Do not use in presence of asthma, diabetes, or mechanical obstruction of the intestine or urogenital tract, and in patients receiving choline esters or depolarizing muscle relaxants.

Principal Adverse Reactions

Cardiovascular: Bradycardia, palpitations
Pulmonary: Bronchospasm, dyspnea, respiratory paralysis
CNS: Seizures, restlessness
GI: Salivation, nausea and vomiting, defecation
Eye: Miosis

PHYTONADIONE-VITAMIN K (AQUAMEPHYTON, KONAKION)

Use(s): Treatment of hypoprothrombinemia, prophylaxis and treatment of hemorrhagic diseases of the newborn; reversal of effects of oral anticoagulants

Dosing: Hemorrhagic diseases of the newborn:
    Prophylaxis:
        Newborns: IM/SC, 0.5-1 mg within 1 hr after birth
        Mother, IM, 1-5 mg 12-24 hr before delivery
    Treatment:
        Newborns: IM/SC, 1 mg. Higher doses may be necessary if the mother has received anticoagulants.
        Failure to respond may indicate another diagnosis or coagulation disorder.
    Hypoprothrombinemia:
        Adults: IV/IM/SC/PO, 2.5-25 mg, intravenous rate of 1 mg/min

Elimination: Hepatic
How Supplied:
Injection, 10 mg/ml
Tablets, 5 mg
Storage: Injection/Tablets: Room temperature (15°-30° C). Protect from light. Do not permit (injection) to freeze.

Pharmacology

Phytonadione is an aqueous dispersion of vitamin K_1, which is necessary for the hepatic synthesis of prothrombin (factor II), proconvertin (factor VII), plasma thromboplastin component (factor IX), and Stuart factor (factor X). The mechanism by which vitamin K promotes formation of these clotting factors in the liver is not known. It is ineffective in severe hypoprothrombinemia and against heparin-induced anticoagulation. Give whole blood or component therapy concurrently when bleeding is severe.

Pharmacokinetics

Onset: IV/IM/SC, 1-2 hr; PO, 6-12 hr
Peak Effect: IV/IM/SC, 3-6 hr (normal prothrombin level within 12 to 14 hr)
Duration: Varies
Interaction/Toxicity: Pharmacologic antagonist to coumarin and indandione derivatives; decreased absorption with concurrent oral administration of cholestyramine or mineral oil.

Guidelines/Precautions

1. Onset of action is slow. Fresh plasma or blood transfusion may be required for severe blood loss or lack of response to vitamin K.

2. Conduct periodic monitoring of prothrombin time. Over-zealous therapy with vitamin K may restore conditions that originally permitted thromboembolic phenomena.
3. Failure to respond to vitamin K may indicate the presence of coagulation defect or that the condition being treated is unresponsive to vitamin K.
4. Anaphylactic shock and death may occur after IV injection. Restrict IV route to situations where other routes of administration are not available.

Principal Adverse Reactions

Cardiovascular: Cardiac arrest, hypotension
Pulmonary: Respiratory arrest, dyspnea
CNS: Dizziness
Dermatologic: Local hemorrhage at injection site
Allergic: Shock, anaphylaxis (with IV injection)
Hematologic: Hyperbilirubinemia at injection site

PIPECURONIUM BROMIDE (ARDUAN)

Use(s): Skeletal muscle relaxation

Dosing: Intubating: IV, 0.07-0.085 mg/kg
Maintenance: IV, 0.01-0.04 mg/kg (10%-50% of intubating dose)
Pretreatment/priming: IV, 10% of intubating dose given 3-5 min before depolarizer/nondepolarizer relaxant dose
Elimination: Renal
How Supplied: Powder for injection, 10 mg
Storage: Temperature of 2°-30° C. Protect from light. When reconstituted with bacteriostatic water for injection, solution may be refrigerated or stored at room temperature

and should be used within 5 days. When reconstituted with sterile water for injection or compatible IV solutions (NS, D_5W, LR, D_5NS), refrigerate vials and use within 24 hr. Single use only. Discard unused solution.

Pharmacology

This long-acting nondepolarizing neuromuscular blocking agent is a piperazinium derivative. It acts by competing for cholinergic receptors at the motor end plate. The time of onset and duration are similar to those of pancuronium at comparable doses. The drug has no clinically significant hemodynamic effects. Histamine release rarely occurs.

Pharmacokinetics

Onset: <3 min
Peak Effect: 3-5 min
Duration: 45-120 min
Interaction/Toxicity: Neuromuscular blockade is potentiated by aminoglycoside, antibiotics, local anesthetics, loop diuretics, magnesium, lithium, ganglionic blocking drugs, hypothermia, hypokalemia, respiratory acidosis, and prior administration of succinylcholine; dosage requirements are decreased (about 30%-45%) and duration of neuromuscular blockade is prolonged (up to 25%) by volatile anesthetics; recurrent paralysis may occur with quinidine, enhanced neuromuscular blockade may occur in patients with myasthenia gravis or inadequate adrenocortical function; effects are antagonized by anticholinesterases such as neostigmine, edrophonium, pyridostigmine; pretreatment doses decrease fasciculations but reduce intensity and shorten duration of succinylcholine neuromuscular blockade; priming doses decrease the time to onset of maximal blockade by about 30-60 sec; resistance to effects is increased or effects are

reversed with use of theophylline and in patients with burn injury and paresis.

Guidelines/Precautions

1. Monitor response with peripheral nerve stimulator to minimize risk of overdosage.
2. Reverse effects with anticholinesterases such as neostigmine, edrophonium, or pyridostigmine bromide in conjunction with atropine or glycopyrrolate.
3. Pretreatment doses may induce a degree of neuromuscular blockade sufficient to cause hypoventilation in some patients.

Principal Adverse Reactions

Cardiovascular: Hypotension, hypertension, bradycardia, myocardial infarction
Pulmonary: Hypoventilation, apnea
CNS: Depression
GU: Anuria
Dermatologic: Rash, urticaria
Musculoskeletal: Inadequate block, prolonged block
Metabolic: Hypoglycemia, hyperkalemia, increased creatinine

POTASSIUM CHLORIDE (POTASSIUM CHLORIDE)

Use(s): Electrolyte replacement, treatment of hypokalemia, treatment of cardiac arrhythmias associated with digitalis toxicity and hypokalemia

Dosing: IV, 10-20 mEq/hr. Dilute before use. Maximum concentration (maintenance infusion) 40 mEq/L of IV fluid. In critical conditions, with close ECG monitoring, higher rates (20-40 mEq/hr and concentrations (60-80 mEq/L) may be administered. Maximum 24 hr dose: 200 mEq with serum potassium >2.5 mEq/L, 400 mEq with serum potassium <2.5 mEq/L. (Children IV infusion up to 3 mEq/kg or 40 mEq/m^2 per day.) Monitoring of the ECG and plasma potassium concentrations is essential during IV administration of potassium.

Do not administer undiluted potassium. Potassium preparations must be diluted with suitable large-volume parenteral solutions (preferably NS), mixed well, and given by slow IV infusion.

PO, 20-100 mEq daily (2-4 divided doses) (Maximum daily requirements for infants, 2-3 mEq/kg or 40 mEq/m^2)

Elimination: Renal
How Supplied:
Injection, 20 mEq/10 ml, 30 mEq/15 ml, 40 mEq/20 ml, 60 mEq/30 ml, 400 mEq/200 ml;
Capsules extended release, 8 mEq, 10 mEq, 20 mEq
Tablets, 8 mEq,10 mEq
For solution, 15 mEq/packet, 20 mEq/packet, 25 mEq/packet
For suspension (extended release), 20 mEq/packet
Solution, 6.7 mEq/5 ml, 10.0 mEq/5 ml, 13.3 mEq/5 ml, 10 mEq/15 ml, 10 mEq/15 ml, 15 mEq/15 ml, 20 mEq/15 ml, 30 mEq/15 ml, 40 mEq/15 ml

Storage:
Tablets/solution/suspension: Room temperature (15°-30° C). Protect from heat.
Injection: Protect from freezing and excessive heat.

Dilution for Infusion:

IV (piggy back, peripheral line), 10-20 mEq in 100 ml D_5W, NS, or LR (0.1-0.2 mEq/ml)

IV (piggy back, central line, cardiac monitor), 10-20 mEq in 50 ml D_5W, NS, or LR (0.2-0.4mEq/ml)

IV (maintenance infusion), 10-40 mEq in 1 L D_5W, NS, or LR (0.01-0.04 mEq/ml)

IV (maintenance infusion, cardiac monitor), 60-80 mEq in 1 L D_5W, NS, or LR (0.06-0.08 mEq/ml)

Pharmacology

Potassium is the major cation of intracellular fluid. It is essential for maintenance of intracellular tonicity and acid-base balance. Potassium is an important activator in many enzymatic reactions and is essential in a number of physiologic processes, including transmission of nerve impulses; contraction of cardiac, skeletal, and smooth muscles; gastric secretion; renal function; tissue synthesis; and carbohydrate metabolism. After absorption, potassium first enters the extracellular fluid and is then actively transported into the cells, where its concentration is up to 40 times that outside the cell. Dextrose, insulin, and oxygen facilitate movement of potassium into cells. In healthy adults, plasma potassium concentrations generally range from 3.5-5 mEq/L. Plasma concentrations up to 7.7 mEq/L may be normal in neonates. Plasma potassium concentrations, however, are not necessarily accurate indications of cellular potassium concentrations; cellular deficits can occur without decreases in plasma potassium concentrations, and hypokalemia may occur without substantial depletion of cellular potassium. Changes in extracellular fluid pH produce reciprocal effects on plasma potassium concentrations. A change of 0.1 unit in plasma pH may produce an inverse change of 0.6 mEq/L in plasma potassium concentration. Potassium concentrations in gastric and intestinal secretions are higher than plasma concentrations.

Pharmacokinetics

Onset: IV, immediate
Peak Effect: IV, varies
Duration: IV, varies
Interaction/Toxicity: Severe or life-threatening hyperkalemia may occur with concomitant administration of angiotensin-converting enzyme (ACE) inhibitors, potassium-sparing diuretics, and salt substitutes; GI toxicity is enhanced by anticholinergic drugs (e.g., atropine, glycopyrrolate), which delay gastric emptying.

Guidelines/Precautions

1. Concentrated potassium solutions are for IV admixtures only; do not use undiluted. Direct injection may be instantaneously fatal.
2. Do not infuse rapidly. Base therapy on close medical supervision with continuous or serial ECG and serum potassium determinations. Plasma levels are not necessarily indicative of tissue levels.
3. Use with caution in the presence of cardiac disease, particularly in digitalized patients (with bradyarrhythmias and potassium levels >3.0 mEq/L) or in the presence of renal disease, metabolic acidosis, Addison's disease, prolonged or severe diarrhea, familial periodic paralysis, hypoadrenalism, hyponatremia, and myotonia congenita.
4. Hypokalemia associated with metabolic acidosis should be treated with an alkalinizing potassium salt

(e.g., potassium bicarbonate, citrate, gluconate, or acetate).

5. In states of dehydration and shock, do not replenish potassium until hydration and diuresis are established.

6. Intestinal and gastric ulceration and bleeding have occurred with extended-release potassium chloride preparations. These dosage forms should be reserved for patients who cannot tolerate or refuse to take liquid or effervescent preparations. Do not use solid oral dosage forms in patients in whom there is a structural, pathologic (e.g., diabetic gastroparesis), and/or pharmacologic (e.g., induced by anticholinergics) cause for arrest or delay in passage of the dosage form through the GI tract; an oral liquid preparation should be used in these patients.

7. High plasma concentrations of potassium may cause death through cardiac depression, arrhythmia, or arrest.

8. Signs and symptoms of hyperkalemia include: paresthesia of extremities, flaccid paralysis, muscle or respiratory paralysis, areflexia, weakness, listlessness, mental confusion, weakness and heaviness of legs, hypotension, cardiac arrhythmias, heart block, and ECG abnormalities such as tall peaked T waves, depression of the ST segment, disappearance of P waves, prolongation of the QT interval, spreading and slurring of the QRS complex with development of a biphasic curve, and cardiac arrest.

9. Treat hyperkalemia by immediate termination of potassium administration. Monitor ECG. Infusion of combined glucose (1/2 g/kg) and insulin (0.15 unit/kg) in a ratio of 3 g glucose to 1 unit regular insulin may be administered to shift potassium into cells. Administer sodium bicarbonate 50 to 100 mEq IV to reverse aci-

dosis and also produce an intracellular shift. Give 10 to 20 ml IV calcium gluconate or calcium chloride 10% to reverse ECG changes. To remove potassium from the body, use sodium polysterene sulfonate resin (kayexalate), hemodialysis, or peritoneal dialysis. In digitalized patients, too-rapid lowering of serum potassium can cause digitalis toxicity.

10. Treat extravasation by discontinuing IV administration at that site and local infiltration with 1% procaine HCl and hyaluronidase.

Principal Adverse Reactions

Cardiovascular: Arrhythmias, cardiac arrest.

CNS: Lethargy, coma

GI: Nausea, vomiting, abdominal pain, esophageal/small bowel ulceration

Dermatologic: Phlebitis at injection site, sloughing, necrosis, abscess formation

Metabolic: Hyperkalemia

PRILOCAINE HCL (CITANEST)

Use(s): Regional anesthesia

Dosing: Intravenous regional:

Upper extremities, 200-250 mg (40-50 ml of 0.5% solution)

Lower extremities, 250- 300 mg (100-120 ml of 0.25% solution)

Do not add epinephrine for intravenous regional block. If desired, add fentanyl 50 μg to enhance the block and/or muscle relaxant (pretreatment doses only) (e.g., pancuronium 0.5 mg).

Rate of onset and potency of local anesthetic action may be enhanced by carbonation. (Add 5 ml of 8.4% sodium bicarbonate with 40 ml of 0.5% prilocaine. Do not use if there is precipitation.)

Topical, 0.6-3 mg/kg (2%-4% solution)

Infiltration/peripheral nerve block, 0.5-6 mg/kg (0.5%-2% solution)

Brachial plexus block: 300-750 mg (30-50 ml of 1%-1.5% solution); children 0.5-0.75 ml/kg.

With high doses add epinephrine 1:200,000 to decrease systemic toxicity (in the absence of any contraindications). Add tetracaine 0.5-1 mg/kg to prolong the block.

Epidural: 200-300 mg (1%-2% solution); maximum safe dose, 6 mg/kg without epinephrine; 9 mg/kg with epinephrine 1:200,000

Solutions containing preservatives should not be used for epidural block. Except where contraindicated, vasoconstrictor drugs may be added to increase effect and prolong local or regional anesthesia. For dosage/route guidelines, see Epinephrine, Dosing or Phenylephrine, Dosing. Do not use vasoconstrictor drugs for IV regional anesthesia or local anesthesia of end organs (digits, penis, ears).

Elimination: Hepatic, pulmonary

How Supplied: Injection, 4% with or without epinephrine 1:200,000

Storage: Room temperature (15°-30° C). Protect from light.

Pharmacology

This amide local anesthetic stabilizes the neuronal membrane and prevents the initiation and transmission of impulses. Prilocaine is equipotent to lidocaine but longer in duration; it is less toxic and undergoes rapid hepatic metabolism to ortho-toludine, which oxidizes hemoglobin to methemoglobin. When the dose of prilocaine exceeds 600 mg, there may be sufficient methemoglobin to cause the patient to appear cyanotic, and oxygen-carrying capacity is reduced. The unique ability to cause dose-related methemoglobinemia limits its clinical usefulness, with the exception of intravenous regional anesthesia.

Pharmacokinetics

Onset: Infiltration, 1-2 min; epidural, 5-15 min
Peak Effect: Infiltration/epidural, <30 min
Duration: Infiltration, 0.5-1.5 hr; with epinephrine, 2-6 hr; epidural, 1-3 hr; prolonged with epinephrine
Interaction/Toxicity: Methemoglobinemia occurs at high doses (greater than 600 mg); clearance is reduced with coadministration of beta blockers or cimetidine; toxic drug concentrations may result in seizures, respiratory depression, and cardiovascular collapse; benzodiazepines, barbiturates, and volatile anesthetics increase seizure threshold; duration of regional anesthesia is prolonged by vasoconstrictor agents (e.g., epinephrine and alpha-2 agonists such as clonidine); alkalinization increases rate of onset and potency of local or regional anesthesia.

Guidelines/Precautions

1. Treat methemoglobinemia with methylene blue (1- 2 mg/kg injected over 5 min).

2. Use with caution in patients with hypovolemia, severe congestive heart failure, shock, and all forms of heart block.

3. Use is contraindicated in infants less than 6 months of age (low dose may cause severe methemoglobinemia) and in patients with hypersensitivity to amide-type local anesthetics.

4. In intravenous regional blocks, deflate the cuff after 40 min and for no less than 20 min. Between 20 and 40 min, the cuff can be deflated, reinflated immediately, and finally deflated after a minute to reduce the sudden absorption of anesthetic into the systemic circulation.

5. Toxic plasma levels (e.g., from accidental intravascular injection) may cause cardiopulmonary collapse and seizures. Premonitory signs and symptoms manifest as numbness of the tongue and circumoral tissues, metallic taste, restlessness, tinnitus, and tremors. Support of circulation (IV fluids, vasopressors, IV sodium bicarbonate 1-2 mEq/kg to treat cardiac toxicity [sodium channel blockade], IV bretylium 5 mg/kg, and DC cardioversion/defibrillation for ventricular arrhythmias) and securing a patent airway (ventilate with 100% oxygen) are paramount. Thiopental (0.5-2 mg/kg IV), midazolam (0.02-0.04 mg/kg IV), or diazepam (0.1 mg/kg IV) may be used for prophylaxis and/or treatment of seizures.

6. The level of sympathetic blockade (bradycardia with block above T5) determines the degree of hypotension (often heralded by nausea and vomiting) after epidural or intrathecal prilocaine. Fluid hydration (10-20 ml/kg NS or lactated Ringer's solution), vasopressor agents (e.g., ephedrine), and left uterine displacement in pregnant patients may be used for prophylaxis and/or treatment. Administer atropine to treat bradycardia.

7. Epidural injections should be avoided when the patient has hypovolemic shock, septicemia, infection at the injection site, or coagulopathy.
8. Monitor for hypoventilation with release of the cuff when a muscle relaxant is added to the local anesthetic solution for intravenous regional blockade.

Principal Adverse Reactions

Cardiovascular: Hypotension, arrhythmia, collapse
Pulmonary: Respiratory depression, paralysis
CNS: Seizures, tinnitus, blurred vision
Hematologic: Methemoglobinemia
Allergic: Urticaria, anaphylactoid reactions
Epidural/Caudal: High spinal, urinary retention, lower extremity weakness and paralysis, loss of sphincter control, headache, backache, cranial nerve palsies, slowing of labor

PROCAINAMIDE HCL (PRONESTYL, PROCAN SR)

Use(s): Arrhythmia control in malignant hyperthermia; treatment of lidocaine-resistant ventricular arrhythmias, atrial fibrillation, or paroxysmal atrial tachycardia

Dosing: Loading:

Slow IV push, 100 mg every 5 min until the arrhythmia is suppressed or hypotension occurs (maximum 1 g). Do not exceed rate of 50 mg/min (children 3-6 mg/kg given over 5 min).

Dilute 1g in 50 ml D_5W),

IM, 100-500 mg

PO, 1.25 g then 750 mg 1 hr later if no changes in ECG

Maintenance:
>> Infusion, 2-6 mg/min (children 0.02-0.08 mg/kg/min)
>> PO, 0.5-1 g q3-6h (q6h with sustained-release tablets) (children 40-60 mg/kg/daily in 4 divided doses)
>> Therapeutic level, 4-12 μg/ml

Elimination: Hepatic (acetylation), renal

How Supplied:

Injection, 100 mg/ml, 500 mg/ml

Tablets, 250 mg, 375 mg, 500 mg

Tablets, sustained release, 250 mg, 500 mg, 750 mg, 1000 mg. Do not use sustained-release tablets for initial oral therapy.

Capsules, 250 mg, 375 mg, 500 mg.

Storage:

Injections: Room temperature (15°-30° C). Refrigeration (2°-8° C) may be preferable because it retards oxidation and associated development of color. Do not use solutions that are darker than light amber or otherwise discolored. Injections diluted in D_5W are stable for 24 hr at room temperature or for 7 days when refrigerated.

Oral Preparations: Room temperature (15°-30° C). Avoid temperatures >40° C.

Dilution for Infusion: 2 g in 500 ml D_5W (4 mg/ml)

Pharmacology

Procainamide, like quinidine and disopyramide, is a class 1A antiarrhythmic (membrane stabilizer). It increases the effective refractory period and reduces impulse conduction velocity in the atria, His-Purkinje fibers, and ventricular muscle. It has a variable effect on AV conduction with a direct slowing action and weaker vagolytic effect on the AV node. Direct myocardial depression may occur at high plasma levels (greater than 8 μg/ml). Antiarrhythmic effect is seen at plasma levels of 4-12 μg/ml. Procainamide undergoes hepatic acetylation to an active metabolite N-acetyl procainamide, which has antiarrhythmic activity. The rate of acetylation is genetically determined. Serum half-life of NAPA is markedly prolonged (from 7 to 70 hr in patients with congestive heart failure and/or renal insufficiency). Procainamide is an effective alternative for acute treatment of lidocaine-resistant ventricular arrhythmias.

Pharmacokinetics

Onset: IV, immediate; IM, 10-30 min
Peak Effect: IV, 5-15 min; IM, 15-60 min
Duration: 2.5 hr, half-life in fast acetylators; 5 hr, half-life in slow acetylators
Interaction/Toxicity: Hypotension may occur with rapid IV administration and is potentiated by use of other antiarrythmics; may cause myocardial depression or ventricular arrhythmias at high plasma levels exaggerated by hyperkalemia; ventricular asystole or fibrillation may occur in the presence of heart block associated with digitalis toxicity; lupus erythematosus-like syndrome may occur; potentiates effect of both nondepolarizing and depolarizing muscle relaxants; serum levels are increased with concomitant administration of cimetidine and ranitidine.

Guidelines/Precautions

1. Reduce doses in the presence of congestive heart failure and renal failure.
2. Use is contraindicated in complete heart block, torsades de pointes, lupus erythematosus.
3. Patients with atrial flutter or fibrillation should be cardioverted or heart rate controlled (e.g., with digitalis, beta blockers, calcium channel blockers) before procain-

amide administration to avoid enhancement of AV conduction and intolerable ventricular rate acceleration.
4. Use cautiously in first-degree heart block and arrhythmias associated with digitalis intoxication.
5. Requires periodic monitoring of plasma levels, vital signs, and ECG (QRS widening of more than 25% may signify overdosage).

Principal Adverse Reactions

Cardiovascular: Hypotension, heart block, arrhythmias
CNS: Seizures, confusion, depression, psychosis
GI: Anorexia, nausea, vomiting, diarrhea (usually with large oral doses)
Dermatologic: Lupus erythematosus, urticaria, pruritus
Hematologic: Thrombocytopenia, neutropenia, hemolytic anemia, agranulocytosis
Allergic: Angioneurotic edema, eosinophilia
Others: Fever, chills

PROCAINE HCL (NOVOCAIN)

Use(s): Regional anesthesia

Dosing: Infiltration, <500 mg 0.5%-2% solution
Epidural, <500 mg 1%-2% solution
Spinal, 50-200 mg 10% solution with glucose 5%
Maximum safe dose: 10 mg/kg (without epinephrine), 15 mg/kg (with epinephrine)
Solutions containing preservatives should not be used for epidural or spinal block. Except where contraindicated, vasoconstrictor drugs may be added to increase effect and prolong local or regional anesthesia. For dosage/route guidelines, see Epinephrine, Dosing or Phenyle-

phrine, Dosing. Do not use vasoconstrictor drugs for IV regional anesthesia or local anesthesia of end organs (digits, penis, nose, ears).

Elimination: Plasma pseudocholinesterase

How Supplied:

Injection, 1%, 2%

Spinal (hyperbaric solution); 10%

Storage: Room temperature (15°-30° C). Protect from light.

Pharmacology

Procaine is a benzoic-acid-ester local anesthetic. It stabilizes the neuronal membrane and prevents the initiation and transmission of impulses. It possesses vasodilator activity and is ineffective as a surface anesthetic. It has a rapid onset of action and a relatively short duration that depends on the anesthetic technique, type of block, concentration, and individual patient. Vasoconstrictor drugs may be added to the procaine solution to delay systemic absorption and prolong the duration of action.

Pharmacokinetics

Onset: Infiltration/spinal, 2-5 min; epidural, 5-25 min

Peak Effect: Infiltration/epidural/spinal, <30 min

Duration: Infiltration, 0.25-0.5 hr; with epinephrine, 0.5-1.5 hr; epidural/spinal, 0.5-1.5 hr; prolonged with epinephrine

Interaction/Toxicity: Prolongs the effect of succinylcholine; metabolite (PABA) inhibits action of sulfonamides and aminosalicylic acid; toxicity is enhanced by anticholinesterases (which inhibit degradation); high plasma levels may cause seizures, respiratory arrest, and cardiovascular collapse; benzodiazepines, barbiturates, and volatile anesthetics increase seizure threshold; duration of regional anesthesia is prolonged by vasoconstrictor agents (e.g., epinephrine) and alpha-2 agonists (e.g., clonidine); alkalinization increases rate of onset and potency of local or regional anesthesia.

Guidelines/Precautions

1. Use with caution in patients with severe disturbances of cardiac rhythm, shock, or heart block.
2. Reduce doses for spinal anesthesia in obstetric, elderly, hypovolemic, and high-risk patients and patients with increased intraabdominal pressure.
3. Use is contraindicated in patients with hypersensitivity to procaine or ester-type local anesthetics, and patients with allergy to suntan lotion (contains PABA derivatives).
4. Toxic plasma levels (e.g., from accidental intravascular injection) may cause cardiopulmonary collapse and seizures. Premonitory signs and symptoms manifest as numbness of the tongue and circumoral tissues, metallic taste, restlessness, tinnitus, and tremors. Support of circulation (IV fluids, vasopressors, IV sodium bicarbonate 1-2 mEq/kg to treat cardiac toxicity [sodium channel blockade], IV bretylium 5 mg/kg, and DC cardioversion/defibrillation for ventricular arrhythmias) and securing a patent airway (ventilate with 100% oxygen) are paramount. Thiopental (0.5-2 mg/kg IV), midazolam (0.02-0.04 mg/kg IV), or diazepam (0.1 mg/kg IV) may be used for prophylaxis and/or treatment of seizures.
5. The level of sympathetic blockade (bradycardia with block above T5) determines the degree of hypotension (often heralded by nausea and vomiting) after epidural or intrathecal procaine. Fluid hydration (10-20 ml/kg NS or lactated Ringer's solution), vasopressor agents (e.g., ephedrine) and left uterine displacement in pregnant patients may be used for prophylaxis and/or treatment. Administer atropine to treat bradycardia.

6. Epidural, caudal, or intrathecal injections should be avoided when the patient has hypovolemic shock, septicemia, infection at the injection site, or coagulopathy.

Principal Adverse Reactions

Cardiovascular: Hypotension, bradycardia, arrhythmias, heart block
Pulmonary: Respiratory depression, arrest
CNS: Tinnitus, seizures, dizziness, restlessness, loss of hearing, euphoria, diplopia, postspinal headache, arachnoiditis, palsies
Allergic: Urticaria, pruritus, angioneurotic edema
Epidural/caudal/spinal: High spinal, loss of bladder and bowel control, permanent motor, sensory, and autonomic (sphincter control) deficit of lower segments

PROCHLORPERAZINE (COMPAZINE)

Use(s): Antiemetic; antipsychotic

Dosing: Antiemetic:
PO, 5-10 mg 3-4 times daily
Rectal, 25 mg twice daily
IV/IM, 5-10 mg (at 5 mg/ml/min)
Do not administer SC because of local irritation.
Elimination: Hepatic
How Supplied:
Tablets, 5 mg, 10 mg, 25 mg
Capsules, extended release, 10 mg, 15 mg, 30 mg
Suppositories, 2.5 mg, 5 mg, 25 mg
Injection, 5 mg/ml
Storage: Injection/tablets: Room temperature (15°-30° C). Protect from light.

Pharmacology

Prochlorperazine is a piperazine phenothiazine. Its antipsychotic activity is thought to result from the drug's central antidopaminergic actions. Its antiemetic action is mediated via the chemoreceptor trigger zone of the medulla. It produces alpha adrenergic blockade, which may result in hypotension. Prochlorperazine interferes with central thermoregulatory mechanisms and may produce tardive dyskinesia and extrapyramidal symptoms secondary to blockade of dopaminergic receptors in the basal ganglia.

Pharmacokinetics

Onset: IV, few min; IM, 10-20 min; PO, 30-40 min; rectal, 60 min
Peak Effect: IV/IM/PO, 15-30 min
Duration: IV/IM/PO/rectal, 3-4 hr; PO extended release, 10-12 hr
Interaction/Toxicity: Potentiates CNS and circulatory depressant effects of alcohol, opioids, barbiturates, and antihistamines; diminishes effects of oral anticoagulants; counteracts antihypertensive effect of propranolol; decreases metabolism of phenytoin; lowers seizure threshold and increases dosage requirements for anticonvulsant agents; acute encephalopathic syndrome may occur in the presence of high serum lithium levels; hypotension may result from rapid IV injection; may induce extrapyramidal symptoms, neuroleptic malignant syndrome.

Guidelines/Precautions

1. Extrapyramidal reactions may consist of dystonic reactions, feelings of motor restlessness (akathisia), and parkinsonian signs and symptoms. Dystonic reactions occur more frequently in children, especially those with

acute infections, whereas parkinsonian symptoms predominate in geriatric patients. Therapy should include discontinuation of prochlorperazine or reduction in dosage, and treatment with an anticholinergic antiparkinsonian agent (e.g., benztropine, trihexyphenidyl) or with diphenhydramine (IV/PO 25 mg). Maintenance of an adequate airway should be instituted if necessary.

2. Use cautiously in geriatric patients; patients with glaucoma, prostatic hypertrophy, and seizure disorders; and children with acute illnesses (e.g., chickenpox, measles).
3. Do not use in pediatric surgery.
4. Neuroleptic malignant syndrome (hyperpyrexia tachycardia, muscle rigidity) should be managed by immediate discontinuation of prochlorperazine and symptomatic and supportive treatment, including correction of fluid and electrolyte imbalances, administration of dantrolene or bromocriptine (PO 2.5-10 mg tid), cooling of the patient, maintenance of renal function, management of cardiovascular instability, and prevention of respiratory complications.
5. Prochlorperazine possesses little or no antimotion sickness activity.
6. Do not crush or chew sustained-release capsules.
7. Do not use epinephrine to treat prochloperazine-induced hypotension. Phenothiazines cause a reversal of epinephrine's vasopressor effects and a further lowering of blood pressure. Treat the drug-induced hypotension with norepinephrine or phenylephrine.

Principal Adverse Reactions

Cardiovascular: Hypotension, hypertension
Pulmonary: Bronchospasm, laryngeal edema
CNS: Drowsiness, dizziness, extrapyramidal reactions, tardive dyskinesia

GI/Hepatic: Cholestatic jaundice, nausea, vomiting
Endocrine: Gynecomastia, amenorrhea, hyperglycemia
Allergic: Angioneurotic edema, anaphylactoid reactions

PROMETHAZINE HCL (PHENERGAN)

Use(s): Antiemetic, premedication, adjunct to analgesics for control of postoperative pain

Dosing: IV/deep IM/PO/rectal, 12.5-50 mg (do not give SC)
Elimination: Hepatic
How Supplied:
Injection, 25 mg/ml, 50 mg/ml
Tablets/suppositories, 12.5 mg, 25 mg, 50 mg
Oral solution, 6.25 mg/5 ml, 25 mg/5 ml
Storage: Injection/tablets: Room temperature (15°-25° C). Protect from light. Do not permit injection to freeze.
Suppositories: Refrigerate (2°-8° C). Do not permit to freeze.

Pharmacology

This phenothiazine derivative does not possess neuroleptic or antipsychotic activity in typical standard doses. It is a good histamine H1-receptor antagonist with sedative, antiemetic, anticholinergic, and anti–motion-sickness effects. Promethazine competitively antagonizes in varying degrees most, but not all, of the pharmacologic effects of histamine mediated at H1 receptors. The drug is not effective in the treatment of bronchial asthma, allergic reactions, or angioedema in which chemical mediators other than histamine are responsible for the symptoms.

Pharmacokinetics

Onset: IV, 2-5 min; IM/PO/rectal, 15-30 min
Peak Effect: IV/IM/PO/rectal, <2 hr
Duration: IV/IM/PO/rectal, 2-8 hr
Interaction/Toxicity: Potentiates CNS and circulatory depressant effect of alcohol, volatile anesthetics, sedative-hypnotics including barbiturates, tranquilizers; intraarterial or subcutaneous injection may result in necrosis and gangrene; may reverse vasopressor effect of epinephrine; extrapyramidal reactions may occur at high doses and with concomitant use of MAO inhibitors.

Guidelines/Precautions

1. Extrapyramidal reactions may consist of dystonic reactions, feelings of motor restlessness (akathisia), and parkinsonian signs and symptoms. Dystonic reactions occur more frequently in children, especially those with acute infections, whereas parkinsonian symptoms predominate in geriatric patients. Therapy should include discontinuation of promethazine or reduction in dosage, and treatment with an anticholinergic antiparkinsonian agent (e.g., benztropine, trihexyphenidyl) or with diphenhydramine (IV/PO 25 mg). Maintenance of an adequate airway should be instituted if necessary.
2. Use with caution in patients with cardiovascular disease, liver dysfunction, asthmatic attack, narrow-angle glaucoma, bone-marrow depression, prostatic hypertrophy, stenosing peptic ulcer, pyloroduodenal and bladder neck obstruction.
3. Use with caution if at all in children.
4. Produces a high degree of drowsiness and sedation at clinically effective doses.

5. Do not use epinephrine to treat promethazine-induced hypotension. Phenothiazines cause a reversal of epinephrine's vasopressor effects and a further lowering of blood pressure. Treat the drug-induced hypotension with norepinephrine or phenylephrine.

Principal Adverse Reactions

Cardiovascular: Hypotension, bradycardia, tachycardia, extrasystoles

Pulmonary: Bronchospasm, nasal stuffiness

CNS: Drowsiness, sedation, dizziness, confusion, tremors

GI: Nausea, vomiting

Hematologic: Leukopenia, agranulocytosis, thrombocytopenia

PROPOFOL (DIPRIVAN)

Use(s): Conscious sedation, induction agent, maintenance of anesthesia, treatment of chemotherapy-induced/postoperative nausea and vomiting

Dosing: Sedation:

　　　IV bolus, 25-50 mg (0.5-1 mg/kg), titrate slowly to the desired effect (e.g., onset of slurred speech).

　　　Infusion, 20-75 μg/kg/min; monitor respiratory and cardiac function continuously.

　　Anesthesia induction: IV, 2-2.5 mg/kg (give slowly over 30 sec in 2-3 divided doses)

　　Anesthesia maintenance:

　　　IV bolus, 25-50 mg

　　　Infusion, 100-200 μg/kg/min

　　Antiemetic: IV, 10 mg

Elimination: Hepatic, extrahepatic (pulmonary)

How Supplied: Injection, 10 mg/ml

Storage: Temperature of 4°-22° C. Refrigeration is not recommended. Protect from light. Shake well before use.

Dilution for Infusion: Use undiluted or dilute with D_5W to concentration of 2 mg/ml or higher. Discard after use or within 6 hours after ampules or vials have been opened; whichever occurs sooner. There is no preservative.

Pharmacology

Propofol is a diisopropylphenol intravenous hypnotic agent that produces rapid induction of anesthesia with minimal excitatory activity (e.g., myoclonus). It undergoes extensive distribution and rapid elimination. Induction doses are associated with apnea and hypotension secondary to direct myocardial depression and a decrease in systemic vascular resistance with minimal change in heart rate. The drug obtunds the hemodynamic response to laryngoscopy and intubation. Propofol does not have any analgesic properties, but unlike barbiturates, it is not antianalgesic. Compared with sodium thiopental, recovery is more rapid and there is less nausea and vomiting. Propofol may have intrinsic antiemetic effects. Subhypnotic doses are effective in treating postoperative and chemotherapy-associated nausea and vomiting. Like etomidate, propofol may suppress the adrenal cortex and decrease plasma cortisol levels. However, unlike etomidate, the adrenal suppression is rapidly reversible and responds to ACTH stimulation. EEG changes on induction include increases in alpha, delta, and theta activity with occasional burst suppression. When used for maintenance of anesthesia, propofol produces dose-dependent decreases in amplitude of somatosensory-evoked potentials. Propofol may have proconvulsant and anticonvulsant activity. Proconvulsant effects may represent activation of epileptogenic foci. Anticonvulsant effects are most likely due to nonspecific cortical depression rather than elevation of the seizure threshold. Propofol reduces cerebral blood flow, intracranial pressure, and cerebral metabolic rate. It may decrease cerebral perfusion pressure because of its effects on mean arterial pressure (CPP = MAP−ICP). Histamine release may occur, and allergic reactions most likely represent anaphylaxis.

Pharmacokinetics

Onset: Within 40 sec
Peak Effect: 1 min
Duration: 5-10 min
Interaction/Toxicity: Potentiates CNS and circulatory depressant effects of narcotics, sedative hypnotics, volatile anesthetics; pulmonary extraction is decreased and plasma levels are increased (up to 50%) with concomitant administration of alfentanil, fentanyl, halothane (concentrate >1.5%); pain may occur on injection into small vein; potentiates the neuromuscular blockade of nondepolarizing muscle relaxants (e.g., atracurium).

Guidelines/Precautions

1. Reduce doses in elderly, hypovolemic, and high risk surgical patients and with concomitant use of narcotics and sedative hypnotics.
2. Minimize pain by injecting into a large vein and/or mixing IV lidocaine (0.1 mg/kg) with the induction dose of propofol.
3. Because of its effects on cerebral perfusion pressure, propofol is not recommended in patients with increased intracranial pressure. It should be administered with caution to patients with a history of epilepsy or seizures disorders.
4. Use with caution in cesarean section. Compared with thiopental, induction doses of propofol may be associated

with high umbilical vein concentrations, muscular hypotonus, and lower neonatal Apgar scores at 1 and 5 min.
5. The soybean-fat emulsion vehicle of propofol supports rapid growth of bacteria, and strict aseptic technique must be maintained during handling. The propofol ampule should be discarded after a single use.
6. Use is contraindicated in patients allergic to eggs or soybean oil.

Principal Adverse Reactions

Cardiovascular: Hypotension, arrhythmia, tachycardia, bradycardia, hypertension
Pulmonary: Respiratory depression, apnea, hiccough, bronchospasm, laryngospasm
CNS: Headache, dizziness, euphoria, confusion, clonic/myoclonic movement, opisthotonus, seizures
GI: Nausea, vomiting, abdominal cramps
Local: Burning, stinging, pain at the injection site
Allergic: Erythema, urticaria, pruritus
Other: Fever, disinhibition, sexual illusions

PROPRANOLOL HCL (INDERAL)

Use(s): Antihypertensive, antianginal, antiarrhythmic (supraventricular and ventricular arrhythmias), treatment of acute myocardial infarction, migraine prophylaxis, symptomatic treatment of thyrotoxicosis, pheochromocytoma, and tremors

Dosing: Hypertension:
IV, 0.5-3.0 mg (10-30 μg/kg) q2min to maximum of 6-10 mg.
PO, 20-80 mg daily in single or divided doses.

Therapeutic concentration, 50-100 ng/ml

Arrhythmia:

PO, 10-30 mg tid-qid

IV, 0.5-3.0 mg (10-30 μg/kg) q2min to maximum of 6-10 mg

Angina: PO, 80-320 mg daily in single or divided doses

Acute myocardial infarction: IV, 1-3 mg; do not exceed 1 mg/min to avoid lowering the blood pressure and causing cardiac standstill; if necessary, give a second dose after 2 min, then PO, 180-240 mg/day in 3 or 4 divided doses

Migraine prophylaxis: PO, 20-80 mg 1 to 4 times daily, maximum dose 240 mg daily; a trial of at least 2 months is indicated

Elimination: Hepatic, pulmonary

How Supplied:

Injection, 1 mg/ml

Tablets, 10 mg, 20 mg, 40 mg, 60 mg, 80 mg, 90 mg

Capsules, extended-release, 60 mg, 80 mg, 120 mg, 160 mg

Oral solution, 20 mg/5ml, 40 mg/5ml,

Oral solution concentrate, 80 mg/ml

Storage: Injection/oral preparations: Room temperature (15°-30° C). Protect from light. Extended-release capsules should be protected from freezing and excessive heat.

Pharmacology

Propranolol is a nonselective beta adrenergic receptor antagonist without intrinsic sympathomimetic activity. The degree of beta blockade depends on the ongoing beta activity at the time of administration. Thus decreases in heart rate and cardiac output (beta 1 receptor blockade) are greater in the presence of increased sympathetic nervous system activity. Blockade of beta-2 receptors increases peripheral and coronary vascular resistance. Reduced cardiac work is the basis for use of the drug after myocardial infarction and in the treatment of angina. Propranolol depresses automaticity and conduction velocity in cardiac muscle. Propranolol may prevent common migraine and reduce the number of attacks in some patients. It is not effective for a migraine attack that has already started. The antimigraine effect may be partly due to inhibition of vasodilation. The drug also may inhibit arteriolar spasm of the pial vessels in the brain. Propranolol increases uterine activity more in the nonpregnant than in the pregnant uterus.

Pharmacokinetics

Onset: Antihypertensive effects: IV, <2 min; PO, <30 min
Peak Effect: Antihypertensive effects: IV, within 1 min; PO, varies
Duration: Antihypertensive effects: IV, 1-6 hr; PO, 6-12 hr
Interaction/Toxicity: Potentiates myocardial depression of inhaled and injected anesthetics; additive effects occur with catecholamine-depleting drugs (e.g., reserpine), calcium channel blockers; antagonizes cardiac-stimulating and bronchodilating effects of sympathomimetics; potentiates vasoconstrictive effect of epinephrine; increased serum levels occur with concomitant use of chlorpromazine, cimetidine, halothane; decreased serum levels occur with enzyme inducers (e.g., phenytoin, phenobarbital, rifampin); potentiates effects of digoxin, succinylcholine, nondepolarizing muscle relaxants (e.g., tubocurarine); produces hypoglycemia, prolongs the hypoglycemic effect of

insulin, and may mask symptoms of hypoglycemia (e.g., tachycardia); may unmask direct negative inotropic effects of ketamine.

Guidelines/Precautions

1. Contraindicated in cardiogenic shock, sinus bradycardia, block greater than first degree, bronchial asthma, and congestive heart failure unless the failure is secondary to a tachyarrhythmia treatable with propranolol.
2. Use with caution in patients with diabetes and nonallergic bronchospastic disease (e.g., bronchitis).
3. Excessive myocardial depression may be treated with IV atropine (1-2 mg), IV isoproterenol (0.02-0.15 μg/kg/min), or a transvenous cardiac pacemaker.
4. Risk of ischemia or infarction is increased in patients with coronary artery disease if drug is withdrawn abruptly.
5. Epinephrine use in patients receiving propranolol may result in rapid blood pressure increase and decreased pulse rate with first- or second-degree heart block. The beta adrenergic activity of epinephrine is blocked, while alpha adrenergic effects are unopposed.

Principal Adverse Reactions

Cardiovascular: Bradycardia, hypotension, congestive heart failure, AV block
Pulmonary: Bronchospasm
CNS: Depression, disorientation, dizziness, memory loss
GI: Nausea, vomiting, mesenteric thrombosis
Hematologic: Agranulocytosis, thrombocytopenic purpura, nonthrombocytopenic purpura

PROSTAGLANDIN E₁-ALPROSTADIL (PROSTIN VR)

Use(s): Maintain patency of patent ductus arteriosus; treatment of severe pulmonary hypertension with right heart failure

Dosing: IV, 0.05-0.4 μg/kg/min (titrate to lowest effective dose)

Elimination: Pulmonary (oxidation)

How Supplied: Injection, 500 μg/ml

Storage: Refrigerate (2°-8° C).

Dilution for Infusion: 500 μg in 250 ml D₅W or NS (2 μg/ml)

Pharmacology

Prostaglandin E_1 relaxes smooth muscle of the ductus arteriosus. This is beneficial in infants who have congenital defects that restrict the pulmonary or systemic blood flow and who depend on a patent ductus arteriosus for adequate blood oxygenation. PGE_1 produces vasodilation and reduces blood pressure, resulting in a reflex increase in cardiac output and heart rate. In infants with restricted systemic blood flow, the drug increases the systemic blood pressure and decreases the ratio of pulmonary artery pressure to aortic pressure. Infants who respond best are less than 4 days old with low pretreatment PO_2 (<40 mm Hg). PGE_1 is metabolized rapidly (70% in one lung passage) and must be administered as a continuous intravenous infusion. In treatment of severe pulmonary hypertension with right-heart failure, PGE_1 may be infused into the right atrium, from which point it proceeds directly to the pulmonary artery and attenuates pulmonary vasoconstriction. Because of lung metabolism, relatively less of the drug passes on to the systemic vasculature. To reverse the systemic vasodilation, norepinephrine is infused into the left atrium simultaneously.

Pharmacokinetics

Onset: Cyanotic heart disease, 5-10 min; acyanotic heart disease, 1.3-3 hr
Peak Effect: Cyanotic heart disease, 30 min; acyanotic heart disease, 1.5-3 hr
Duration: 1-2 hr (postinfusion)
Interaction/Toxicity: Inhibits platelet aggregation; apnea may occur at high doses

Guidelines/Precautions

1. Use with caution in neonates with bleeding tendencies.
2. Do not use in respiratory distress syndrome.
3. Measure efficacy by monitoring blood oxygenation as well as arterial pressure and blood pH.
4. Apnea occurs in 10%-12% of neonates weighing less than 2 kg at birth.

Principal Adverse Reactions

Cardiovascular: Hypotension, bradycardia, arrhythmias, congestive heart failure
Pulmonary: Apnea, bronchial wheezing, respiratory depression
CNS: Seizures, cerebral bleeding, lethargy, hypothermia
GI: Diarrhea, gastric regurgitation, hyperbilirubinemia
Hematologic: Disseminated intravascular coagulation, anemia, thrombocytopenia
Renal: Anuria, hematuria
Skeletal: Cortical proliferation of the long bones
Other: Hyperkalemia, hypokalemia, hypoglycemia, peritonitis

PROTAMINE SULFATE (PROTAMINE SULFATE)

Use(s): Heparin antagonist

Dosing: Slow IV, 1 mg neutralizes 90 USP units heparin (lung) or 115 USP units heparin (intestinal mucosa). Do not exceed 50 mg in any 10 min period. Dose is determined by dose of heparin given, route of administration, and time elapsed since it was given. Give half dose if 30-60 min has elapsed since IV injection of heparin and quarter dose if 2 or more hr has elapsed.

Elimination: Hepatic
How Supplied: Injection, 10 mg activity/ml
Storage:

Powder for injection: Room temperature (15°-30° C). When reconstituted with sterile water for injection, solution should be used immediately and unused portions discarded. When reconstituted with bacteriostatic water for injection (containing benzyl alcohol), solution is stable at room temperature for 72 hours.

Injection: Refrigerate (2°-8° C). Do not permit to freeze.

Pharmacology

This low-molecular-weight protein is rich in arginine and strongly basic. Protamine is prepared from the sperm or mature testes of salmon or related species. It neutralizes heparin by combining with it to form a stable complex that is devoid of anticoagulant activity. Despite the formation of this complex, the effect of heparin may persist and be responsible for continued bleeding, especially after cardiopulmonary bypass. In the absence of heparin, protamine has a weak anticoagulant effect. Rapid intravenous injection is associated with histamine release, peripheral vasodilation, decrease in blood pressure, and increase in pulmonary vascular resistance.

Pharmacokinetics

Onset: 30 sec-1 min
Peak Effect: <5 min
Duration: 2 hr (dependent on body temperature)
Interaction/Toxicity: Potentiates vasodilators; severe hypotension and anaphylactoid reactions may occur with rapid IV administration; chemically incompatible with solutions of cephalosporins and penicillin.

Guidelines/Precautions

1. Hyperheparinemia or bleeding may occur 30 min-18 hr after complete neutralization of heparin.
2. Giving more than 100 mg over a short time is unwise unless one has certain knowledge of a larger requirement.
3. Rapid administration of protamine may result in severe hypotension and anaphylaxis.
4. Risk of allergic reactions is increased in patients who are allergic to fish or who have been previously treated with protamine-containing insulin preparations, and in the presence of antiprotamine antibodies in the serum of infertile or vasectomized men.
5. Patients known to be allergic to protamine and requiring heparin anticoagulation may be pretreated with histamine receptor antagonists followed by a slow trial intravenous infusion of protamine; may be allowed to recover from the heparin effect requiring multiple blood transfusions; or may be given hexadimethrine, an alter-

nate heparin antagonist (not available commercially in the United States).

6. Protamine may be inactivated by blood. When it is used to neutralize large doses of heparin, a heparin "rebound" may occur. More protamine should be administered in this instance.

Principal Adverse Reactions

Cardiovascular: Hypotension, hypertension, bradycardia
Pulmonary: Pulmonary hypertension, dyspnea, bronchospasm
Allergic: Anaphylactoid reactions, anaphylaxis, flushing
GI: Nausea, vomiting, thrombocytopenia

PYRIDOSTIGMINE BROMIDE (REGONAL, MESTINON)

Use(s): Reversal of nondepolarizing muscle relaxants, treatment of myasthenia gravis

Dosing: Reversal: Slow IV, 0.25 mg/kg (maximum dose 30 mg) with atropine or glycopyrrolate (atropine IV, 0.015 mg/kg, or glycopyrrolate IV, 0.01 mg/kg)

Myasthenia gravis:

PO, 60-1500 mg/day (average 600 mg/day), space doses to provide maximum relief; children, 7 mg/kg/day divided into 5 or 6 doses

PO sustained release, 180 to 540 mg once or twice daily

To supplement oral dosage preoperatively and postoperatively, during labor and postpar-

tum, during myasthenic crisis, or when oral
therapy is impractical, give one thirtieth the
oral dose IM or very slow IV.

Neonates of myasthenic mothers: 0.05-0.15
mg/kg IM. Differentiate between cholinergic
and myasthenic crisis in the neonate.

Administration of pyridostigmine 1 hr before
completion of the second stage of labor
enables patients to have adequate strength during labor and provides protection to infants in
the immediate postnatal state.

Elimination: Hepatic, renal
How Supplied:
Injection, 5 mg/ml
Tablets, 60 mg
Tablets, sustained release, 180 mg
Oral solution, 60 mg/5 ml
Storage: Injection/tablets: Room temperature (15°-25°
C). Solution: Protect from light.

Pharmacology

This pyridine analog of neostigmine is an anticholinesterase agent and blocks the enzyme responsible for
the hydrolysis of acetylcholine. Acetylcholine levels build,
thereby facilitating the transmission of impulses across the
myoneural junction. In myasthenia gravis, there is an
increased response of skeletal muscle to repetitive impulses
caused by increased availability of acetylcholine. Pyridostigmine has a slower onset and longer duration of action
than neostigmine. When used for reversal of neuromuscular
blockade, the muscarinic cholinergic effects (bradycardia,
salivation, gastrointestinal stimulation) are prevented by the
concurrent use of atropine or glycopyrrolate.

Pharmacokinetics

Onset: Reversal: IV, 2-5 min; myesthenia: IM, <15 min; PO, 20-30 min
Peak Effect: Reversal: IV, 15 min; myesthenia: IM, 15 min
Duration: Reversal: IV, 90 min; myesthenia: PO, 3-6 hr; IM, 2-4 hr
Interaction/Toxicity: Does not antagonize and may prolong the phase-1 block of succinylcholine; antagonizes the effects of nondepolarizing muscle relaxants such as tubocurarine, atracurium, vecuronium, pancuronium; antagonism of neuromuscular blockade is reduced by aminoglycoside antibiotics, hypothermia, hypokalemia, respiratory and metabolic acidosis; may produce bradycardia, salivation, fasciculations, gastrointestinal stimulation.

Guidelines/Precautions

1. Use is contraindicated in patients with peritonitis or mechanical obstruction of the intestines or urinary tract.
2. Pyridostigmine overdosage may induce a cholinergic crisis characterized by nausea, vomiting, bradycardia or tachycardia, excessive salivation and sweating, bronchospasm, weakness, and paralysis.
3. Treatment of a cholinergic crisis includes discontinuation of pyridostigmine and administration of atropine (10 μg/kg IV q3-10min until muscarinic symptoms disappear) and if necessary pralidoxime (15 mg/kg IV over 2 min) for reversal of nicotinic symptoms. Give other supportive treatment as indicated (e.g., artificial respiration, tracheostomy, oxygen).
4. Use with caution in patients with bradycardia, bronchial asthma, cardiac arrhythmias, or peptic ulcer.

Principal Adverse Reactions

Cardiovascular: Bradycardia, AV block, nodal rhythm, hypotension

Pulmonary: Increased bronchial secretions, bronchospasm, respiratory depression

GI: Nausea, vomiting, diarrhea, abdominal cramps, increased peristalsis, increased salivation

Musculoskeletal: Muscle cramps, fasciculations, weakness

Other: Miosis, diaphoresis

RANITIDINE (ZANTAC)

Use(s): Treatment of duodenal ulcer, gastroesophageal reflux, pathologic hypersecretory conditions; prophylaxis against acid pulmonary aspiration, stress ulcers, upper GI bleeding in critically ill patients

Dosing: PO, 150 mg twice daily, alternately 150-300 mg at bedtime.

IV/IM, 50 mg q6-8h (dilute IV dose in 20 ml NS and give over 5-15 min).

Infusion, 6.25 mg/hr (10.7 ml/hr of 0.6 mg/ml solution)

Elimination: Hepatic

How Supplied:

Tablet, 150 mg, 300 mg

Oral solution, 15 mg/ml

Injection, 25 mg/ml

Storage: Tablets/solution/injection: Temperature of 4°-30° C. Protect from light. Avoid freezing and excessive heat. When reconstituted with normal saline, D_5W, $D_{10}W$, or LR, the injection is stable for 48 hr at room temperature.

Dilution for Infusion: 150 mg (6 ml) in 250 ml D_5W or NS (0.6 mg/ml)

Pharmacology

This histamine H_2 receptor antagonist blocks histamine-, pentagastrin- and acetylcholine-induced secretion of hydrogen ions by gastric parietal cells. Nocturnal and food-induced gastric secretion also are inhibited. Ranitidine has no significant effect on gastric emptying time, volume, or pancreatic secretions. A single oral dose of 150 mg will provide acid inhibition for a period of 8 to 12 hr. Ranitidine also suppresses histamine-induced peripheral vasodilation and inotropic effects. The drug has minimal entrance into the central nervous system and thus, in contrast with cimetidine, produces fewer side effects such as CNS dysfunction in elderly patients. It is also reported to produce less inhibition of microsomal drug metabolizing enzymes and less antiandrogen effects than cimetidine.

Pharmacokinetics

Onset: IV/IM, <15 min; PO, <30 min
Peak Effect: IV/IM, 1-2 hr; PO, 2-3 hr
Duration: IV/IM, 6-8 hr; PO, 8-12 hr
Interaction/Toxicity: Absorption is decreased by concurrent antacids; may decrease absorption of diazepam; may increase hypoglycemic effect of glipizide; may interfere with warfarin clearance; may antagonize neuromuscular blockade of nondepolarizing muscle relaxants (by an intrinsic anticholinesterase effect); may potentiate succinylcholine depolarizing blockade.

Guidelines/Precautions

1. Use with caution in elderly patients.
2. Full daily dose may be given once a day.

Principal Adverse Reactions

Cardiovascular: Tachycardia, bradycardia, premature ventricular beats with rapid IV injection
Pulmonary: Bronchospasm
CNS: Headache, depression, dizziness, confusion
GI/Hepatic: Nausea, vomiting, hepatitis, diarrhea
Hematologic: Leukopenia, granulocytopenia, thrombocytopenia
Dermatologic: Erythema multiforme, alopecia

RITODRINE HCL (YUTOPAR)

Use(s): Uterine relaxation; threatened or spontaneous abortion

Dosing: Infusion: 0.05-0.3 mg/min (titrate upward by 0.05 mg/min every 10 min until desired response). Continue infusion for at least 12 hr after cessation of uterine contractions.

PO, 10 mg every 2 hr for 24 hr then 10-20 mg every 4-6 hr. Maximum dose, 120 mg daily.
Elimination: Hepatic
How Supplied:
Injection, 10 mg/ml, 15 mg/ml
Tablets, 10 mg
Storage: Injection/tablets: Room temperature (15°-30° C). Protect from heat.
Dilution for Infusion: 150 mg in 500 ml NS (0.3 mg/ml)

Pharmacology

This beta-2 adrenergic receptor agonist increases the levels of cyclic AMP in uterine smooth muscle. Calcium cellular balance is altered, resulting in relaxation. Beta-1 effects manifest as tachycardia, hypertension, and fluid overload caused by increased sodium and water retention. Pulmonary edema also may be secondary to excessive tachycardia. Intravenous infusion is associated with transient elevations of blood glucose, insulin, and fatty acids, and a decrease in serum potassium. Ritodrine readily crosses the placenta, and the concentration of insulin in cord blood may be increased, resulting in neonatal hypoglycemia.

Pharmacokinetics

Onset: IV, immediate
Peak Effect: IV, <50 min; PO, 30-60 min
Duration: 1.7-2.6 hr (half-life)
Interaction/Toxicity: Incidence of pulmonary edema is increased with concomitant administration of cortico-steroids; potentiates cardiovascular depression of volatile anesthetics, magnesium, narcotics, diazoxide; additive effects (hypertension) occur with sympathomimetics and in the presence of parasympatholytics such as atropine; hypo-kalemia is associated with infusion and also use of potassi-um-depleting diuretics; may increase insulin requirements in insulin-dependent diabetics; action is antagonized by beta adrenergic blocking drugs.

Guidelines/Precautions

1. Monitor glucose and electrolytes during infusions.
2. Use is contraindicated before the twentieth week of pregnancy and in those conditions in which continuation of the pregnancy is hazardous to the mother or fetus, specifically, antepartum hemorrhage that demands immediate delivery, eclampsia, severe preeclampsia, intrauterine fetal death, chorioamnionitis, maternal car-

diac disease, pulmonary hypertension, maternal hyperthyroidism, uncontrolled maternal diabetes mellitus, preexisting maternal medical conditions such as pheochromocytoma, hypovolemia, and bronchial asthma already treated by beta mimetics and/or steroids.
3. Frequent monitoring of maternal uterine contractions, heart rate, blood pressure, and fetal heart rate is required.
4. Monitor fluid intake. To avoid pulmonary edema, limit fluid intake to 1.5-2 L/24 hr.
5. Pulmonary edema is especially common in patients taking corticosteroids.

Principal Adverse Reactions

Cardiovascular: Tachycardia, palpitations, arrhythmias, hypertension, angina, bradycardia after drug withdrawal
Pulmonary: Dyspnea, hyperventilation, pulmonary edema
CNS: Tremors, headache, anxiety
GI: Nausea, vomiting, diarrhea
Metabolic: Hypokalemia, hyperglycemia, hyperinsulinemia
Neonatal: Tachycardia, hypoglycemia, ileus

ROCURONIUM BROMIDE (ZEMURON)

Use(s): Skeletal muscle relaxation

Dosing: Intubation: IV, 0.6-1.2 mg/kg
Maintenance: IV, 0.06-0.6 mg/kg (10%-50% of intubating dose)
Infusion: 5-15 μg/kg/min
Pretreatment/priming: IV, 10% of intubating dose given 3-5 min before depolarizer/nondepolarizer relaxant dose

In obese patients, rocuronium dosage should be based on actual body weight (and not ideal body weight as with most drugs).

Elimination: Renal, hepatic
How Supplied: Injection, 10 mg/ml
Storage: Refrigerate at 2° to 8° C. Use within 30 days upon removal from refrigeration to room temperature.
Dilution for Infusion: 200 mg in 100 ml D_5W, NS, or LR (2 mg/ml)

Pharmacology

Rocuronium is a rapidly acting steroidal nondepolarizing neuromuscular blocking agent with a duration of action similar to that of vecuronium. Rocuronium is 8 times less potent than vecuronium and competes for cholinergic receptors at the motor end plate. Onset time is decreased and duration prolonged with increasing doses. There are no clinically significant changes in hemodynamic parameters. Unlike vecuronium, rocuronium has slight vagolytic activity and may occasionally produce tachycardia. Rocuronium does not release clinically significant concentrations of histamine.

Pharmacokinetics

Onset: 45-90 sec
Peak Effect: 1-3 min
Duration: 15-150 min (dose dependent)
Interaction/Toxicity: Neuromuscular blockade is potentiated by aminoglycoside, antibiotics, local anesthetics, volatile anesthetics, loop diuretics, magnesium, lithium, ganglionic blocking drugs, hypothermia, hypokalemia, respiratory acidosis, and prior administration of succinylcholine; dosage requirements are decreased (about 30%-

45%) and duration of neuromuscular blockade is prolonged (up to 25%) by volatile anesthetics; recurrent paralysis may occur with quinidine; enhanced neuromuscular blockade may occur in patients with myasthenia gravis or inadequate adrenocortical function; effects are antagonized by anticholinesterase inhibitors such as neostigmine, edrophonium, pyridostigmine; pretreatment doses of rocuronium decrease fasciculations but reduce intensity and shorten duration of succinylcholine neuromuscular blockade; priming doses decrease the time to onset of maximal blockade by about 30-60 sec; resistance is increased or effects are reversed with use of theophylline, anticonvulsants (e.g., phenytoin, carbamazepine), and in patients with burn injury and paresis.

Guidelines/Precautions

1. Monitor response with peripheral nerve stimulator to minimize risk of overdosage.
2. Reverse effects with anticholinesterases such as neostigmine, edrophonium, or pyridostigmine bromide in conjunction with atropine or glycopyrrolate.
3. Pretreatment doses may induce a degree of neuromuscular blockade sufficient to cause hypoventilation in some patients.
4. Rocuronium does not appear to trigger malignant hyperthermia.

Principal Adverse Reactions

Cardiovascular: Tachycardia, arrhythmia
Pulmonary: Hypoventilation, apnea, bronchospasm, pulmonary hypertension
Musculoskeletal: Inadequate block, prolonged block
Dermatologic: Rash, injection-site edema, pruritus

SCOPOLAMINE HYDROBROMIDE (SCOPOLAMINE HBr)

Use(s): Premedication, sedation, amnesia, vagolysis, treatment of motion sickness.

Dosing: PO, 0.4-0.8 mg

IV/IM/SC, 0.2-0.65 mg (Children 0.006 mg/kg, maximum dose 0.3 mg). Dilute with sterile water for IV administration.

Transdermal patch, 1.5 mg, apply to postauricular skin

Elimination: Hepatic, renal
How Supplied:
Capsules, 0.25 mg
Injection, 0.3 mg/ml, 0.4 mg/ml, 0.86 mg/ml, 1 mg/ml
Transdermal patch, 1.5 mg, delivers 5 μg/hr for 72 hr
Ophthalmic solution, 0.25%
Storage: Injection/solution/transdermal: Room temperature (15°-30° C). Do not permit injection to freeze.

Pharmacology

This ester of the organic base scopine antagonizes the action of acetylcholine at cholinergic postganglionic nerve endings. Scopolamine has greater antisialogogue and ocular effects than atropine and lesser effects on the heart (tachycardia), bronchial smooth muscle (bronchodilation), and gastrointestinal tract. The decrease in heart rate caused by small doses reflects a weak peripheral muscarinic cholinergic effect. It is a tertiary amine and may readily cross the blood-brain barrier, exerting effects on the central nervous system. Scopolamine produces a more marked and longer-lasting sedative effect than atropine, and therapeutic doses may cause drowsiness, euphoria, amnesia, and fatigue. It prevents motion sickness by inhibition of vestibular input to the CNS and a direct action on the vomiting center within the reticular formation of the brainstem.

Pharmacokinetics

Onset: IV, almost immediate; IM/PO/TD, within 30 min
Peak Effect: IV, 50-80 min; IM/PO, 2 hr; TD, 3 hr
Duration: IV, 2 hr; IM/PO, 4-6 hr; TD, 3 days
Interaction/Toxicity: Central anticholinergic syndrome; potentiates sedative effects of narcotics, benzodiazepines, anticholinergics, antihistamines, volatile anesthetics.

Guidelines/Precautions

1. Central anticholinergic syndrome may be due to blockade of muscarinic cholinergic receptors in the CNS. Symptoms include hallucinations, delirium, and coma. Treat central anticholinergic syndrome with intravenous physostigmine 15-60 μg/kg.
2. Use with great caution in patients with narrow-angle glaucoma, coronary artery disease, urinary bladder neck, and pyloric or intestinal obstruction.
3. May cause confusion and restlessness, particularly in the elderly (>65 years) and young (<13 years).
4. Use is not recommended in obstetrics. May be associated with fetal tachycardia and decreased beat-to-beat variability.

Principal Adverse Reactions

Cardiovascular: Tachycardia, bradycardia (with small doses)
Pulmonary: Tachypnea
CNS: Drowsiness, confusion, disorientation, restlessness
GI: Constipation, paralytic ileus, nausea, vomiting, dry mouth
Eye: Blurred vision, impairment of accommodation
Allergic: Urticaria, anaphylaxis

SECOBARBITAL (SECONAL)

Use(s): Premedication, sedation, hypnosis, anticonvulsant

Dosing: Premedication/sedation:

> IM, 4-5 mg/kg (inject deep and not more than 250 mg in any one site)
>
> PO, 100-300 mg (Children 2-6 mg/kg, maximum dose 100 mg)
>
> Rectal, 4-5 mg/kg (dilute injectable solution with water to a concentration of 10-15 mg/ml)

> Hypnosis: IV titrate, average dose 50-100 mg, do not exceed 50 mg per 15 min period, total dosage in excess of 250 mg is not recommended
>
> Anticonvulsant: Slow IV/IM: 250-350 mg (5.5 mg/kg); repeat q3-4 hr as indicated

Elimination: Hepatic

How Supplied:

Injection, 50 mg/ml

Tablets, 100 mg

Capsules, 50 mg and 100 mg

Rectal injection, 50 mg/ml

Storage: Injection/rectal injection: Refrigerate (2°-8° C). Protect from light.

Tablets/capsules: Room temperature (15°-30° C).

Pharmacology

This short-acting barbiturate depresses the sensory cortex, decreases motor activity, alters cerebellar function, and produces dose-dependent drowsiness, sedation, and hypnosis. It may induce paradoxic excitement in elderly persons and children and in the presence of acute or chronic pain.

Induction doses produce respiratory depression and decreases in peripheral vascular resistance, arterial pressure, cardiac output, and coronary perfusion pressure.

Pharmacokinetics

Onset: IV, almost immediate; PO, 10-30 min; IM/rectal, 15-30 min
Peak Effect: IV, 1 min
Duration: IV, 15 min (awakening), 3-4 hr (sedative effect); PO/IM/rectal, 6-8 hr (sedative effect)
Interaction/Toxicity: Potentiates CNS and circulatory depressant effects of narcotics, sedative hypnotics, alcohol, and volatile anesthetics; decreases effects of oral anticoagulants, digoxin, beta blockers, corticosteroids, quinidine, theophylline; actions are prolonged by MAO inhibitors, chloramphenicol; arterial or extravascular injection produces necrosis, gangrene.

Guidelines/Precautions

1. Use is contraindicated in patients with a history of manifest or latent porphyria or status asthmaticus and in the presence of acute or chronic pain.
2. Use with caution in patients with hypertension, hypovolemia, ischemic heart disease, acute adrenocortical insufficiency, uremia, and septicemia, and for obstetric delivery.
3. Reduce doses in elderly, hypovolemic, and high-risk surgical patients and with concomitant use of narcotics and other sedatives.
4. Treat intraarterial injection by local infiltration of phentolamine (5-10 mg in 10 ml NS) and, if necessary, sympathetic block.
5. Use IV route only in emergency.

Principal Adverse Reactions

Cardiovascular: Bradycardia, hypotension
Pulmonary: Respiratory depression, apnea, laryngospasm, bronchospasm
CNS: Somnolence, paradoxic excitement, ataxia, confusion
GI: Nausea, vomiting, constipation, diarrhea
Allergic: Rash, urticaria, angioneurotic edema
Dermatologic: Necrosis, gangrene with intraarterial injection

SODIUM BICARBONATE (SODIUM BICARBONATE)

Use(s): Correction of metabolic acidosis and urinary alkalinization; enhancement of rate of onset and potency of local anesthetics; adjunct treatment of acute symptomatic hyponatremia

Dosing: Acidosis in cardiac arrest: IV, 1 mEq/kg (followed by 0.5 mEq/kg every 10 min of arrest depending on arterial blood gases). Because of absence of proof of efficacy and the numerous adverse effects, use sodium bicarbonate only after application of more definitive and better substantiated interventions, such as prompt defibrillation, effective chest compression, endotracheal intubation and hyperventilation with 100% oxygen, and the use of drugs such as epinephrine and lidocaine. These interventions usually will take approximately 10 min.

Acidosis: Body weight (kg) × base deficit (mEq/L) × 0.3 (0.4 in infants) = Bicarbonate dose (mEq). Give one half of calculated estimate. Further doses should depend on clinical response. In the presence of normal renal function, achieving a total CO_2 content of about 20 mEq/L will be associated with a normal blood pH. (Neonates and children (under 2 years): slow IV administration of a 4.2% solution of the calculated dose. Maximum dose: 8 mEq/kg/day.)

Bicarbonation of local anesthetics:

　Add 1 ml of 8.4% sodium bicarbonate with 20 ml of 0.25%-0.5% bupivacaine.

　Add 1 ml of 8.4% sodium bicarbonate with 30 ml of 2%-3% chloroprocaine.

　Add 1 ml of 8.4% sodium bicarbonate with 10 ml of 0.5%-2% lidocaine.

　Add 1 ml of 8.4% sodium bicarbonate with 10 ml of 1%-3% mepivacaine.

　Add 1 ml of 8.4% sodium bicarbonate with 10 ml of 0.5%-2% prilocaine.

　Do not use if the local anesthetic precipitates out of the solution.

Alkalinization of urine: 48 mEq (4 g) initially, then 12-24 mEq (1-2 g) every 4 hr. Dosage of 30-48 mEq (2.5-4 g) every 4 hr may be required in some patients.

Acute symptomatic hyponatremia: Slow IV 1 mEq/kg. Use sodium bicarbonate (which is a 6% solution of sodium) if 3% saline is not immediately available. Repeat if sodium level is less than 120 mEq/L and patient remains symptomatic. Rapid elevation of serum sodium is contraindicated in patients with chronic asymptomatic hyponatremia.

Elimination: Renal

How Supplied:

Injection:

  Adult, 8.4% (1 mEq/ml)

  Pediatric, 7.5% (0.892 mEq/ml), 5% (0.6 mEq/ml)

  Children younger than 2 years and neonates, 4.2% (0.5 mEq/ml)

Solution sterile to adjust pH of injections 4.2% (0.5 mEq/ml), 4% (0.48 mEq/ml)

Tablets, 300 mg, 325 mg, 600 mg, 650 mg

Storage: Injection/tablets: Room temperature (15°-30° C). Avoid freezing.

Pharmacology

Dissociates in water to provide sodium (Na^+) and bicarbonate ($HCO3^-$) ions. Buffers excess hydrogen ion concentration and raises blood pH. One gram provides 11.9 mEq sodium and 11.9 mEq bicarbonate. Urinary alkalinization is useful in the treatment of certain drug intoxications (i.e., barbiturates, salicylates, lithium, methyl alcohol), in hemolytic reactions to diminish nephrotoxicity of blood pigments, and in methotrexate therapy to prevent nephrotoxicity. Bicarbonation of local anesthetics increases the pH and enhances rate of onset and potency. A big increase in pH may precipitate the local anesthetic out of solution as drug base.

Pharmacokinetics

Onset: 2-10 min

Peak Effect: 10-30 min

Duration: 30-60 min

Interaction/Toxicity: Increases risks of solute overload with coadministration of parenteral fluids, especially those containing sodium, in patients receiving corticosteroids or corticotropin; chemical incompatibility occurs with solutions containing calcium; increases end-tidal CO_2; urinary alkalinization increases half-lives and duration of action of quinidine, amphetamines, ephedrine, and pseudoephedrine; increases renal clearance of tetracyclines, especially doxycycline; extravasation may cause tissue necrosis, sloughing; metabolic acidosis may occur with excessive, too-rapid administration and in patients with hypokalemia or hypochloremia; carpopedal spasms may occur as pH rises in patients with coexistent hypocalcemia; hypokalemia from intracellular shift of potassium may occur with excessive administration and predispose to cardiac arrhythmias.

Guidelines/Precautions

1. Avoid overdosage and alkalosis by giving repeated small doses and monitoring pH.
2. Use cautiously in patients with congestive heart failure or other edematous or sodium-retaining states as well as in patients with oliguria or anuria.
3. Treat electrolyte imbalances before or concomitantly with administration of bicarbonate.
4. In neonates and children (under 2 years), rapid injection of hypertonic sodium bicarbonate solutions may produce hypernatremia, a decrease in cerebrospinal fluid, and possibly intracranial hemorrhage.
5. Unlike the other drugs used in resuscitation (e.g., epinephrine, atropine, lidocaine), sodium bicarbonate should never be given via an endotracheal tube because inactivation of surfactant renders the lung atelectatic.
6. Treat extravasation by prompt elevation of the part, warmth, and local injection of lidocaine or hyaluronidase.
7. Control symptoms of alkalosis (tetany, hyperirritability) by parenteral injection of calcium gluconate or, if severe, IV infusion of 2.14% ammonium chloride solution. Sodium chloride (0.9%) IV or potassium chloride

may be indicated if there is hypokalemia.

8. Liberation of carbon dioxide and its rapid intracellular diffusion after sodium bicarbonate administration may worsen intracellular acidosis during cardiopulmonary resuscitation. Increased arterial P_{CO_2} (and the paradoxic acidosis) is a rapidly acting and potent negative inotrope. On the other hand, the negative inotropic effect of metabolic acidosis is slower in onset and may not be fully manifest until 30 min have elasped from onset of acidosis to a magnitude equivalent to that induced more rapidly by carbon dioxide.

9. Rapid elevation of serum sodium in patients with chronic asymptomatic hyponatremia may result in the osmotic demyelination syndrome.

Principal Adverse Reactions

Cardiovascular: Peripheral edema, arrhythmias, myocardial depression

Pulmonary: Pulmonary edema

CNS: Intracranial hemorrhage

Metabolic: Alkalosis, hypernatremia, hypokalemia, hyperosmolality, intracellular/cerebrospinal fluid/central venous acidosis, inhibition of oxygen release to the tissues

Dermatologic: Necrosis, sloughing with extravasation

SODIUM CITRATE (SHOHL'S SOLUTION, BICITRA)

Use(s): Antacid, premedication (aspiration prophylaxis), systemic alkalinization, anticoagulant for banked blood (for transfusion)

Dosing: Antacid/premedication: PO, 15-30 ml diluted with 15-30 ml water as single dose.

Systemic alkalinization: PO, 10-30 ml diluted with 15-90 ml water after meals and at bedtime. Each milliliter contains 1 mEq sodium and is equivalent to 1 mEq bicarbonate.

Elimination: Hepatic

How Supplied: Unit dose, 15 ml, 30 ml, 120 ml, 1 pint, 1 gallon

Storage: Protect from excessive heat.

Pharmacology

Sodium citrate is a nonparticulate acid-neutralizing buffer. The alkalinizing activity depends on oxidation to bicarbonate in the body. Sodium citrate is fast-acting and produces a rapid rise in the pH value of gastric acid. 15 ml will neutralize and buffer 117 ml of 0.1N HCl to a pH value of 2.5. Sodium citrate also has anticoagulant activity. It forms an undissociated calcium citrate complex, making calcium unavailable to the clotting mechanism. The sterile solution is added to banked blood to prevent clotting and the crenation or swelling of cells.

Pharmacokinetics

Onset: Almost immediate
Peak Effect: Few minutes
Duration: 2 hr
Interaction/Toxicity: May induce alkalosis, especially in the presence of hypocalcemia.

Guidelines/Precautions

1. Contraindicated in patients on sodium-restricted diet or with severe renal impairment.
2. Because of high sodium content (1 mEq/ml), use cautiously in patients with cardiac failure, hypertension, impaired renal function, peripheral and pulmonary edema, and toxemia of pregnancy.

Principal Adverse Reactions

CNS: Seizures
GI: Nausea, vomiting, diarrhea
Metabolic: Alkalosis

SODIUM NITROPRUSSIDE (NIPRIDE, NITROPRESS)

Use(s): Antihypertensive, controlled hypotension, treatment of cardiogenic pulmonary edema, precardiac transplant evaluation

Dosing: Infusion, 10-300 μg/min (0.25-10 μg/kg/min) (maximum dose 10 μg/kg/min for 10 min or chronic infusion of 0.5 μg/kg/min). Wrap infusion bag in aluminium foil or opaque material to protect from light.
Elimination: Hepatic
How Supplied: Sterile powder for infusion, 5 ml vial containing 50 mg
Storage: Powder: Room temperature (15°-30° C). Protect from light. Reconstituted solutions are stable for 24 hr at room temperature when adequately protected from light.
Dilution for Infusion: 50 mg in 2-3 ml D_5W then in 250 ml D_5W (200 μg/ml)

Pharmacology

Nitroprusside is a potent peripheral vasodilator that acts on both arterial and venous smooth muscle. Its vasodilating properties may result from the generation of nitric oxide, which may be endothelial derived relaxing factor (EDRF). It lacks significant effects on other smooth muscle, such as the uterus or duodenum. The decrease in peripheral vascular resistance is associated with a decrease in blood pressure and activation of baroreceptor-mediated reflex tachycardia. It may alter pulmonary ventilation:perfusion ratio (thus increasing shunting) and increases cerebral blood flow. Uterine blood flow is decreased. Nitroprusside is rapidly metabolized to cyanide, which is converted to thiocyanate by the enzyme rhodanase in the liver and kidney. This detoxification reaction depends on the availability of a sulfur donor (endogenous thiosulfate).

Pharmacokinetics

Onset: 30-60 sec
Peak Effect: 1-2 min
Duration: 1-10 min
Interaction/Toxicity: Hypotensive effects are potentiated by volatile anesthetics, ganglionic blocking agents, and other antihypertensive and circulatory depressants; cyanide toxicity is manifested by tachyphylaxis, elevated mixed venous Po_2, and metabolic acidosis; thiocyanate toxicity (above 10 mg/100 ml) is manifested by skeletal muscle weakness, nausea, mental confusion, and hypothyroidism.

Guidelines/Precautions

1. There is risk of cyanide toxicity even at relatively low doses, and appropriate monitoring is required. Treat cyanide toxicity by immediate discontinuation of nitroprusside. Administer B_{12} (1 g /50 mg nitroprusside) or amyl nitrite inhalation for 15-30 sec each minute until a slow IV administration of sodium nitrite 5 mg/kg (3% solution) over 5 min to convert hemoglobin to methemoglobin. Then follow with intravenous sodium thiosulfate (150 mg/kg in 50 ml D_5W over 15 min).
2. Monitor plasma thiocyanate concentrations in any patient receiving therapy for longer than 48 hr. Thiocyanate retention is more likely in patients with impaired

renal function or hyponatremia and may present with symptoms of hypothyroidism. The thiocyanate ion is readily removed by peritoneal dialysis or hemodialysis.

3. In pregnant hypertensive patients, sodium nitroprusside is not recommended after induction of general anesthesia because of the risk of fetal cyanide toxicity.

4. Use is contraindicated in patients with compensatory hypertension (e.g., arteriovenous shunts, coarctation of the aorta) and those with inadequate cerebral circulation.

5. Administer with a calibrated infusion pump.

Principal Adverse Reactions

Cardiovascular: Hypotension, collapse, palpitations, tachycardia
CNS: Headache, apprehension, raised intracranial pressure
GI: Nausea, retching
Hematologic: Methemoglobinemia
Other: Cyanide toxicity, hypothyroidism, antiplatelet effect, methemoglobinemia

---

SUCCINYLCHOLINE CHLORIDE (ANECTINE, SUCOSTRIN, QUELICIN)

Use(s): Skeletal muscle relaxation

Dosing: IV, 0.7-1 mg/kg (1.5 mg/kg with nondepolarizer pretreatment), neonates and infants, 2-3 mg/kg, children, 1-2 mg/kg
Deep IM, 2.5-4 mg/kg, max IM dose, 150 mg
Infusion, 0.5-10 mg/min (10-200 μg/kg/min), titrate to desired response
Max total dose (to avoid prolonged phase 2 block) <5 mg/kg.

Elimination: Plasma pseudocholinesterase
How Supplied:
Injection, 20 mg/ml, 50 mg/ml, 100 mg/ml
Powder for injection, 100 mg, 500 mg, 1 g per vial with
diluent
Storage:
Injection: Refrigerate (2°-8° C) to avoid loss of potency.
Anectine multidose vial may be stable for 14 days at
room temperature (15°-30° C) without significant loss of
potency.
Powder: Stable indefinitely at room temperature (15°-30°
C). Use within 24 hr of reconstitution. Discard unused
solutions.
Dilution for Infusion: 250 mg in 250 ml D_5W or NS
(1 mg/ml)

Pharmacology

Succinylcholine is an ultrashort-acting depolarizing skeletal muscle relaxant. Like acetylcholine, it combines with
cholinergic receptors of the motor end plate to produce
depolarization observed as fasciculations. Neuromuscular
transmission is then inhibited as long as an adequate concentration of succinylcholine remains at the receptor site;
the neuromuscular block produces a flaccid paralysis. Succinylcholine has no effect on consciousness, pain threshold,
or cerebration and no direct effect on the uterus or other
smooth muscles. It increases intraocular pressure. Barrier
pressure is maintained, with elevation of both intragastric
and lower esophageal sphincter pressure. When given over
a long period of time, the characteristic depolarizing neuromuscular block (phase-1 block) may change to a block that
superficially resembles a nondepolarizing block. (phase-II
block). This may be associated with prolonged hypoventi-

lation. After confirmation of phase-II block by peripheral nerve stimulation (train-of-four fade, posttetanic facilitation), observe spontaneous recovery of the twitch for 20-30 min, then reverse with anticholinesterase (e.g., neostigmine) combined with an anticholinergic agent (e.g., glycopyrrolate or atropine). A phase-I block will be potentiated. Histamine release occurs but rarely is of clinical significance. Initial cardiac effects reflect actions at autonomic ganglia (elevations in heart rate and blood pressure). Subsequent cardiac effects at higher doses (sinus bradycardia, junctional rhythm) reflect actions at cardiac muscarinic cholinergic receptors.

Pharmacokinetics

Onset: IV, 30-60 sec; IM, 2-3 min
Peak Effect: IV, 60 sec
Duration: IV, 4-6 min; IM, 10-30 min
Interaction/Toxicity: Prolonged neuromuscular blockade may occur in patients with hypokalemia or hypocalcemia, or low plasma pseudocholinesterase, and patients receiving phenelzine, beta adrenergic blockers, procainamide, metoclopramide, lidocaine, magnesium, oxytocin, trimethaphan, volatile anesthetics, and anticholinesterases (e.g., neostigmine, echothiopate); blockade is prolonged by pretreatment with pancuronium; blockade is antagonized and fasciculations are decreased by pretreatment with other nondepolarizing muscle relaxants (e.g., tubocurarine [most effective]); response is unpredictable in myasthenia gravis; bradycardia may occur after second IV injection, especially in children; sensitivity to succinylcholine is increased during pregnancy secondary to decreased pseudocholinesterase; succinylcholine is incompatible with alkaline solutions and will precipitate sodium thiopental.

Guidelines/Precautions

1. Monitor response with peripheral nerve stimulator.

2. Abrupt onset of malignant hyperthermia may be triggered by succinylcholine. Early premonitory signs include muscle rigidity, especially jaw muscles, tachycardia and tachypnea unresponsive to increased depth of anesthesia, evidence of increased oxygen consumption and carbon dioxide production (change in color and increased temperature of the CO_2 absorber), rising body temperature, and metabolic acidosis.

3. Development of masseter muscle spasm after administration of succinylcholine may be associated with malignant hyperthermia susceptibility. However, it may be due to an insufficient dose of succinylcholine (especially in children). The anesthetic may be continued without triggering agents and the patient evaluated for malignant hyperthermia. The development of an increase in muscle tone, rising body temperature, and cardiac arrhythmias suggests that the patient is undergoing a hypermetabolic episode. The anesthetic needs to be abandoned and treatment begun for malignant hyperthermia.

4. Use with caution in patients with fractures and muscle spasm caused by additional trauma from fasciculations and those with cardiovascular, hepatic, pulmonary, metabolic, or renal disorders.

5. Repeated administration at short intervals (less than 5 min) is associated with bradycardia. Bradycardia may be prevented by atropine, thiopental, ganglionic blocking drugs, and nondepolarizing muscle relaxants.

6. Succinylcholine elevates serum potassium (0.3-0.5 mEq/L in normal patients). Alarming levels of potassium (as high as 11 mEq/L) along with cardiovascular

collapse may occur when succinylcholine is used in patients with severe burns, hyperkalemia, electrolyte imbalance, severe trauma, paraplegia, spinal-cord injury, upper-motor-neuron injury, and degenerative or dystrophic neuromuscular disease. The risks of hyperkalemia in these patients increases over time and usually peaks at 7 to 10 days after the injury. The precise time of onset and the duration of the risk period are not known.

7. Succinylcholine increases both intragastric and gastroesophageal sphincter pressure. Fasciculations may increase potential for regurgitation and aspiration.

8. Administration of succinylcholine soon after an anticholinesterase (e.g., neostigmine, pyridostigmine) will produce a prolonged neuromuscular blockade (up to 60 min). This is partly due to inhibition of plasma pseudocholinesterase and delayed metabolism of succinylcholine.

9. Prolonged respiratory paralysis may occur in patients with low plasma pseudocholinesterase, as in severe liver disease or cirrhosis, burns, cancer, pregnancy, dehydration, collagen disease, and abnormal body temperatures; in patients receiving pancuronium, MAO inhibitors, neostigmine, echothiophate, oral contraceptives, and chlorpromazine; or those with a recessive hereditary trait. Administer minimal doses (test dose of 5-10 mg) with extreme care. Echothiophate should be discontinued 4 weeks before anesthesia with succinylcholine.

10. Use is contraindicated in patients with genetic disorders of plasma pseudocholinesterases, familial history of malignant hyperthermia, myopathies associated with elevated creatine phosphokinase (CPK) values, acute narrow-angle glaucoma, penetrating eye injuries, or hypersensitivity to succinylcholine.

11. Apparently healthy children and adolescents may have undiagnosed myopathies, and administration of succinylcholine may result in acute rhabdomyolysis, hyperkalemia, and cardiac arrest. Succinylcholine is indicated in these age groups only for emergency tracheal intubation or in instances where immediate securing of the airway is necessary.

Principal Adverse Reactions

Cardiovascular: Hypotension, bradycardia, arrhythmias, tachycardia, hypertension
Pulmonary: Hypoventilation, apnea, bronchospasm
GI: Excess salivation, increased intragastric and lower esophageal sphincter tone.
Allergic: Anaphylactic reactions, rash
Musculoskeletal: Prolonged block, inadequate block, muscle soreness, increase in masseter muscle tone
Other: Hyperkalemia, malignant hyperthermia, myoglobinemia, increased intraocular pressure

SUFENTANIL CITRATE (SUFENTA)

Use(s): Analgesia, anesthesia

Dosing: Analgesia
IV/IM, 10-30 μg (0.2-0.6 μg/kg)
Intranasal, 1.5-3 μg/kg
Use undiluted injectate solution for intranasal route.
Induction:
IV bolus, 2-10 μg/kg
Infusion, 0.1-0.5 μg/kg/min for $\leq$20 min.

Titrate dose to patient response.To avoid chest-wall rigidity, administer muscle relaxant simultaneously with induction doses.

Anesthesia supplement:

IV bolus, 0.6-4 μg/kg

Infusion, 0.005-0.05 μg/kg/min

Sole anesthetic:

IV, 10-30 μg/kg (average total dosage—titrate to effect) or

Infusion, 0.05-0.1 μg/kg/min

Epidural:

Bolus, 10-50 μg (0.2-0.7) μg/kg

Infusion: 5-30 μg/hr (0.1-0.6 μg/kg/hr)

Spinal: 1-10 μg (0.02-0.08 μg/kg)

Patient-controlled analgesia–IV:

Bolus, 2-10 μg (0.04-0.2 μg/kg)

Infusion, 2-20 μg/hr (0.04-0.4 μg/kg/hr)

Lockout interval, 3-10 min

Patient-controlled analgesia–epidural:

Bolus, 4 μg (0.08 μg/kg)

Infusion, 6 μg/hr (0.12 μg/kg)

Lockout interval, 10-20 min

Elimination: Hepatic

How Supplied: Injection, 50 μg/ml

Storage: Room temperature (15°-30° C). Protect from light.

Dilution for Infusion:

IV, 500 μg in 100 ml NS (5 μg/ml);

Epidural

Bolus, 10-30 μg in 15-20 ml local anesthetic or (preservative-free) NS

Infusion,100 μg in 100 ml local anesthetic or (preservative-free) NS (1 μg/ml)

Pharmacology

This drug is a thiamyl analog of fentanyl with 5-7 times the analgesic potency. Sufentanil attenuates the hemodynamic response to endotracheal intubation and surgical manipulation (e.g., incision). Cardiovascular effects are generally similar to those of fentanyl. Sufentanil may produce a dose-dependent bradycardia, probably by stimulation of the vagal nucleus in the medulla. This may be sufficient to decrease cardiac output. Depression of ventilation is due to a decrease in response of the respiratory centers in the brainstem to increases in CO_2. The drug causes a decrease in cerebral metabolic requirements for oxygen. Sufentanil, like alfentanil or fentanyl, has no clinically significant effect on cerebral blood flow or intracranial pressure.

Pharmacokinetics

Onset: IV, 1-3 min; intranasal, <5 min; epidural/spinal, 4-10 min

Peak Effect: IV, 3-5 min; intranasal, 10 min; epidural/spinal, <30 min

Duration: IV, 20-45 min; IM, 2-4 hr; epidural/spinal, 2-4 hr

Interaction/Toxicity: Circulatory and ventilatory depressant effects are potentiated by other narcotics, sedatives, nitrous oxide, volatile anesthetics; ventilatory depressant effects are potentiated by MAO inhibitors, phenothiazines, and tricyclic antidepressants; analgesia is enhanced and prolonged by alpha-2 agonists (e.g., clonidine, epinephrine); addition of epinephrine to intrathecal/epidural sufentanil results in increased side effects (e.g., nausea) and prolonged motor block; skeletal muscle rigidity may occur in higher dosages sufficient to interfere with ventilation; incidence of bradycardia is increased with use of vecuronium.

Guidelines/Precautions

1. In hemodynamically stable patients, analgesic doses may be given 2-4 min before laryngoscopy to attenuate the pressor response to intubation. Requirements for induction agents (e.g., sodium thiopental) may be decreased.

2. Reduce doses in elderly, hypovolemic, or high-risk surgical patients and with concomitant use of sedatives and other narcotics. Incremental doses should be determined from effect of initial dose.

3. Narcotic effect is reversed with naloxone (IV 0.2-0.4 mg or higher). Duration of reversal may be shorter than duration of narcotic effect.

4. May produce a dose-related rigidity of skeletal muscles.

5. Crosses the placental barrier, and usage in labor may produce depression of respiration in the neonate. Resuscitation may be required; have naloxone available.

6. Undesirable side effects of epidural, caudal, or intrathecal sufentanil include delayed respiratory depression (up to 8 hr), pruritus, nausea and vomiting, and urinary retention. Naloxone (IV 0.2-0.4 mg prn or infusion 5 - 10 μg/kg/hr) is effective for prophylaxis and/or treatment. Ventilatory support for respiratory depression must be readily available. Antihistamines (e.g., diphenhydramine 12.5-25 mg IV/IM q6hr prn) may be used in treating pruritus. Metoclopramide (10 mg IV q6hr prn) may be used in treating nausea and vomiting. Urinary retention that does not respond to naloxone may require straight bladder catheterization.

7. Epidural, caudal, or intrathecal injections should be avoided when the patient has septicemia, infection at the injection site, or coagulopathy.

Principal Adverse Reactions

Cardiovascular: Hypotension, bradycardia.
Pulmonary: Respiratory depression, apnea
CNS: Dizziness, sedation, euphoria, dysphoria, anxiety
GI: Nausea, vomiting, delayed gastric emptying, biliary tract spasm
Eye: Miosis
Musculoskeletal: Muscle rigidity

TERBUTALINE SULFATE (BRETHAIRE, BRICANYL)

Use(s): Bronchodilator, inhibition of premature labor

Dosing: Bronchodilator:

SC, 0.25 mg, may repeat in 15-30 min, do not exceed 0.5 mg in 4 hr

Inhalation, 2 breaths separated by 60 sec every 4 to 6 hr

PO, 2.5-5 mg 3 times daily

Inhibition of premature labor (unlabeled use):

Infusion IV, 10-80 μg/min, titrate upward, maintain minimum effective doses for 4 hr

PO, 2.5 mg q4-6hr

Elimination: Hepatic
How Supplied:
Injection, 1 mg/ml
Aerosol, each actuation delivers 0.2 mg
Tablets, 2.5 mg, 5 mg
Storage: Injection/tablets/aerosol: Room temperature (15°-30° C). Protect injection from light. Aerosol container should not punctured, used or stored near heat or an open flame, or placed into a fire or incinerator for disposal.

Pharmacology

This beta-2 adrenergic receptor agonist relieves acute bronchospasm in acute and chronic obstructive pulmonary disease. Beta-1 effects are manifest as tachycardia and hypertension. Continuous intravenous infusion, as used to stop uterine contractions in premature labor, has been associated with maternal tachycardia, pulmonary edema, hypoglycemia, hypokalemia, and neonatal hypoglycemia.

Pharmacokinetics

Onset: SC, 5-15 min; PO, <30 min; inhalation, 5-30 min
Peak Effect: SC, 30-60 min; PO, 2-3 hr; inhalation, 1-2 hr
Duration: SC, 90 min-4 hr; PO, 4-8 hr; inhalation, 3-6 hr
Interaction/Toxicity: Effects are antagonized by beta blockers; risk of arrhythmias is increased in patients receiving volatile anesthetics; risk of hypokalemia is increased in patients receiving potassium-depleting diuretics; pulmonary edema is associated with continuous infusion.

Guidelines/Precautions

1. Terbutaline has an unlabeled use for management of preterm labor.
2. Use with caution in patients with hypertension, ischemic heart disease, arrhythmias, diabetes mellitus, hyperthyroidism, and seizures, and those susceptible to hypokalemia.
3. Paradoxic bronchoconstriction has occasionally occurred with repeated excessive use of inhalation preparations.
4. Excessive use may lead to beta agonist cardiomyopathy.
5. Use is contraindicated in patients with hypersensitivity to terbutaline or other sympathomimetic amines.

Principal Adverse Reactions

Cardiovascular: Tachycardia, palpitations, hypertension, arrhythmias
Pulmonary: Dyspnea, pulmonary edema
CNS: Tremors, dizziness, headache
GI: Nausea, vomiting, diarrhea
Metabolic: Hypokalemia, hypoglycemia, hyperinsulinemia

TETRACAINE (PONTOCAINE)

Use(s): Regional and topical anesthesia

Dosing: Spinal: bolus/infusion, 5-20 mg (Children 0.4 mg/kg with a minimum of 1 mg) (1% solution). Dilute dose with equal volume of supplied dextrose solution (hyperbaric), or cerebrospinal fluid (isobaric), or sterile water (hypobaric).

Brachial plexus block: Combine 0.5-1 mg/kg tetracaine with 30-50 ml (0.5-0.75 ml/kg) of bupivacaine (0.25%-0.375%), lidocaine (1%), or mepivacaine (1%).

Spray (topical): 2% solution: Apply for 1 sec (never more than 2 sec). Average expulsion rate of residue from spray is 200 mg/sec.

Maximum safe dose: 1-1.5 mg/kg (without epinephrine), 2.5 mg/kg (with epinephrine).

Solutions containing preservatives should not be used for spinal block. Except where contraindicated, vasoconstrictor drugs may be added to increase effect and prolong local or regional anesthesia. For dosage/route guidelines, see Epinephrine, Dosing or

> Phenylephrine, Dosing. Do not use vasoconstrictor drugs for IV regional anesthesia or local anesthesia of end organs (digits, penis, nose, ears).

Elimination: Plasma cholinesterase

How Supplied:

Injection, 1% with 10% dextrose, 0.2% in 6% dextrose, 0.3% in 6% dextrose

Powder for reconstitution, 20 mg

Storage: Room temperature (15°-30° C). Protect from light.

Pharmacology

This ester of para-amino benzoic acid is a potent long-acting local anesthetic. It stabilizes the neuronal membrane and prevents initiation and transmission of nerve impulses. It has a prolonged duration of action compared with procaine and chloroprocaine secondary to a much slower rate of hydrolysis by plasma cholinesterase. The duration of action may be further prolonged by the addition of vasoconstrictor drugs to delay systemic absorption. High plasma levels may produce seizures and cardiovascular collapse secondary to a decrease in peripheral vascular resistance and direct myocardial depression.

Pharmacokinetics

Onset: Infiltration: 15 min; spinal, <10 min

Peak Effect: Infiltration/spinal, 15 min-1 hr

Duration: Infiltration, 2-3 hr; spinal, 1.25-3.0 hr

Interaction/Toxicity: Prolongs the effect of succinylcholine; metabolite (PABA) inhibits the action of sulfonamides and aminosalicylic acid; toxicity enhanced by cimetidine, anticholinesterases (which inhibit degradation);

plasma levels >8 μg/ml are associated with seizures, respiratory and cardiac depression; benzodiazepines, barbiturates, and volatile anesthetics increase seizure threshold; duration of regional anesthesia is prolonged by vasoconstrictor agents (e.g., epinephrine) and alpha-2 agonists (e.g., clonidine); alkalinization increases rate of onset and potency of local or regional anesthesia.

Guidelines/Precautions

1. Do not use as injection.
2. Do not use on eyes.
3. To minimize systemic absorption, do not apply topically to large areas of denuded or inflamed tissue.
4. Use with caution in patients with severe disturbances of cardiac rhythm, shock, or heart block.
5. Reduce doses for spinal anesthesia in obstetric, elderly, hypovolemic, and high-risk patients and those with increased intraabdominal pressure.
6. Cauda equina syndrome with permanent neurologic deficit has occured in patients receiving greater than 20 mg of a 1% tetracaine solution with a continuous spinal technique.
7. There is potential for allergic reaction with repeated use.
8. Use is contraindicated in patients with hypersensitivity to tetracaine or ester-type local anesthetics and patients with allergy to suntan lotion (contains PABA derivatives).
9. Toxic plasma levels (e.g., from accidental intravascular injection) may cause cardiopulmonary collapse and seizures. Premonitory signs and symptoms manifest as numbness of the tongue and circumoral tissues, metallic taste, restlessness, tinnitus, and tremors. Support of circulation (IV fluids, vasopressors, IV sodium bicar-

bonate 1-2 mEq/kg to treat cardiac toxicity [sodium channel blockade], IV bretylium 5 mg/kg, and DC cardioversion/defibrillation for ventricular arrhythmias) and securing a patent airway (ventilate with 100% oxygen) are paramount. Thiopental (0.5-2 mg/kg IV), midazolam (0.02-0.04 mg/kg IV), or diazepam (0.1 mg/kg IV) may be used for prophylaxis and/or treatment of seizures.

10. The level of sympathetic blockade determines the degree of hypotension after intrathecal administration of tetracaine. Blocks above T5 affect cardiac sympathetic nerves and are associated with bradycardia and decreased cardiac output. Fluid hydration (10-20 ml/kg NS or lactated Ringer's solution), vasopressor agents (e.g., ephedrine), and left uterine displacement in pregnant patients may be used for prophylaxis and/or treatment. Administer atropine to treat bradycardia.

11. Caudal or intrathecal injections should be avoided when the patient has hypovolemic shock, septicemia, infection at the injection site, or coagulopathy.

Principal Adverse Reactions

Cardiovascular: Hypotension, bradycardia, heart block, arrhythmias, peripheral vasodilation
Pulmonary: Respiratory impairment or paralysis
CNS: Postspinal headache, tinnitus, seizures, blurred vision, restlessness
Allergic: Urticaria, erythema, angioneurotic edema
Spinal: High spinal, loss of perineal sensation and sexual function, backache, weakness and paralysis of the lower extremities, loss of sphincter control, slowing of labor, cranial nerve palsies, meningitis

THIOPENTAL SODIUM (PENTOTHAL)

Use(s): Induction agent, supplementation of regional anesthesia, anticonvulsant, reduction of elevated intracranial pressure, cerebral protection (barbiturate narcosis)

Dosing: Induction: IV, 3-5 mg/kg (children 5-6, mg/kg; infants 7-8 mg/kg)

       Anesthesia supplementation: IV, 0.5-1 mg/kg

       Rectal induction: 25 mg/kg

       Anticonvulsant: IV, 0.5-2 mg/kg, repeat as necessary

       Reduction of ICP: IV, 1-4 mg/kg

       Barbiturate narcosis:

          IV bolus, 8 mg/kg prn to maintain EEG burst suppression (mean total dose 40 mg/kg)

          Infusion, 0.05-0.35 mg/kg/min; inotropic and respiratory support are required at high doses

Elimination: Hepatic

How Supplied:

Injection, 250 mg, 400 mg, and 500 mg syringes

Vials with diluent, 500 mg and 1 g

Kits with 1, 2.5, 5 g

Rectal suspension, 400 mg/g of suspension

Storage: Powder: Room temperature (15°-30° C). Reconstituted solutions should be used promptly. Solutions are stable for 24 hr either refrigerated (2°-8° C) or at room temperature.

Dilution for Infusion: Barbiturate narcosis: IV, 5000 mg in 250 ml sterile water or NS (20 mg/ml).

Pharmacology

This ultrashort-acting thiobarbiturate depresses the central nervous system and induces hypnosis and anesthesia but not analgesia. Recovery after a short dose is rapid (because of redistribution from the brain to other body tissues), with some somnolence and anterograde amnesia. Because of the high lipid solubility and slow elimination, repeated intravenous doses lead to a cumulative drug effect. The drug produces respiratory depression and hemodynamic effects, including a decrease in systemic vascular resistance, arterial pressure, cardiac output, and coronary perfusion pressure. Uterine blood flow is decreased. Induction doses of thiopental may suppress the adrenal cortex and decrease plasma cortisol levels. However, unlike etomidate, the adrenal suppression is rapidly reversible and responds to ACTH stimulation. Thiopental decreases cerebral blood flow, cerebral metabolic rate, and intracranial pressure. Cerebral perfusion pressure is maintained. The nonspecific late latency waves of somatosensory, brainstem auditory, and visual evoked potentials are uniformly depressed. EEG changes include an initial increase in the alpha amplitude followed by a progressive decrease in activity. High doses of thiopental that induce burst suppression to the isoelectric point may provide protection during profound controlled hypotension and reduce infarct size in patients with cerebral emboli and temporary focal ischemia. Thiopental narcosis does not affect outcome in patients with severe head injuries or after cardiac arrest. Histamine release can occur, and allergic reactions most likely represent anaphylaxis.

Pharmacokinetics

Onset: IV, 10-20 sec; rectal, 8-10 min (variable)
Peak Effect: IV, 30-40 sec
Duration: IV, 5-15 min (awakening)

Interaction/Toxicity: Potentiates CNS and circulatory depressant effects of narcotics, sedative hypnotics, alcohol, volatile anesthetics; decreases effects of oral anticoagulants, digoxin, beta blockers, corticosteroids, quinidine, theophylline; actions are prolonged by MAO inhibitors, chloramphenicol; use is incompatible with solutions of succinylcholine, tubocurarine, or other drugs with an acid pH; arterial or extravascular injection (especially with concentrations above 5%) produce necrosis, gangrene.

Guidelines/Precautions

1. Treat intraarterial or extravascular injection by local infiltration of phentolamine (5 to 10 mg in 10 ml NS), or injection into the artery of a dilute solution of papaverine (40 to 80 mg) or 10 ml of 1% procaine to inhibit smooth muscle spasm. Urokinase 75,000 IU may be injected into the artery for lysis of clot emboli. If necessary, perform sympathetic block of the brachial plexus or stellate ganglion.
2. Shivering after pentothal anesthesia is a thermal reaction caused by increased sensitivity to cold. Treatment consists of warming the patient with blankets, maintaining room temperature and administering meperidine, chlorpromazine, or methylphenidate.
3. Use is contraindicated in patients with status asthmaticus, acute intermittent porphyria, variegate porphyria, and hereditary coproporphyria.
4. Use with caution in patients with hypertension, hypovolemia, ischemic heart disease, acute adrenocortical insufficiency, uremia, septicemia.
5. Reduce doses in elderly, hypovolemic, and high-risk surgical patients and with concomitant use of narcotics and sedatives.

6. Most incidences of coughing and airway spasm during thiopental induction are due to manipulation of the airway during light levels of anesthesia rather than to a direct drug effect. In patients with active bronchospasm, ketamine may be preferable to thiopental for intravenous induction.

Principal Adverse Reactions

Cardiovascular: Circulatory depression, arrhythmias
Pulmonary: Respiratory depression, apnea, laryngospasm, bronchospasm
CNS: Emergence delirium, prolonged somnolence and recovery, headache
GI: Nausea, emesis, salivation
Dermatologic: Thrombophlebitis, necrosis, gangrene
Allergic: Erythema, pruritus, urticaria, anaphylactic reactions
Other: Skeletal muscle hyperactivity, shivering

TRIMETHAPHAN CAMSYLATE (ARFONAD)

Use(s): Vasodilator, controlled hypotension, acute treatment of hypertensive emergencies

Dosing: Infusion, 0.5-4 mg/min (Children 10-150 μg/kg/min)
Elimination: Plasma cholinesterase
How Supplied: Injection, 50 mg/ml
Storage: Refrigerate (2°-8° C). Stable for 14 days at up to 25° C. When reconstituted with NS or D_5W, solutions are stable for 24 hr at room temperature.
Dilution for Infusion: 1500 mg in 500 ml D_5W (3 mg/ml); do not use other diluents.

Pharmacology

Trimethaphan blocks nicotinic ganglionic receptors. It acts rapidly but so briefly that it must be given by continuous intravenous infusion. Directly relaxes capacitance vessels, blocks autonomic nervous system reflexes, and lowers blood pressure by decreasing cardiac output and reducing peripheral vascular resistance. Histamine release does not contribute to the reduction in blood pressure, and there is no association with increases in plasma concentrations of catecholamines and renin, reflecting the effect of ganglionic blockade. Increases in heart rate most likely reflect parasympathetic blockade. Ganglionic blockade is due to occupation of receptors normally responsive to acetylcholine as well as stabilization of postsynaptic membranes against the actions of acetylcholine released from presynaptic nerve endings. Trimethaphan decreases cerebral blood flow and evokes smaller increases in intracranial pressure compared with nitroprusside or nitroglycerin.

Pharmacokinetics

Onset: Immediate
Peak Effect: 1-2 min
Duration: 10-30 min
Interaction/Toxicity: Additive hypotensive effects with other antihypertensives, volatile and spinal anesthetics, sedative hypnotics, narcotics, diuretics; inhibits plasma cholinesterase and may prolong the duration of succinylcholine; potentiates nondepolarizing muscle relaxants (e.g., vecuronium).

Guidelines/Precautions

1. Use is contraindicated when there is inadequate availability of fluids or inability to replace blood for techni-

cal reasons and in conditions when hypotension may subject the patient to undue risk (e.g., hypovolemia, anemia, shock, respiratory insufficiency).

2. Use with caution in patients with arteriosclerosis, cardiac disease, hepatic or renal disease, degenerative disease of the CNS, Addison's disease, or diabetes mellitus, or those receiving corticosteroids.

3. Mydriasis produced by trimethaphan may interfere with neurologic evaluation of the patient after neurosurgery.

4. Tachyphylaxis may occur, requiring increasing doses to maintain effect.

5. Pregnant women are overly sensitive to this ganglionic blocker, and placental transfer of the drug can result in fetal toxicity.

Principal Adverse Reactions

Cardiovascular: Hypotension, tachycardia
Pulmonary: Respiratory depression, arrest
CNS: Decreased cerebral blood flow
GU: Urinary retention
GI: Ileus
Eye: Mydriasis
Allergic: Urticaria, pruritus, anaphylactic reaction

VASOPRESSIN (PITRESSIN)

Use(s): Diagnosis and treatment of diabetes insipidus; treatment of GI hemorrhage, hemophilia; control of postoperative ileus

Dosing: Diabetes insipidus: SC/IM, 5-10 units 2-3 times daily as needed
GI hemorrhage: infusion, 0.2-0.4 units/min, maximum dose 0.9 units/min

Elimination: Renal, hepatic

How Supplied: Injection: vasopressin 20 units/ml; vasopressin tannate, 5 units/ml (not for IV use)

Storage: Injection: Room temperature (15°-30° C). Avoid freezing.

Dilution for Infusion: 200 units of vasopressin in 250 ml D$_5$W or NS (0.8 unit/ml)

Pharmacology

Commercially available vasopressin injection contains antidiuretic hormone (ADH) and the water soluble pressor principle of bovine and porcine posterior pituitaries. The drug is relatively free of oxytocic activity. The potency of vasopressin is standardized according to the pressor activity and expressed in USP Posterior Pituitary (pressor) units. The antidiuretic action is due to increased reabsorption of water by the renal tubules. Vasopressin produces contraction of the smooth muscle of the GI tract and vascular bed. Enhanced GI motility may manifest as abdominal pain, nausea, and vomiting. Direct effect on vascular smooth muscle is not antagonized by denervation or adrenergic blocking drugs. Generalized vasoconstriction and increased blood pressure occur only with doses that are much larger than those administered for the treatment of diabetes insipidus. Small doses may produce selective vasoconstriction of coronary arteries, myocardial ischemia, and in some instances myocardial infarction. Ventricular arrhythmias may accompany these cardiac effects. Increases circulating plasma concentration of factor VIII and may be beneficial in the management of severe hemophilia, particularly to reduce bleeding associated with surgery. Prolonged use may result in antibody formation and a shorter duration of action. Vasopressin is inactivated by trypsin in the GI tract and thus must be administered parenterally. Compared with the synthetic analog desmopressin, absorption through the nasal mucosa is relatively poor.

Pharmacokinetics

Onset: IM/SC, almost immediate (antidiuretic effect)
Peak Effect: IM/SC, 30-60 min (antidiuretic effect)
Duration: IM/SC, 2-8 hr (antidiuretic effect); infusion, 30-60 min (pressor response)
Interaction/Toxicity: Antidiuretic effect is potentiated by carbamazepine, chlorpropamide, clofibrate, urea, fludrocortisone, tricyclic antidepressants; effect is decreased by demeclocycline, norepinephrine, lithium, heparin, alcohol; sensitivity to pressor effect is increased by ganglionic blocking agents.

Guidelines/Precautions

1. Use cautiously in the presence of epilepsy, migraine, asthma, heart failure, or any state in which a rapid addition to extracellular water may constitute a hazard.
2. Water intoxication may be treated with water restriction and temporary withdrawal of vasopressin until polyuria occurs. Severe water intoxication may require osmotic diuresis with mannitol, hypertonic dextrose, or urea alone or with furosemide.

Principal Adverse Reaction

Pulmonary: Cardiac arrest, circumoral pallor
CNS: Tremors, vertigo, "pounding" in head
GI: Abdominal cramps, nausea, vomiting
Allergic: Anaphylaxis
Other: Water intoxication

VECURONIUM BROMIDE (NORCURON)

Use(s): Skeletal muscle relaxation

Dosing: Intubating: IV, 0.08-0.1 mg/kg
      Maintenance:
          IV, 0.01-0.05 mg/kg (10%-50% of intubating dose)
          Infusion, 1-2 μg/kg/min
      Pretreatment/priming: IV, 10% of intubating dose given 3-5 min before depolarizer/nondepolarizer relaxant dose

Elimination: Renal, hepatic

How Supplied: Powder for injection, 10 mg/5 ml, 10 mg/10 ml with diluent

Storage: Powder: Room temperature (15°-30° C). Protect from light. When reconstituted with sterile water for injection, solution is stable for 24 hr either refrigerated or at room temperature. When reconstituted with D_5W, NS, or D_5NS, solution is stable for 24 hr when refrigerated (2°-8° C).

Dilution for Infusion: 20 mg in 100 ml D_5W (0.2 mg/ml)

Pharmacology

This monoquaternary analog of pancuronium is a nondepolarizing neuromuscular blocking agent of intermediate duration. Vecuronium competes for cholinergic receptors at the motor end plate. It is a third more potent than pancuronium, but its duration of neuromuscular activity is shorter and recovery more rapid. With continuous infusions (>6 hr), recovery may be prolonged because of the accumulation of active metabolites. Onset time is decreased and duration prolonged with increasing doses. There are no clinically significant changes in hemodynamic parameters. Vagotonic effects may result in bradycardia when vecuronium is combined with potent opioids (e.g., sufentanil, fentanyl). Vecuronium does not release clinically significant concentrations of histamine.

Pharmacokinetics

Onset: <3 min
Peak Effect: 3-5 min
Duration: 25-30 min
Interaction/Toxicity: Neuromuscular blockade is potentiated by aminoglycoside, antibiotics, local anesthetics, loop diuretics, magnesium, lithium, ganglionic blocking drugs, hypothermia, hypokalemia, respiratory acidosis, and prior administration of succinylcholine; dosage requirements are decreased (about 30%-45%) and duration of neuromuscular blockade is prolonged (up to 25%) by volatile anesthetics; recurrent paralysis may occur with quinidine; enhanced neuromuscular blockade may occur in patients with myasthenia gravis or inadequate adrenocortical function; effects are antagonized by anticholinesterases such as neostigmine, edrophonium, pyridostigmine; pretreatment doses of vecuronium decrease fasciculations but reduce intensity and shorten duration of succinylcholine neuromuscular blockade; priming doses decrease the time to onset of maximal blockade by about 30-60 sec; increased resistance or reversal of effects may occur with use of theophylline and in patients with burn injury and paresis.

Guidelines/Precautions

1. Monitor response with peripheral nerve stimulator to minimize risk of overdosage.
2. Reverse effects with anticholinesterases such as neostigmine, edrophonium, or pyridostigmine bromide in conjunction with atropine or glycopyrrolate.

3. Pretreatment doses may induce a degree of neuromuscular blockade sufficient to cause hypoventilation in some patients.

4. Prolonged paralysis (days to months) may occur after termination of long-term infusions in intensive care patients, especially those with renal failure, electrolyte imbalance (hypokalemia, hypocalcemia, hypermagnesemia), and concomitant corticosteroids and/or aminoglycosides. This is due to development of acute myopathy and persistent neuromuscular blockade secondary to accumulation of active metabolites, particularly 3-desacetyl vecuronium (which has 60% of the activity of vecuronium and is excreted by the kidneys).

Principal Adverse Reactions

Cardiovascular: Bradycardia
Pulmonary: Hypoventilation, apnea
Musculoskeletal: Inadequate block, prolonged block

VERAPAMIL HCL (CALAN, ISOPTIN)

Use(s): Treatment of supraventricular tachyarrhythmias, angina; antihypertensive

Dosing: Arrhythmia:

   IV, 5-10 mg (0.075 - 0.25 mg/kg) (give over 2 min), may repeat dose 30 min later if necessary.

   Digitalized patients, PO, 240-320 mg/day in divided doses 3 or 4 times/day every 6-8 hr

   Nondigitalized patients, PO, 240-480 mg/day in divided doses 3 or 4 times/day every 6-8 hr

   Angina: PO, 40-120 mg 3 times a day

Antihypertensive:
>PO, 40-80 mg 3 times a day
>PO sustained release, 120-240 mg daily
>IV, 2.5-10 mg (0.05-0.2 mg/kg), titrate to patient response

Elimination: Renal
How Supplied: Injection, 2.5 mg/ml; tablets, 40 mg, 80 mg, 120 mg; tablets, SR, 120 mg, 180 mg, 240 mg
Storage: Room temperature (15°-30° C). Do not permit to freeze. Protect from light.

Pharmacology

Verapamil is a calcium channel blocker that selectively inhibits the transmembrane influx of calcium ions into cardiac muscle and smooth muscle. The antiarrhythmic effect is due to inhibition of calcium influx through the slow channel in cells of the cardiac conduction system. It slows AV conduction and prolongs the effective refractory period within the AV node in a rate-related manner. It reduces ventricular rate in atrial flutter or fibrillation, interrupts reentry at the AV node, and restores normal sinus rhythm in patients with paroxysmal supraventricular tachycardia (PSVT). Verapamil increases antegrade conduction across accessory bypass tracts, which may result in an increase in the ventricular response rate. It decreases myocardial contractility, systemic vascular resistance, and arterial pressure. Decreased myocardial demand accounts for the effectiveness in the treatment of angina pectoris. It increases intracranial pressure and may decrease uterine blood flow.

Pharmacokinetics

Onset: IV, 2-5 min; PO, 30 min
Peak Effect: IV, within 10 min; PO, 1.2-2 hr

Duration: IV, 30-60 min; PO, 3-7 hr (half-life)

Interaction/Toxicity: Potentiates effects of depolarizing and nondepolarizing muscle relaxants; additive cardiovascular depressant effects may occur with use of volatile anesthetics, other antihypertensives such as diuretics, angiotensin-converting enzyme inhibitors, and vasodilators; increases toxicity of digoxin, benzodiazepines, carbamazepine, oral hypoglycemics, and possibly quinidine and theophylline; cardiac failure, AV conduction disturbances, and sinus bradycardia may occur with concurrent use of beta blockers; severe hypotension and bradycardia may occur with bupivacaine; concomitant use of IV verapamil and IV dantrolene may result in cardiovascular collapse; decreases lithium effect and neurotoxicity; decreased clearance may occur with cimetidine; verapamil is chemically incompatible with solutions of bicarbonate or nafcillin; may be displaced from binding sites by, or may displace from binding sites, other highly protein-bound drugs such as oral anticoagulants, hydantoins, salicylates, sulfonamides, and sulfonylureas.

Guidelines/Precautions

1. May worsen heart failure in patients with poor left ventricular function.
2. Excessive bradycardia, AV block may be treated with isoproterenol, calcium chloride, norepinephrine, atropine, or cardiac pacing.
3. Rapid ventricular rate (caused by antegrade conduction in flutter/fibrillation with Wolff-Parkinson-White [WPW] may be treated with procainamide, lidocaine, or DC cardioversion.

4. Use with caution in patients receiving any highly protein-bound drug such as oral anticoagulants, hydantoins, salicylates, sulfonamides, and sulfonylureas.
5. Do not chew or divide sustained-release tablets.

Principal Adverse Reactions

Cardiovascular: Hypotension, bradycardia, tachycardia
Pulmonary: Bronchospasm, laryngospasm
CNS: Dizziness, headache, seizures
GI: Nausea, abdominal discomfort
Allergic: Urticaria, pruritus

Volatile Anesthetics

II

DESFLURANE (SUPRANE)

Use(s): Inhalation anesthesia

Dosing: Titrate to effect for induction or maintenance of anesthesia

Elimination: Pulmonary, hepatic, renal

How Supplied: Volatile liquid

Storage: Room temperature (15°-30° C).

Pharmacology

Desflurane is a nonflammable fluorinated methyl ethyl ether. It differs from isoflurane by the substitution of a fluorine atom for chlorine. Desflurane has a vapor pressure of approximately 673 mm Hg at 20° C and boils at 23.5° C. Unlike other volatile anesthetics, the low boiling point of desflurane precludes its delivery by standard vaporizers. Maintenance of a stable inspired concentration requires the use of electrically heated and pressurized vaporizers and flow meters calibrated in ml/min vapor output. Desflurane is less potent than isoflurane with a MAC in oxygen of 6% atm and in 60% nitrous oxide of 2.8% atm. The blood/gas partition coefficient at 37° C is 0.42. This low solubility in blood means a rapid induction of anesthesia. After 30 min of administration, the ratio of alveolar concentrations to the inspired concentration is 0.91 compared with 0.85 for

359

sevoflurane, 0.99 for nitrous oxide, and 0.73 for isoflurane. Unlike sevoflurane, desflurane may cause coughing and excitation, which may limit the speed of induction. The low tissue solubility of desflurane (fat/blood partition coefficient, 18.7) results in rapid elimination and awakening. After 5 min, the ratio of the alveolar concentration relative to the concentration present at the conclusion of administration is 0.12, compared with 0.22 for isoflurane and 0.25 for halothane. Because of the fast washout rate for desflurane, addition of nitrous oxide does not confer any kinetic advantages (unlike the other volatile anesthetics). Desflurane is very resistant to degradation by soda lime and thus can be used in low-flow or closed-system anesthesia. Compared with isoflurane, desflurane undergoes significantly less metabolism to fluoride and nonvolatile organic fluoride compounds. A 1-MAC hour does not result in any change in the serum fluoride concentration. Like isoflurane, desflurane causes a moderate increase in $Paco_2$ (approximately 20%) reflecting an increase in the rate of breathing insufficient to offset a decrease in tidal volume. Depression of ventilation reflects a direct depressant effect on the medullary ventilatory center and perhaps peripheral effects on intercostal muscle function. Bronchial smooth muscle relaxation may be produced by a direct effect or indirectly by reductions in afferent nerve traffic or central medullary depression of bronchoconstriction reflexes. Desflurane produces dose-dependent reductions of arterial blood pressure principally through peripheral vasodilation. Mean arterial pressure is preserved to a greater degree than with equipotent doses of isoflurane. At light levels of anesthesia, there is little effect on heart rate. Deeper levels of desflurane may be associated with transient increases in plasma catecholamines, heart rate, and blood pressure. Desflurane attenuates baroreceptor reflex responses (tachycardia) to hypotension and vasomotor reflex responses (increased peripheral resistance) to hypovolemia. At equipotent concentrations, desflurane produces less direct decreases in myocardial contractility than isoflurane. Like isoflurane, desflurane does not sensitize the heart to catecholamines. In one study, the dose of submucosally injected epinephrine necessary to produce ventricular cardiac arrhythmias in 50% of patients anesthetized with a 0.8 MAC concentration of desflurane was 6.9 μg/kg, compared with an epinephrine dosage of 5.7 μg/kg with a 0.7 MAC concentration of isoflurane. Unlike isoflurane, desflurane does not cause coronary artery vasodilation that may lead to coronary artery steal syndrome. Decrease in cerebral metabolic rate is closely linked to cerebral electrical activity. Increased anesthetic concentrations decrease EEG wave frequency and increase voltage with electrical silence at high concentrations. Desflurane, like isoflurane, may produce a dose-related decrease in the amplitude and increase in the latency of cortical components of somatosensory-evoked potentials. The latencies of certain peaks of brainstem auditory evoked potentials may be increased. Cerebral vasodilation produced by desflurane causes an increase in cerebral blood flow and cerebral blood volume. Elevation of intracranial pressure parallels increase in cerebral blood flow. The increase in cerebral blood flow is attenuated with time and reflects a return of cerebral vascular autoregulation. Like isoflurane, CO_2 reactivity is preserved and hyperventilation of the lungs ($Paco_2 \leq 30$) may decrease cerebral blood flow and intracranial pressure. Desflurane produces uterine vasodilation and dose-dependent decrease in uterine blood flow. Desflurane has a direct muscle-relaxant effect, and potentiation of neuromuscular blocking drugs may involve desensitization of the postjunctional membrane. Desflurane potentiates muscle relaxants to an extent similar to isoflurane or enflurane and to a greater extent than halothane or nitrous oxide. Unlike isoflurane, desflurane does not increase muscle blood flow. Desflurane can trigger malignant hyperthermia in susceptible swine.

Pharmacokinetics

Onset: Loss of eyelid reflex (2.5 MAC desflurane), 1.2 min
Peak Effect: Dose dependent
Duration: Emergence time (response to commands) after thiopental for induction and 60% nitrous oxide plus 0.65 MAC desflurane, 8.8 min
Interaction/Toxicity: Ventilatory and circulatory depressant effects are decreased by nitrous oxide substitution; circulatory depressant effects are potentiated by arterial hypoxemia, antihypertensives, beta adrenergic antagonists, calcium channel blockers; potentiates depolarizing and nondepolarizing muscle relaxants; minimum alveolar concentration (MAC) decreased by nitrous oxide, clonidine, lithium, ketamine, pancuronium, narcotic agonists, narcotic agonist-antagonist, physostigmine, neostigmine, sedative-hypnotics, chlorpromazine, verapamil, hypothermia, hyponatremia, hypo-osmolality, pregnancy, Δ-9-tetrahydrocannabinol; minimum alveolar concentration (MAC) is increased by MAO inhibitors, ephedrine, levodopa, chronic ethanol abuse, hypernatremia, hyperthermia, acute cocaine and acute amphetamine ingestion.

Guidelines/Precautions

1. Patients with stenotic lesions of the aortic or mitral valves poorly tolerate changes in blood pressure and systemic vascular resistance.

2. The minimum alveolar concentration (MAC) is highest in the first 6 months of life and is slightly lower in neonates. Beyond adolescence, anesthetic requirements decrease with age so that an 80-year-old patient should require only three fourths the alveolar concentration for anesthesia required for a young adult.

3. Produces dose-related depression of uterine contractility and tone, which can contribute to perioperative blood loss. However, the uterine response to oxytocic drugs is blocked only at high concentrations (>0.5%)

4. Desflurane crosses the placental barrier, and the degree of fetal and neonatal depression (hypotension, hypoxia, acidosis) is directly proportional to the depth and duration of maternal anesthesia.

5. Changes in mental function may persist beyond the period of anesthetic administration and the immediate postoperative period. Psychomotor performance and driving skills may be altered.

6. Use is contraindicated in patients with known or suspected genetic susceptibility to malignant hyperthermia.

7. Abrupt onset of malignant hyperthermia may be triggered by desflurane. Early premonitory signs include muscle rigidity, especially jaw muscles, tachycardia and tachypnea unresponsive to increased depth of anesthesia, evidence of increased oxygen consumption and carbon dioxide production (change in color and increased temperature of the CO_2 absorber), rising body temperature, and metabolic acidosis.

Principal Adverse Reactions

Cardiovascular: Hypotension, arrhythmias
Pulmonary: Respiratory depression, apnea

CNS: Dizziness, euphoria, increased cerebral blood flow and intracranial pressure
GI/Hepatic: Nausea, vomiting, ileus, hepatic dysfunction
GU: Renal dysfunction
Metabolic: Malignant hyperthermia

ENFLURANE (ETHRANE)

Use(s): Inhalation anesthesia

Dosing: Titrate to effect for induction or maintenance of anesthesia
Elimination: Pulmonary, hepatic, renal
How Supplied: Volatile liquid, 125 ml, 250 ml
Storage: Room temperature (15°-30° C).

Pharmacology

Enflurane is a nonflammable fluorinated ethyl methyl ether. It has a vapor pressure of approximately 175 mm Hg at 20° C and boils at 56.5° C. In this respect it is similar to other volatile anesthetics and can be delivered by standard vaporizers. It is less potent than isoflurane with a MAC in oxygen of 1.7% atm and in 70% nitrous oxide of 0.65% atm. The blood/gas partition coefficient at 37° C is 1.91. This intermediate solubility in blood combined with a high potency produces a rapid induction of anesthesia. After 30 min of administration, the ratios of alveolar concentrations to the inspired concentration is 0.65, compared with 0.99 for nitrous oxide and 0.73 for isoflurane. The intermediate tissue solubility of enflurane (fat/blood partition coefficient, 36.0) results in rapid elimination and awakening. After 5 min, the ratio of the alveolar concentration relative to the concentration present at the conclusion of administration is 0.24 compared with 0.22 for isoflurane. Enflurane is slowly metabolized by the hepatic mixed-function oxidase system. Biotransformation releases fluoride ions by oxidative dehalogenation. Peak plasma fluoride concentrations after a 2.5-MAC-hr exposure to enflurane are about 20 μmol/L, which is approximately one third the level considered to be potentially nephrotoxic. Enflurane is resistant to degradation by soda lime and thus can be used in low-flow or closed-system anesthesia. Like isoflurane, enflurane causes a moderate increase in $Paco_2$ (approximately 20%), reflecting an increase in the rate of breathing insufficient to offset a decrease in tidal volume. Depression of ventilation reflects a direct depressant effect on the medullary ventilatory center and perhaps peripheral effects on intercostal muscle function. Bronchial smooth-muscle relaxation may be produced by a direct effect or indirectly by reductions in afferent nerve traffic or central medullary depression of bronchoconstriction reflexes. Enflurane inhibits the hypoxic pulmonary vasoconstrictor response (HPV) in a dose-related manner. It has little or no effect on pulmonary vascular smooth muscle. Enflurane produces dose-dependent reductions of arterial blood pressure in part or whole, a consequence of decreases in myocardial contractility and cardiac output. It produces dose-dependent elevations in heart rate. Enflurane attenuates baroreceptor reflex responses (tachycardia) to hypotension and vasomotor reflex responses (increased peripheral resistance) to hypovolemia. Like isoflurane, enflurane does not sensitize the heart to catecholamines. In one study, the dose of submucosally injected epinephrine necessary to produce ventricular cardiac arrhythmias in 50% of patients anesthetized with a 1.25 MAC concentration of enflurane was 10.9

μg/kg, compared with 1.5 μg/kg for halothane and 6.5 μg/kg for isoflurane. Unlike isoflurane, enflurane does not cause coronary artery vasodilation that may lead to coronary artery steal syndrome. Decrease in cerebral metabolic rate is closely linked to cerebral electrical activity. Increased anesthetic concentrations decrease EEG wave frequency and increase voltage. Electrical silence does not occur, but a high-voltage repetitive-spiking activity may be produced. This activity may be attenuated or abolished by decreasing the enflurane dose or increasing the arterial carbon dioxide partial pressure ($Paco_2$ >30 mm Hg). Enflurane does not enhance preexisting epileptic foci, with the possible exceptions being certain types of myoclonic epilepsy and photosensitive epilepsy. Enflurane, compared with isoflurane or halothane, produces the greatest dose-related decrease in the amplitude and increase in the latency of cortical components of somatosensory-evoked potentials. The latencies of certain peaks of brainstem auditory evoked potentials may be increased. Cerebral vasodilation produced by enflurane causes an increase in cerebral blood flow and cerebral blood volume. Elevation of intracranial pressure parallels increase in cerebral blood flow. Unlike isoflurane or halothane, hyperventilation does not attenuate such increase but on the contrary increases the risk of seizure activity, which could lead to an elevation in cerebral metabolic oxygen requirements, carbon dioxide production, increased cerebral blood flow, and increased intracranial pressure. Enflurane increases both the rate of production and resistance to reabsorption of cerebrospinal fluid, which may contribute to sustained increases in intracranial pressure associated with administration of this drug. Enflurane produces uterine vasodilation and dose-dependent decrease in uterine blood flow. Enflurane has a direct muscle-relaxant effect, and potentiation of neuro-muscular blocking drugs may involve desensitization of the postjunctional membrane. Enflurane potentiates muscle relaxants to an extent similar to isoflurane or desflurane and to a greater extent than halothane or nitrous oxide. Enflurane can trigger malignant hyperthermia in suscepti-ble swine.

Pharmacokinetics

Onset: Loss of eyelid reflex (2.4 MAC enflurane plus 66% N_2O): 2.9 min

Peak Effect: Surgical anesthesia, 2% to 4.5% produces anesthesia in 7-10 min

Duration: Emergence time (response to commands) after thiopental for induction and 66% nitrous oxide plus 0.9 MAC enflurane, 15.1 min

Interaction/Toxicity: Ventilatory and circulatory depres-sant effects are decreased by nitrous oxide substitution; cir-culatory depressant effects are potentiated by arterial hypoxemia, antihypertensives, beta adrenergic antagonists, calcium channel blockers; potentiates depolarizing and nondepolarizing muscle relaxants; decreases pulmonary extraction and increases serum levels of propofol and nor-epinephrine; minimum alveolar concentration (MAC) is decreased by nitrous oxide, clonidine, lithium, ketamine, pancuronium, narcotic agonists, narcotic agonist-antago-nist, physostigmine, neostigmine, sedative-hypnotics, chlor-promazine, verapamil, hypothermia, hyponatremia, hypoos-molality, pregnancy, Δ-9-tetrahydrocannabinol; minimum alveolar concentration (MAC) is increased by MAO inhibitors, ephedrine, levodopa, chronic ethanol abuse, hypernatremia, hyperthermia, and acute cocaine and acute amphetamine ingestion.

Guidelines/Precautions

1. Patients with stenotic lesions of the aortic or mitral valves poorly tolerate changes in blood pressure and systemic vascular resistance.
2. The minimum alveolar concentration (MAC) is highest in the first 6 months of life and is slightly lower in neonates. Beyond adolescence, anesthetic requirements decrease with age so that an 80-year-old patient should require only three fourths the alveolar concentration for anesthesia required for a young adult.
3. Enflurane produces dose-related depression of uterine contractility and tone, which can contribute to perioperative blood loss. However, the uterine response to oxytocic drugs is blocked only at high concentrations (>1.0%).
4. Enflurane crosses the placental barrier, and the degree of fetal and neonatal depression (hypotension, hypoxia, acidosis) is directly proportional to the depth and duration of maternal anesthesia.
5. Changes in mental function may persist beyond the period of anesthetic administration and the immediate postoperative period. Psychomotor performance and driving skills may be altered.
6. Use is contraindicated in patients with seizure disorders and known or suspected genetic susceptibility to malignant hyperthermia.
7. Abrupt onset of malignant hyperthermia may be triggered by enflurane. Early premonitory signs include muscle rigidity, especially jaw muscles, tachycardia and tachypnea unresponsive to increased depth of anesthesia, evidence of increased oxygen consumption and carbon dioxide production (change in color and increased temperature of the CO_2 absorber), rising body temperature, and metabolic acidosis.

Principal Adverse Reactions

Cardiovascular: Hypotension, arrhythmias
Pulmonary: Respiratory depression, apnea
CNS: Seizures, dizziness, euphoria, increased cerebral blood flow and intracranial pressure
GI: Nausea, vomiting, hepatic dysfunction
GU: Renal dysfunction, renal failure
Musculoskeletal: Motor activity of various muscle groups
Metabolic: Malignant hyperthermia, glucose elevation

HALOTHANE (FLUOTHANE)

Use(s): Inhalation anesthesia

Dosing: Titrate to effect for induction or maintenance of anesthesia
Elimination: Pulmonary, hepatic, renal
How Supplied: Volatile liquid, 125 ml, 250 ml
Storage: Room temperature (15°-25° C). Protect from light.

Pharmacology

A nonflammable halogenated alkene, halothane is 2-bromo-2chloro-1,1,1-trifluoroethane. It has a vapor pressure of approximately 241 mm Hg at 20° C and boils at 50.2° C. In this respect it is similar to other volatile anesthetics and can be delivered by standard vaporizers. It is more potent than isoflurane with a MAC in oxygen of 0.77% atm and in 66% nitrous oxide of 0.29% atm. The blood/gas partition coefficient at 37° C is 2.3. The intermediate solubility in blood combined with a high potency permits rapid onset and recovery from anesthesia. After 30 min of administration, the ratio of alveolar concentration to the inspired concentration in adults is 0.58, compared with 0.99 for nitrous oxide and 0.73 for isoflurane. The alveolar rate of rise of halothane is more rapid in children, with a ratio of alveolar concentration to the inspired concentration of 0.8 after 30 min. This probably results from the greater ventilation and perfusion per kilogram of tissue in children and the fact that the increased perfusion is devoted mainly to the vessel-rich group. After the first few minutes of emergence, with alveolar concentration less than 0.01 MAC, rapid decline of alveolar concentrations depends more on metabolism and less on blood solubility. The intermediate tissue solubility (fat/blood partition coefficient, 60.0) and considerable metabolism of halothane result in rapid elimination and awakening. After 5 min the ratios of the alveolar concentration relative to the concentration present at the conclusion of administration is 0.25, compared with 0.22 for isoflurane. Halothane is susceptible to decomposition to hydrochloric acid, hydrobromic acid, chloride, bromide, and phosgene. For this reason, it is stored in amber-colored bottles, and thymol is added as a preservative to prevent spontaneous oxidative decomposition. Thymol that remains in vaporizers after vaporization of halothane can cause vaporizer turnstiles or temperature-compensating devices to malfunction. Halothane does not decompose in contact with warm soda lime and thus can be used in low-flow or closed-system anesthesia. When moisture is present, the vapor attacks aluminium, brass, and lead, but not copper. Rubber, some plastics, and similar materials are soluble in halothane (rubber/gas partition coefficient of 120 for halothane compared with 62 for isoflurane, 74 for enflurane, and 1.2 for nitrous oxide) and will deteriorate rapidly in contact with halothane liquid or vapor. Like isoflurane, halothane causes a moderate increase in PaCO$_2$ (approximately 20%), reflecting an increase in the rate of breathing insufficient to offset a decrease in tidal volume. Depression of ventilation reflects a direct depressant effect on the medullary ventilatory center and perhaps peripheral effects on intercostal muscle function. Bronchial smooth-muscle relaxation may be produced by a direct effect or indirectly by reductions in afferent nerve traffic or central medullary depression of bronchoconstriction reflexes. Halothane inhibits the hypoxic pulmonary vasoconstrictor response (HPV) at inspired concentrations of 3% or greater. It has little or no effect on pulmonary vascular smooth muscle. Halothane produces dose-dependent reductions of arterial blood pressure in part or whole, a consequence of decreases in myocardial contractility and cardiac output. Halothane frequently decreases heart rate (reversible with atropine) and may slow the conduction of cardiac impulses through the atrioventricular node and His-Purkinje system. This increases the likelihood of cardiac arrhythmias caused by a reentry mechanism. Junctional rhythm leading to reductions of blood pressure may occur during administration of halothane and most likely reflects suppression of sinus node activity. Halothane attenuates baroreceptor reflex responses (tachycardia) to hypotension and vasomotor reflex responses (increased peripheral resistance) to hypovolemia. It sensitizes the myocardium to the action of epinephrine and norepinephrine; the combination may cause serious cardiac arrhythmias. In one study, the dose of submucosally injected epinephrine necessary to produce ventricular cardiac arrhythmias in 50% of patients anesthetized with a 1.25 MAC concentration of halothane was 1.5 μg/kg, compared with 6.5 μg/kg for isoflurane and 10.9 μg/kg for enflurane. In contrast to adults, children tolerate higher doses of subcutaneous epinephrine (7.8-10 μg/kg) injected with or without lidocaine during halothane anesthesia. Unlike isoflurane, halothane does not cause coronary artery vasodilation that may lead to coronary artery steal syndrome. Decrease in cerebral metabolic rate is closely linked to cerebral electrical activity. Increased anesthetic concentrations decrease EEG wave frequency and increase voltage, with electrical silence at high concentrations (3.5 MAC). Halothane, like isoflurane or enflurane but to a lesser degree, may produce a dose-related decrease in the amplitude and increase in the latency of cortical components of somatosensory-evoked potentials. The latencies of certain peaks of brainstem auditory evoked potentials may be increased. Cerebral vasodilation and increase in cerebral blood flow and cerebral blood volume produced by halothane are greater than those produced by isoflurane or enflurane (200% increase in cerebral blood flow at 1.1 MAC of halothane compared with 30%-50% increase with enflurane and no change with isoflurane.) Elevation of intracranial pressure parallels increase in cerebral blood flow. The increase in cerebral blood flow is attenuated with time (within 2 hr for halothane) and reflects a return of cerebral vascular autoregulation. Hyperventilation of the lungs ($Paco_2 \leq 30$) before introduction of halothane opposes the increase in intracranial pressure. Halothane decreases the rate of CSF production but increases resistance to reabsorption. The increase in CSF pressure returns to normal with time. Halothane produces uterine vasodilation and dose-dependent decrease in uterine blood flow. Halothane has a direct muscle-relaxant effect, and potentiation of neuromuscular blocking drugs may involve desensitization of the postjunctional membrane. Halothane potentiates muscle relaxants to a lesser extent than isoflurane or desflurane but to a greater extent than nitrous oxide. Halothane can trigger malignant hyperthermia in susceptible swine.

Pharmacokinetics

Onset: Dose dependent
Peak Effect: Dose dependent; decrease in intellectual function, 2 days
Duration: Dose dependent; decrease in intellectual function, 8 days
Interaction/Toxicity: Ventilatory and circulatory depressant effects are decreased by nitrous oxide substitution; circulatory depressant effects are potentiated by arterial hypoxemia, antihypertensives, beta adrenergic antagonists, and calcium channel blockers; tachycardia, arrhythmias, and hypertension may occur with concomitant use of cocaine and sympathomimetics (e.g., epinephrine); potentiates depolarizing and nondepolarizing muscle relaxants; decreases pulmonary extraction and increases serum levels of norepinephrine and propofol (halothane concentration >1.5%); minimum alveolar concentration (MAC) is decreased by nitrous oxide, clonidine, lithium, ketamine, pancuronium, narcotic agonists, narcotic agonist-antagonist, physostigmine, neostigmine, sedative-hypnotics, chlorpromazine, verapamil, hypothermia, hyponatremia, hypoosmolality, pregnancy, Δ-9-tetrahydrocannabinol; minimum alveolar concentration (MAC) is increased by MAO inhibitors, ephedrine, levodopa, chronic ethanol abuse, hypernatremia, hyperthermia, and acute cocaine and acute amphetamine ingestion.

Guidelines/Precautions

1. Patients with stenotic lesions of the aortic or mitral valves poorly tolerate changes in blood pressure and systemic vascular resistance.

2. The minimum alveolar concentration (MAC) is highest in the first 6 months of life and is slightly lower in neonates. Beyond adolescence, anesthetic requirements decrease with age so that an 80-year-old patient should require only three fourths the alveolar concentration for anesthesia required for a young adult.

3. Halothane is not recommended for obstetric anesthesia except when uterine relaxation is required. It is a potent uterine relaxant and can contribute to perioperative blood loss. However, the uterine response to oxytocic drugs is blocked only at concentrations above 0.25%-0.5%.

4. Halothane crosses the placental barrier, and the degree of fetal and neonatal depression (hypotension, hypoxia, acidosis) is directly proportional to the depth and duration of maternal anesthesia.

5. Halothane administration has been associated with hepatic dysfunction. There may be two types: one characterized by transient elevations in serum levels of liver transaminase enzymes (20%-25% of patients) and the other, fulminant hepatic failure (1 in 7,000 to 1 in 30,000). Patients at particular risk appear to be middle-aged obese females with previous closely spaced halothane administration.

6. Concomitant use with epinephrine, cocaine, or sympathomimetics may be associated with cardiac arrhythmias. These arrhythmias may occur independent of the dose of halothane at alveolar concentrations of 0.5%-2%. Treatment may require therapeutic intervention in addition to decreasing the inhaled concentrations of halothane.

7. Changes in mental function may persist beyond the period of anesthetic administration and the immediate postoperative period. Psychomotor performance and driving skills may be altered.

8. Use is contraindicated in patients with known or suspected genetic susceptibility to malignant hyperthermia.
9. Abrupt onset of malignant hyperthermia may be triggered by halothane. Early premonitory signs include muscle rigidity, especially jaw muscles, tachycardia and tachypnea unresponsive to increased depth of anesthesia, evidence of increased oxygen consumption and carbon dioxide production (change in color and increased temperature of the CO_2 absorber), rising body temperature, and metabolic acidosis.

Principal Adverse Reactions

Cardiovascular: Hypotension, bradycardia, arrhythmias.
Pulmonary: Respiratory depression, apnea
CNS: Dizziness, euphoria, increased cerebral blood flow and intracranial pressure
GI/Hepatic: Nausea, vomiting, ileus, hepatic dysfunction, fulminant hepatic failure
Metabolic: Malignant hyperthermia

ISOFLURANE (FORANE)

Use(s): Inhalation anesthesia

Dosing: Titrate to effect for induction or maintenance of anesthesia
Elimination: Pulmonary, hepatic, renal
How Supplied: Volatile liquid, 100 ml
Storage: Room temperature (15°-30° C).

Pharmacology

Isoflurane is a nonflammable halogenated methyl ethyl ether. It has a vapor pressure of approximately 238 mm Hg at 20° C and boils at 48.5° C (760 mm Hg atmospheric pressure). In this respect it is similar to other volatile anesthetics and can be delivered by standard vaporizers. It has a MAC in oxygen of 1.15% atm and in 70% nitrous oxide of 0.5% atm. The blood/gas partition coefficient is 1.4. This intermediate solubility in blood combined with a high potency means a rapid induction of anesthesia. After 30 min of administration, the ratio of alveolar concentrations to the inspired concentration is 0.73. The intermediate tissue solubility of isoflurane (fat/blood partition coefficient, 45.0) results in rapid elimination and awakening. After 5 min, the ratio of the alveolar concentration relative to the concentration present at the conclusion of administration is 0.22 for isoflurane. Isoflurane is resistant to degradation by soda lime and thus can be used in low-flow or closed-system anesthesia. Isoflurane causes a moderate increase in $Paco_2$ (approximately 20%), reflecting an increase in the rate of breathing insufficient to offset a decrease in tidal volume. Unlike other inhaled anesthetics, above a 1 MAC concentration isoflurane does not produce a further increase in the rate of breathing. Depression of ventilation reflects a direct depressant effect on the medullary ventilatory center and perhaps peripheral effects on intercostal muscle function. Bronchial smooth-muscle relaxation may be produced by a direct effect or indirectly by reductions in afferent nerve traffic or central medullary depression of bronchoconstriction reflexes. Isoflurane inhibits the hypoxic pulmonary vasoconstrictor response (HPV) in a dose-related manner. It has little or no effect on pulmonary vascular smooth muscle. Isoflurane produces dose-dependent reductions of arterial blood pressure principally through peripheral vasodilation. It elevates heart rate 20% above awake levels and independent of dose above 1 MAC. Heart rate increases are more likely to occur in young than elderly patients or neonates and may be accentuated by the presence of other drugs (atropine, meperidine, pancuronium) that independently increase heart rate. Depression of baroreceptor reflex responses (tachycardia) to hypotension and vasomotor reflex responses (increased peripheral resistance) to hypovolemia is less pronounced with isoflurane compared with halothane or enflurane. Decreases in stroke volume are offset by an increase in heart rate such that cardiac output is unchanged. At equipotent concentrations, isoflurane and desflurane produce equivalent direct decreases in myocardial contractility. Isoflurane does not sensitize the heart to catecholamines. In one study, the dose of submucosally injected epinephrine necessary to produce ventricular cardiac arrhythmias in 50% of patients anesthetized with a 1.25 MAC concentration of isoflurane was 6.5 μg/kg, compared with 1.5 μg/kg for halothane and 10.9 μg/kg for enflurane. It causes coronary artery vasodilation that may lead to coronary artery steal syndrome. However, there is no evidence of different outcomes for coronary revascularization operations in patients anesthetized primarily with isoflurane compared with enflurane, halothane, or sufentanil. Isoflurane undergoes minimal metabolism, reflecting its chemical stability and low solubility in tissues. Trifluoroacetic acid is the principal organic fluoride metabolite. The minimal changes in plasma concentrations of fluoride resulting from metabolism of isoflurane plus the absence of reductive metabolism render nephrotoxicity or hepatotoxicity after administration of isoflurane unlikely. Decrease in cerebral metabolic rate is closely linked to cerebral electrical activity. Increased anesthetic concentrations decrease EEG wave frequency and increase voltage, with electrical silence at high concentrations. Isoflurane may produce a dose-related decrease in the amplitude and increase in the latency of cortical components of somatosensory-evoked potentials. The latencies of certain peaks of brainstem auditory evoked potentials may be increased. At 1.1 MAC isoflurane, cerebral vasodilation is minimal or unchanged. Increased concentrations cause an increase in cerebral blood flow and cerebral blood volume. Elevation of intracranial pressure parallels an increase in cerebral blood flow. The increase in cerebral blood flow is attenuated with time and reflects a return of cerebral vascular autoregulation. Hyperventilation of the lungs ($PaCO_2$ ≤30) simultaneous with introduction of isoflurane opposes the increase in intracranial pressure. Isoflurane does not alter production of cerebrospinal fluid and at the same time decreases resistance to its reabsorption. This is consistent with minimal increases in intracranial pressure observed. Isoflurane produces uterine vasodilation and dose-dependent decrease in uterine blood flow. Isoflurane has a direct muscle-relaxant effect, and potentiation of neuromuscular blocking drugs may involve desensitization of the postjunctional membrane and increased muscle blood flow. Isoflurane potentiates muscle relaxants to an extent similar to enflurane or desflurane and to a greater extent than halothane or nitrous oxide. Isoflurane can trigger malignant hyperthermia in susceptible swine.

Pharmacokinetics

Onset: Few minutes (dose dependent)
Peak Effect: Surgical anesthesia, 1.5% to 3.0% produces anesthesia in 7-10 min
Duration: Emergence time (response to commands) after thiopental for induction and 60% nitrous oxide plus 0.65 MAC isoflurane, 15.6 min
Interaction/Toxicity: Ventilatory and circulatory depres-

sant effects are decreased by nitrous oxide substitution; circulatory depressant effects are potentiated by arterial hypoxemia, antihypertensives, beta adrenergic antagonists, calcium channel blockers; potentiates depolarizing and nondepolarizing muscle relaxants; decreases pulmonary extraction and increases serum levels of propofol and norepinephrine; minimum alveolar concentration (MAC) is decreased by nitrous oxide, clonidine, lithium, ketamine, pancuronium, narcotic agonists, narcotic agonist-antagonist, physostigmine, neostigmine, sedative-hypnotics, chlorpromazine, verapamil, hypothermia, hyponatremia, hypo-osmolality, pregnancy, Δ-9-tetrahydrocannabinol; minimum alveolar concentration (MAC) is increased by MAO inhibitors, ephedrine, levodopa, chronic ethanol abuse, hypernatremia, hyperthermia, and acute cocaine and acute amphetamine ingestion.

Guidelines/Precautions

1. Patients with stenotic lesions of the aortic or mitral valves poorly tolerate changes in blood pressure and systemic vascular resistance.
2. The minimum alveolar concentration (MAC) is highest in the first 6 months of life and is slightly lower in neonates. Beyond adolescence, anesthetic requirements decrease with age so that an 80-year-old patient should require only three fourths the alveolar concentration for anesthesia required for a young adult.
3. Produces dose-related depression of uterine contractility and tone, which can contribute to perioperative blood loss. However, the uterine response to oxytocic drugs is blocked only at high concentrations (>0.75%)
4. Crosses the placental barrier, and the degree of fetal and neonatal depression (hypotension, hypoxia, acidosis) is

directly proportional to the depth and duration of maternal anesthesia.

5. Changes in mental function may persist beyond the period of anesthetic administration and the immediate postoperative period. Psychomotor performance and driving skills may be altered.

6. Use is contraindicated in patients with known or suspected genetic susceptibility to malignant hyperthermia.

7. Abrupt onset of malignant hyperthermia may be triggered by isoflurane. Early premonitory signs include muscle rigidity, especially jaw muscles, tachycardia and tachypnea unresponsive to increased depth of anesthesia, evidence of increased oxygen consumption and carbon dioxide production (change in color and increased temperature of the CO_2 absorber), rising body temperature, and metabolic acidosis.

Principal Adverse Reactions

Cardiovascular: Hypotension, tachycardia, arrhythmias, coronary artery steal
Pulmonary: Respiratory depression, apnea
CNS: Dizziness, euphoria, increased cerebral blood flow and intracranial pressure
GI/Hepatic: Nausea, vomiting, ileus, hepatic dysfunction
Metabolic: Malignant hyperthermia, glucose elevation

NITROUS OXIDE (NITROUS OXIDE)

Use(s): Inhalation analgesic, supplementation of anesthesia

Dosing: Titrate to effect for analgesia, induction or maintenance of anesthesia
Elimination: Pulmonary, renal, gastrointestinal tract
How Supplied: Blue cylinders

Storage: Room temperature (15°-30° C).

Pharmacology

Nitrous oxide is a strong analgesic and weak anesthetic usually used in combination with other anesthetics. Although nitrous oxide is nonflammable, it will support combustion. It has a vapor pressure of approximately 39,000 mm Hg at 20° C and boils at -88.0° C. It has a minimum alveolar concentration (MAC) with oxygen of 104% atm. The blood/gas partition coefficient for nitrous oxide is 0.47, compared with 1.4 for isoflurane. This very low solubility in blood means a rapid induction of anesthesia. After 30 min of administration, the ratio of alveolar concentration to the inspired concentration is 0.99, compared with 0.73 for isoflurane. The very low tissue solubility of nitrous oxide (fat/blood partition coefficient, 2.3, compared with fat/blood partition coefficient of 45.0 for isoflurane) results in rapid elimination and awakening. After 5 min, the ratio of the alveolar concentration relative to the concentration present at the conclusion of administration is 0.14, compared with 0.22 for isoflurane. Administration of high concentrations of a rapidly absorbed first gas will facilitate the rate of rise in alveolar concentration of a concomitantly administered second gas, a phenomenon called the second-gas effect. This effect is most pronounced when nitrous oxide is combined with a volatile anesthetic. Nitrous oxide is resistant to degradation by soda lime and thus can be used in low-flow or closed-system anesthesia. Unlike the inhaled anesthetics, nitrous oxide does not increase the $Paco_2$. It increases the rate of breathing more than other inhaled anesthetics at concentrations above 1 MAC. Depression of ventilation occurs at high concentrations (>50%) and reflects a direct depressant effect on the medullary ventilatory center and perhaps peripheral effects on intercostal muscle function. Like other inhaled anesthetics, nitrous oxide decreases functional residual capacity. Bronchial smooth-muscle relaxation may be produced by a direct effect or indirectly by reductions in afferent nerve traffic or central medullary depression of bronchoconstriction reflexes. Nitrous oxide does not inhibit the hypoxic pulmonary vasoconstrictor response (HPV). It may produce increases in pulmonary vascular resistance that are exaggerated in patients with preexisting pulmonary hypertension. Alone in a 40% concentration, nitrous oxide directly depresses the myocardium. When it is given to patients with heart disease, particularly in combination with opioids, it will cause hypotension and a decrease in cardiac output. Combined with other inhaled anesthetics (e.g., desflurane, enflurane, halothane, isoflurane, servoflurane), nitrous oxide is sympathomimetic and has mild cardiac depressant effects. There is decreased cardiac output, increased systemic vascular resistance, and increased arterial pressure. Reduction of concentration and substitution of some of the required volatile anesthetic with nitrous oxide leads to less depression of the circulation at a given MAC level than with either agent alone. There is little effect on heart rate. Nitrous oxide attenuates baroreceptor reflex responses (tachycardia) to hypotension and vasomotor reflex responses (increased peripheral resistance) to hypovolemia. Nitrous oxide enhances isoflurane-induced coronary artery vasodilation that may lead to coronary artery steal syndrome. However, 50% nitrous oxide plus a low concentration of isoflurane (about 0.4 MAC) administered to patients with coronary artery disease improves tolerance to pacing-induced myocardial ischemia. Nitrous oxide probably is not metabolized by human tissue. An estimated

0.04% undergoes reductive metabolism to nitrogen in the gastrointestinal tract. Anaerobic bacteria, such as *Pseudomonas*, are responsible for this reductive metabolism. Reductive products of some nitrogen compounds include free radicals that could produce toxic effects on cells. The potential toxic role of these metabolites, however, remains undocumented. Nitrous oxide inhibits methionine synthetase activity by oxidizing the cobalt atom in vitamin B_{12} from an active to an inactive state. Inhibition of enzyme activity results in decreased availability of tetrahydrofolate, which is necessary for the synthesis of DNA. Interference with DNA synthesis could manifest as spontaneous abortions, congenital anomalies, depression of bone marrow function, and polyneuropathy resembling pernicious anemia in individuals chronically exposed to high concentrations of nitrous oxide. Decrease in cerebral metabolic rate is closely linked to cerebral electrical activity. Increased anesthetic concentrations decrease EEG wave frequency and increase voltage, with electrical silence at high concentrations. Nitrous oxide may produce greater attenuations of somatosensory-evoked potentials than low concentrations of enflurane or isoflurane. Cortical responses are more affected than subcortical responses. Nitrous oxide can increase the latency and decrease amplitude of cortical components of visual and auditory evoked potentials. To a modest degree, cerebral vasodilation produced by nitrous oxide causes an increase in cerebral blood flow and cerebral blood volume. Elevation of intracranial pressure parallels increase in cerebral blood flow. The increase in cerebral blood flow is attenuated with time and reflects a return of cerebral vascular autoregulation. Hyperventilation of the lungs ($Pa_{CO_2} \leq 30$) opposes the increase in intracranial pressure. Nitrous oxide does not relax skeletal muscles, and in doses that exceed 1 MAC, may produce skeletal muscle rigidity. It does not have significant effects on uterine contractility. Nitrous oxide, compared with volatile anesthetics, is a weak trigger for malignant hyperthermia.

Pharmacokinetics

Onset: Few minutes (dose dependent)
Peak Effect: Dose dependent
Duration: Varies (dose dependent); emergence time (response to commands) after thiopental for induction and 60% nitrous oxide plus 0.65 MAC isoflurane, 15.6 min; memory impairment, 24 hr or more
Interaction/Toxicity: Ventilatory depressant effects are potentiated by volatile anesthetics; circulatory depressant effects are potentiated by arterial hypoxemia, volatile anesthetics, antihypertensives, beta adrenergic antagonists, calcium channel blockers; increases toxicity of methotrexate (e.g., leukopenia); decreases pulmonary extraction and increases serum levels of propofol and norepinephrine; facilitates uptake of other inhalation anesthetics (second-gas effect); reduces requirements for volatile anesthetics approximately equal to 1% of the MAC value for each volume-percentage alveolar nitrous oxide concentration.

Guidelines/Precautions

1. The chief danger in the use of nitrous oxide is hypoxia; at least 30% oxygen should be used.
2. Nitrous oxide, which is 34 times more soluble than nitrogen, diffuses into air-containing cavities faster than nitrogen can leave, causing potentially dangerous pressure accumulation (e.g., middle ear abnormalities, bowel obstruction, pneumothorax). Nitrous oxide (to a greater extent than other gases) diffuses into air-inflat-

ed endotracheal tube cuffs and increases intracuff volume and pressure, which may result in significant glottic or subglottic trauma. Therefore during general anesthesia, intracuff volume and pressure should be periodically readjusted. Rapid absorption of nitrous oxide after administration is discontinued can produce negative pressures in the middle ear, manifesting as serous otitis or transient postoperative hearing loss.

3. During the first 5 to 10 min of recovery from anesthesia, the outpouring of large volumes of nitrous oxide may displace alveolar oxygen and produce diffusion hypoxia. Displacement of alveolar carbon dioxide may decrease respiratory drive and hence ventilation. It is prudent to administer 100% oxygen at this critical time of recovery.

4. In healthy patients undergoing surgery, megaloblastic bone marrow changes may be seen after about 12 hr of exposure to 50% N_2O and earlier in seriously ill patients. These changes may be preventable by pretreating patients with large doses of folinic acid. Folinic acid is converted to tetrahydrofolate, which is necessary for the synthesis of DNA.

5. An increased risk of renal and hepatic diseases has been reported in dental personnel who work in areas where nitrous oxide is used. Nitrous oxide may precipitate neurologic disease in patients with unrecognized vitamin B_{12} deficiency.

6. Patients with stenotic lesions of the aortic or mitral valves poorly tolerate changes in blood pressure and systemic vascular resistance.

7. Nitrous oxide crosses the placental barrier, and the degree of fetal and neonatal depression (hypotension, hypoxia, acidosis) is directly proportional to the depth and duration of maternal anesthesia.

8. The newborn with or without preexisting pulmonary hypertension may be uniquely vulnerable to the pulmonary-vascular-constricting effects of nitrous oxide. In patients with congenital heart disease, these increases in pulmonary vascular resistance may increase the magnitude of right-to-left intracardiac shunting of blood and further jeopardize arterial oxygenation.

9. Changes in mental function may persist beyond the period of anesthetic administration and the immediate postoperative period. Psychomotor performance and driving skills may be altered.

10. Use only with extreme caution and vigilant monitoring in patients with known or suspected genetic susceptibility to malignant hyperthermia.

11. Abrupt onset of malignant hyperthermia may be triggered by nitrous oxide. Early premonitory signs include muscle rigidity, especially jaw muscles, tachycardia and tachypnea unresponsive to increased depth of anesthesia, evidence of increased oxygen consumption and carbon dioxide production (change in color and increased temperature of the CO_2 absorber), rising body temperature, and metabolic acidosis.

Principal Adverse Reactions

Cardiovascular: Hypotension, arrhythmias.

Pulmonary: Respiratory depression, apnea, diffusion hypoxia

CNS: Dizziness, euphoria, increased cerebral blood flow and intracranial pressure, peripheral neuropathy, subacute combined degeneration of the spinal cord (with chronic abuse and gross exposure)

GI/Hepatic: Nausea, vomiting, ileus

Hematologic: Megaloblastic anemia, bone marrow depression
Metabolic: Malignant hyperthermia
Other: Disinhibition, sexual illusions (at concentration >50%)

SEVOFLURANE (SEVOFLURANE)

Use(s): Inhalation anesthesia

Dosing: Titrate to effect for induction or maintenance of anesthesia
Elimination: Pulmonary, hepatic, renal
How Supplied: Volatile liquid
Storage: Room temperature (15°-30° C).

Pharmacology

Sevoflurane is a nonflammable fluorinated isopropyl ether. It has a vapor pressure of approximately 162 mm Hg at 20° C and boils at 58.5° C. In this respect it is similar to other volatile anesthetics and can be delivered by standard vaporizers. It is less potent than isoflurane, with a MAC in oxygen of 1.71% atm and in 63.5% nitrous oxide of 0.66% atm. The blood/gas partition coefficient at 37° C is 0.59. This low solubility in blood produces a rapid induction of anesthesia. Sevoflurane is less of an irritant to the upper respiratory tract than desflurane, causing less coughing and laryngospasm on induction. After 30 min of administration, the ratio of alveolar concentrations to the inspired concentration is 0.85, compared with 0.9 for desflurane, 0.99 for nitrous oxide, and 0.73 for isoflurane. The low tissue solubility of sevoflurane (fat/blood partition coefficient, 53.4) results in rapid elimination and awakening. After 5 min, the ratio of the alveolar concentration relative to the concentration present at the conclusion of administration is 0.16, compared with 0.22 for isoflurane. Sevoflurane undergoes temperature-dependent degradation by soda lime and baralyme and thus may not be used in low-flow or closed-system anesthesia. Like isoflurane, sevoflurane causes a moderate increase in $PaCO_2$ (approximately 20%), reflecting an increase in the rate of breathing insufficient to offset a decrease in tidal volume. Depression of ventilation reflects a direct depressant effect on the medullary ventilatory center and perhaps peripheral effects on intercostal muscle function. Bronchial smooth muscle relaxation may be produced by a direct effect or indirectly by reductions in afferent nerve traffic or central medullary depression of bronchoconstriction reflexes. Sevoflurane produces dose-dependent reductions of arterial blood pressure principally through peripheral vasodilation. There is little effect on heart rate. Sevoflurane attenuates baroreceptor reflex responses (tachycardia) to hypotension and vasomotor reflex responses (increased peripheral resistance) to hypovolemia. At equipotent concentrations, sevoflurane and isoflurane produce equivalent direct decreases in myocardial contractility. Like isoflurane, sevoflurane does not sensitize the heart to catecholamines. The arrhythmogenic threshold is intermediate between enflurane and isoflurane. In one study, the dose of submucosally injected epinephrine necessary to produce ventricular cardiac arrhythmias in 50% of patients anesthetized with a 1.3 MAC concentration of sevoflurane was 8.57 μg/kg, compared with 5.17 μg/kg for enflurane and 9.81 μg/kg for isoflurane. Unlike isoflurane, sevoflurane may not cause coronary artery vasodilation that may lead to coronary artery steal syndrome. Sevoflurane undergoes oxidative metabolism in the liver with a serum fluoride concentration of approximately 22

μmol/L after a 1-MAC-hr exposure. The magnitude of sevoflurane metabolism resembles that of enflurane (peak plasma fluoride concentrations after a 2.5-MAC-hr exposure to enflurane are about 20 μmol/L). Decrease in cerebral metabolic rate is closely linked to cerebral electrical activity. Increased anesthetic concentrations decrease EEG wave frequency and increase voltage, with electrical silence at high concentrations. Sevoflurane, like isoflurane, may produce a dose-related decrease in the amplitude and increase in the latency of cortical components of visual and auditory evoked potentials. Cerebral vasodilation produced by sevoflurane causes an increase in cerebral blood flow and cerebral blood volume. Elevation of intracranial pressure parallels increase in cerebral blood flow. The increase in cerebral blood flow is attenuated with time and reflects a return of cerebral vascular autoregulation. Hyperventilation of the lungs (Paco$_2$ $\leq$30) opposes the increase in intracranial pressure. Sevoflurane produces uterine vasodilation and dose-dependent decrease in uterine blood flow. Sevoflurane has a direct muscle-relaxant effect, and potentiation of neuromuscular blocking drugs may involve desensitization of the postjunctional membrane. Sevoflurane can trigger malignant hyperthermia in susceptible swine.

Pharmacokinetics

Onset: Loss of eyelid reflex (1.8 MAC sevoflurane plus 66% N$_2$O), 1.6 min
Peak Effect: Dose dependent
Duration: Emergence time (response to commands) after thiopental for induction and 66% nitrous oxide plus 0.9 MAC servoflurane, 14.3 min
Interaction/Toxicity: Ventilatory and circulatory depressant effects are decreased by nitrous oxide substitution; cir-

culatory depressant effects are potentiated by arterial hypoxemia, antihypertensives, beta adrenergic antagonists, calcium channel blockers; potentiates depolarizing and nondepolarizing muscle relaxants; minimum alveolar concentration (MAC) is decreased by nitrous oxide, clonidine, lithium, ketamine, pancuronium, narcotic agonists, narcotic agonist-antagonist, physostigmine, neostigmine, sedative-hypnotics, chlorpromazine, verapamil, hypothermia, hyponatremia, hypoosmolality, pregnancy, Δ-9-tetrahydro-cannabinol; minimum alveolar concentration (MAC) is increased by MAO inhibitors, ephedrine, levodopa, chronic ethanol abuse, hypernatremia, hyperthermia, and acute cocaine and acute amphetamine ingestion.

Guidelines/Precautions

1. Patients with stenotic lesions of the aortic or mitral valves poorly tolerate changes in blood pressure and systemic vascular resistance.

2. The minimum alveolar concentration (MAC) is highest in the first 6 months of life and is slightly lower in neonates. Beyond adolescence, anesthetic requirements decrease with age so that an 80-year-old patient should require only three fourths the alveolar concentration for anesthesia required for a young adult.

3. Produces dose-related depression of uterine contractility and tone, which can contribute to perioperative blood loss.

4. Crosses the placental barrier, and the degree of fetal and neonatal depression (hypotension, hypoxia, acidosis) is directly proportional to the depth and duration of maternal anesthesia.

5. Changes in mental function may persist beyond the period of anesthetic administration and the immediate post-

operative period. Psychomotor performance and driving skills may be altered.

6. Use is contraindicated in patients with known or suspected genetic susceptibility to malignant hyperthermia.

7. Abrupt onset of malignant hyperthermia may be triggered by sevoflurane. Early premonitory signs include muscle rigidity, especially jaw muscles, tachycardia and tachypnea unresponsive to increased depth of anesthesia, evidence of increased oxygen consumption and carbon dioxide production (change in color and increased temperature of the CO_2 absorber), rising body temperature, and metabolic acidosis.

Principal Adverse Reactions

Cardiovascular: Hypotension, arrhythmias
Pulmonary: Respiratory depression, apnea
CNS: Dizziness, euphoria, increased cerebral blood flow and intracranial pressure
GI/Hepatic: Nausea, vomiting, ileus
GU: Renal dysfunction
Metabolic: Malignant hyperthermia

Bibliography

American Hospital Formulary Service, Drug Information, Bethseda, American Society of Hospital Pharmacists, 1994.

Attia RR, et al (editors): *Practical anesthetic pharmacology*, Norwalk, Appleton-Century-Crofts, 1987.

Barash P, et al (editors): *Clinical anesthesia*, Philadelphia, JB Lippincott, 1992.

Berk JL, et al (editors): *Handbook of critical care*, Boston, Little Brown and Company, 1990.

Berry FA, et al (editors): *Anesthetic management of difficult and routine pediatric patients*, New York, Churchill Livingstone, 1990.

Clark W, Brater DC, Johnson AR: *Goth's medical pharmacology*, ed 13, St. Louis, Mosby, 1992.

Drug facts and comparisons, Philadelphia, JB Lippincott, 1994.

Estefanous FG (editor): *Opioids in anesthesia*, Boston, Butterworth Publishers, 1991.

Gilman AG, Goodman LS, Rall TW, et al (editors): *Goodman and Gilman's the pharmacological basis of therapeutics*, New York, Macmillan, 1990.

Hensley FA, et al (editors): *The practice of cardiac anesthesia*, Boston, Little Brown and Company, 1990.

Kaplan JA (editor): *Cardiac anesthesia*, Philadelphia, WB Saunders, 1994.

Miller RD, et al (editors): *Anesthesia*, New York, Churchill Livingstone, 1994.

Omoigui S: *The pain drugs handbook*, St. Louis, Mosby, 1995.

Opie LH, et al (editors): *Drugs for the heart*, Philadelphia, WB Saunders, 1987.

Physician's desk reference, Oradell, Medical Economics Company, 1994.

Ryan JF, et al (editors): *A practice of anesthesia for infants and children*, Philadelphia, WB Saunders, 1986.

Scott DB, et al (editors): *Techniques of regional anesthesia*, Norwalk, Appleton and Lange/Mediglobe, 1989.

Shnider SM, et al (editors): *Anesthesia for obstetrics*, Baltimore, Williams and Wilkins, 1993.

Stoelting RK (editor): *Pharmacology and physiology in anesthetic practice*, Philadelphia, JB Lippincott, 1991.

Wood M (editor): *Drugs and anesthesia*, Baltimore, Williams and Wilkins, 1990.

APPENDICES

Appendix 1

MALIGNANT HYPERTHERMIA PROTOCOL

1. Discontinue all inhalational anesthetics.
2. Hyperventilate with 100% oxygen (15-20 liters/minute).
3. Change the anesthesia circuit and soda lime canister.
4. If possible, get another machine and use a nonrebreathing circuit.
5. Establish lines—a wide bore cannula for CVP, arterial line (if not already in place), Foley catheter, nasogastric tube. Replace all potassium-containing IV fluids (e.g., lactated Ringer's) with normal saline.
6. Administer dantrolene (initial intravenous dose 2.5 mg/kg; titrate further doses as required; maximum dose 10 mg/kg).
   • Dantrolene must be mixed with sterile distilled water.
   • A 70 kg patient will require 9-10 vials (20 mg in each vial) immediately.
   • Remember each vial of dantrolene also contains mannitol 3 g.
7. Start cooling techniques for rapidly increasing temperatures and for those above 40° C:
   • Surface cooling with the patient on a cooling blanket and packed with ice
   • Gastric, rectal, or peritoneal lavage with iced saline
   • Iced IV fluids
   • Pump bypass with a heat exchanger
   Cooling should be stopped when the patient's temperature falls below 38° C in order to prevent inadvertent hypothermia.
8. Treat acidosis with sodium bicarbonate (1-2 mEq/kg initial dose and titrate as necessary).
9. Treat hyperkalemia with sodium bicarbonate, insulin (0.15 μ/kg), and 20% dextrose (500 mg/kg).

10. Treat arrhythmias with procainamide, slow IV 3 mg/kg start, maximum 15 mg/kg.
11. Maintain urine output with mannitol or furosemide.
12. Provide energy substrate with 20% to 50% dextrose with insulin.
13. Provide cardiorespiratory support.
14. Monitor urine output, serum potassium, calcium, arterial blood gases, and clotting studies.
15. Monitor patients in the ICU for at least 24 hr.
16. Follow creatine phosphokinase, calcium, and potassium until they return to normal.
17. Observe patients for disseminated intravascular coagulation.
18. Convert to oral dantrolene when extubated and stable (PO 4-8 mg/kg/day in three divided doses for up to 3 days after the crisis).
19. Counsel patient.

MALIGNANT HYPERTHERMIA HOTLINE
(209) 634-4917
ASK FOR INDEX ZERO
MALIGNANT HYPERTHERMIA CONSULTANT
LIST

Appendix 2

INCOMPATIBILITY TABLE

Physical and Chemical Compatibility for Mixing and Infusing Medications*†

	Aminophylline	Ampicillin	Atropine sulfate	Bretylium	Calcium chloride	Calcium gluconate	Cefazolin	Cimetidine	Diazepam	Diazoxide	Digoxin	Dobutamine	Dopamine	Epinephrine HCl	Furosemide	Gentamicin	Heparin	Hydralazine	Insulin, regular	Isoproterenol
Verapamil	P	P	P	P	P	P	P	P	N	N	P	—	P	P	P	P	P	S	P	P
Tobramycin	N	N	N	N	—	—	N	N	N	N	N	N	N	N	N	N	—	N	N	N
Streptokinase	N	Z	Z	Z	N	Z	Z	Z	Z	Z	Z	Z	Z	Z	Z	Z	Z	N	Z	Z
Sodium bicarbonate	B	Z	—	C	—	—	N	P	N	Z	Z	—	—	—	Z	N	P	N	—	—
Quinidine	Z	Z	Z	P	—	—	Z	Z	P	—	Z	Z	—	—	—	Z	—	Z	—	—
Propranolol	Z	Z	Z	Z	Z	Z	Z	Z	Z	—	Z	Z	Z	Z	Z	Z	Z	Z	Z	Z
Procainamide	Z	Z	P	—	—	Z	Z	Z	Z	Z	Z	Z	Z	Z	Z	Z	Z	Z	Z	Z
Potassium chloride	P	P	P	P	P	P	S	D	D	Z	N	Y	—	P	P	P	P	Y	Z	P
Phytonadione	Z	—	Z	Z	Z	Z	Z	Z	Z	Z	Z	Z	Z	Z	Z	Z	Z	P	Z	Z
Phenytoin	Z	Z	Z	Z	Z	Z	Z	Z	Z	Z	Z	Z	H	Z	Z	Z	Z	Z	Z	Z
Norepinephrine	—	P	Z	Z	P	P	D	Z	D	Z	Z	P	H	P	N	P	P	N	P	—
Nitroprusside	Z	Z	Z	Z	Z	Z	Z	Z	Z	Z	Z	Z	Z	Z	Z	Z	Z	Z	Z	Z
Nitroglycerin	G	Z	Z	Z	G	Z	Z	Z	Z	Z	Z	Z	G	Z	G	Z	Z	G	Z	Z
Netilmicin	Z	Z	P	P	Z	Z	Z	P	Z	Z	Z	Z	Z	Z	Z	Z	Z	Z	Z	Z
Morphine sulfate	—	P	Z	Z	Z	Z	P	Z	Z	Z	Z	Z	Z	H	—	Z	Z	—	Z	—
Lidocaine	P	P	Z	C	P	D	—	D	Z	Z	P	P	—	N	P	Z	P	P	L	—
Isoproterenol	—	P	Z	—	P	P	P	A	P	Z	Z	Z	—	P	P	N	P	P	P	Z
Insulin, regular	—	N	Z	P	Z	Z	Z	A	Z	Z	—	Z	Z	N	Z	P	P	—	Z	N
Hydralazine	—	—	Z	P	Z	Z	Z	Z	Z	Z	H	—	Z	S	Z	N	—	—	P	P
Heparin	P	H	P	Z	Z	Z	P	S	P	Z	Z	Z	P	A	P	D	N	—	P	P
Gentamicin	P	—	P	M	Z	Z	Z	—	P	Z	Z	Z	Z	B	A	P	P	—	Z	Z
Furosemide	B	Z	D	Z	Z	Z	Z	Z	P	P	Z	Z	Z	S	D	N	—	Z	N	N
Epinephrine HCl	—	—	D	Z	—	—	Z	Z	Z	P	P	—	Z	Z	P	—	P	D	Z	Z
Dopamine	P	—	N	C	D	P	Z	Z	P	Z	Z	Z	Z	S	D	P	A	P	N	N
Dobutamine	B	Z	N	P	—	—	Z	Z	M	P	N	Z	Z	Z	S	D	N	B	D	S
Digoxin	Z	Z	Z	D	P	Z	Z	Z	M	Z	Z	Z	Z	Z	Z	Z	Z	H	—	Z
Diazoxide	Z	Z	Z	Z	Z	Z	Z	Z	Z	Z	Z	Z	Z	Z	Z	Z	Z	—	Z	Z
Diazepam	Z	Z	N	Z	Z	Z	Z	Z	P	Z	Z	Z	Z	Z	Z	Z	Z	Z	Z	Z
Cimetidine	—	A	P	Z	Z	Z	P	—	Z	Z	Z	M	Z	P	Z	P	S	P	N	A
Cefazolin	S	S	N	Z	Z	Z	—	P	N	Z	Z	Z	Z	Z	Z	Z	S	N	Z	N
Calcium gluconate	P	P	S	D	—	—	—	Z	Z	Z	Z	Z	Z	Z	P	S	N	Z	N	—
Calcium chloride	Z	N	N	C	—	Z	Z	Z	Z	Z	P	C	D	Z	Z	Z	N	Z	P	P
Bretylium	D	N	Z	N	C	D	N	Z	Z	Z	D	—	N	Z	N	M	N	N	P	—
Atropine sulfate	Z	Z	N	N	C	—	S	N	P	Z	N	D	Z	N	H	P	N	N	Z	N
Ampicillin	N	Z	N	—	S	S	A	Z	Z	Z	N	—	Z	N	—	P	—	N	P	P
Aminophylline	P	Z	N	D	N	P	S	—	Z	Z	P	B	—	P	B	P	—	—	—	—

Lidocaine	P	P	N	C	P	D	I	D	B	B	P	P	P	I	N	P	P	P	L	I		N	N	D	N	P
Morphine sulfate	I	N	P	N		N	N	N	N	N	N	N	N	N	N	N	N	N	N	Y		N	N	N	N	N
Netilmicin	N	P	N	P		N	N	N	N	N	N	N	N	G	N	B	B	N	N	N		N	B	B	N	N
Nitroglycerin	G	N	G	N	N	G	N	D		N	G	G	N	N	N	N	N	G	N	N		N	B	N	N	N
Nitroprusside	N	N	N	N		N	N	N	H	P	N		N	N	N	N	N	N	N	N		N	B	N	N	N
Norepinephrine	I	P	N	N	P	D	N	P		P	H	P	N	N	N	N	N	N	N	N		N	N	N	N	N
Phenytoin	N	N	N	N	N	P		N	N		P	I	N		N	N	N	N	N	N		N	N	N	N	N
Phytonadione	N	I	N	P	N	N	P		I		P	P	P	N	P	N	N	N	N	N		P	N	N	N	N
Potassium chloride	P	P	P	P	S	D	N		P	P	P	P	Y	P	N	N	N	P	N	P		N	N	N	N	N
Procainamide	N	N	P	I		N	N	N	N	P	N		N	N	N	N	N	N	N	N		N	N	N	N	N
Propranolol	N	N	N	N		N	N	N		N	P	N	P	N	N	N	N	N	N	N		N	N	N	N	N
Quinidine	N	N	N	P		I	N		N	N	N	N	I	D	I	N	N	N	N	N		N	N	N	N	N
Sodium bicarbonate	B	N	I	C		N	P	N	N	N	N	N	N	N	N	N	I	N	N	N		N	N	N	N	N
Streptokinase	N	N	N	N		N	N	N	N	N	N	N	N	N	N	N	N	N	N	N		N	N	N	N	N
Tobramycin	N	N	N	I		N	N		N	N	N	N	N	N	N	N	N	N	N	N		N	N	P	N	N
Verapamil	P	P	P	P	P	P	P	P	P	S	P	P	S	P	P	P	P	P	P	P		N	P	P	N	P

*From Zeller FP, Anders R: *Drug Intell Clin Pharm* 1986; 20:349–352. Used with permission.

†C = physically and chemically compatible; P = physically compatible; D = physically compatible only in 0.9% NaCl; G = physically compatible only in a glass bottle; H = physically compatible for 24 hr; A = physically compatible for 4–8 hr; B = physically compatible for 4–8 hr only in D_5W; Y = physically compatible through Y-site for at least 6 hr; L = regular insulin compatible with preservative-free lidocaine solution; M = manufacturer claims medication should not be mixed with other medications but some compatibility data are available; I = incompatible; N = information on compatibility is not available.

Appendix 3

INFUSION TABLES

Sota Omoigui, MD
Didaciane Gatete, RN

Epidural Alfentanil 1500 µg in 150
mL (10 µg/ml)*

µg/hr	ml/hr
100	10
110	11
120	12
130	13
140	14
150	15
160	16
170	17
180	18
190	19
200	20
210	21
220	22
230	23
240	24
250	25

*Data from *The Criticare Drug Dose and Infusion Calculator Software*. Mt Vernon, Ill, Med-Pharm Information Systems, 1991.

Intravenous Alfentanil, 10 mg in 250 mL (40 µg/mL)*†

Dose, µg/kg/min	Patient's Weight (lb/kg)														
	66/30	77/35	88/40	99/45	110/50	121/55	132/60	143/65	154/70	165/75	176/80	187/85	198/90	209/95	220/100
	Infusion Rate, ml/hr														
0.1	5	5	6	7	8	8	9	10	11	11	12	13	14	14	15
0.2	9	11	12	14	15	17	18	20	21	23	24	26	27	29	30
0.3	14	16	18	20	23	25	27	29	32	34	36	38	41	43	45
0.4	18	21	24	27	30	33	36	39	42	45	48	51	54	57	60
0.5	23	26	30	34	38	41	45	49	53	56	60	64	68	71	75
0.6	27	32	36	41	45	50	54	59	63	68	72	77	81	86	90
0.7	32	37	42	47	53	58	63	68	74	78	84	89	95	100	105
0.8	36	42	48	54	60	66	72	78	84	90	96	102	108	114	120
0.9	41	47	54	61	68	74	81	88	95	101	108	115	122	128	135
1.0	45	53	60	68	75	83	90	98	105	113	120	128	135	143	150
2.0	90	105	120	135	150	165	180	195	210	225	240	255	270	285	300
3.0	135	158	180	202	225	248	270	293	315	338	360	383	405	428	450

*Data from *The Criticare Drug Dose and Infusion Calculator Software*, Mt Vernon, Ill, Med-Pharm Information Systems, 1991.
†Infusion rate is found at intersection of "Dose" and Patient's Weight columns.

Aminocaproic Acid, 15 g in 500
mL (30 mg/mL)*

g/hr	mL/hr
0.5	17
0.6	20
0.7	23
0.8	27
0.9	30
1	33
1.1	37
1.2	40
1.25	42

*Data from *The Criticare Drug Dose and Infusion Calculator Software*. Mt Vernon, Ill, Med-Pharm Information Systems, 1991.

Aminophylline, 500 mg in 500 mL (1 mg/mL)†

Dose, mg/kg/hr	Patient's Weight (lb/kg)														
	66/30	77/35	88/40	99/45	110/50	121/55	132/60	143/65	154/70	165/75	176/80	187/85	198/90	209/95	220/100
	Infusion Rate, mL/hr														
0.1	3	4	4	5	5	6	6	6	7	8	8	9	9	10	10
0.2	6	7	8	9	10	11	12	13	14	15	16	17	18	19	20
0.3	9	11	12	14	15	17	18	20	21	23	24	26	27	29	30
0.4	12	14	16	18	20	22	24	26	28	30	32	34	36	38	40
0.5	15	18	20	23	25	28	30	33	35	38	40	43	45	48	50
0.6	18	21	24	27	30	33	36	39	42	45	48	51	54	57	60
0.7	21	25	28	32	35	39	42	46	49	53	56	60	63	67	70
0.8	24	28	32	36	40	44	48	52	56	60	64	68	72	76	80
0.9	27	32	36	41	45	50	54	59	63	68	72	77	81	86	90
1.0	30	35	40	45	50	55	60	65	70	75	80	85	90	95	100

*Data from *The Criticare Drug Dose and Infusion Calculator Software.* Mt Vernon, Ill, Med-Pharm Information Systems, 1991.
†Infusion rate is found at intersection of "Dose" and Patient's Weight columns.

Amrinone, 500 mg in 500 mL (1 mg/mL)*†

Dose, µg/kg/min	Patient's Weight (lb/kg)														
	66/30	77/35	86/40	99/45	110/50	121/55	132/60	143/65	154/70	165/75	176/80	187/85	198/90	209/95	220/100
	Infusion Rate, mL/hr														
1	2	2	2	3	3	3	4	4	4	5	5	5	5	6	6
2	4	4	5	5	6	7	7	8	8	9	10	10	11	11	12
3	5	6	7	8	9	10	11	12	13	14	14	15	16	17	18
4	7	8	10	11	12	13	14	16	17	18	19	20	22	23	24
5	9	11	12	14	15	17	18	20	21	23	24	26	27	29	30
6	11	13	14	16	18	20	22	23	25	27	29	31	32	34	36
7	13	15	17	19	21	23	25	27	29	32	34	36	38	40	42
8	14	17	19	22	24	26	29	31	34	36	38	41	43	46	48
9	16	19	22	24	27	30	32	35	38	41	43	46	49	51	54
10	18	21	24	27	30	33	36	39	42	45	48	51	54	57	60
11	20	23	26	30	33	36	40	43	46	50	53	56	59	63	66
12	22	25	29	32	36	40	43	47	50	54	58	61	65	68	72
13	23	27	31	35	39	43	47	51	55	59	62	66	70	74	78
14	25	29	34	38	42	46	50	55	59	63	67	71	76	80	84
15	27	32	36	41	45	50	54	59	63	68	72	77	81	86	90
16	29	34	38	43	48	53	58	62	67	72	77	82	87	91	96
17	31	36	41	46	51	56	61	66	71	77	82	87	92	97	102
18	32	38	43	49	54	59	65	70	76	81	86	92	97	103	108
19	34	40	46	51	57	63	68	74	80	86	91	97	103	108	114

*The Criticare Drug Dose and Infusion Calculator Software. Mt Vernon, Ill, Med-Pharm Information Systems, 1991.
†Found at intersection of "Dose" and Patient's Weight columns.

Atracurium, 20 mg in 100 mL (0.2 mg/mL)*†

Dose, μg/kg/min	Patient's Weight (lb/kg)														
	66/30	77/35	88/40	99/45	110/50	121/55	132/60	143/65	154/70	165/75	176/80	187/85	198/90	209/95	220/100
	Infusion Rate, mL/hr														
1	9	11	12	14	15	17	18	20	21	22	24	26	27	29	30
2	18	21	24	27	30	33	36	39	42	45	48	51	54	57	60
3	27	32	36	41	45	50	54	59	63	68	72	77	81	86	90
4	36	42	48	54	60	66	72	78	84	90	96	102	108	114	120
5	45	53	60	68	75	83	90	98	105	113	120	128	135	143	150
6	54	63	72	81	90	99	108	117	126	135	144	153	162	171	180
7	63	74	84	95	105	116	126	137	147	158	168	179	189	200	210
8	72	84	96	108	120	132	144	156	168	180	192	204	216	228	240
9	81	95	108	122	135	149	162	176	189	203	216	230	243	257	270
10	90	105	120	135	150	165	180	195	210	225	240	255	270	285	300
11	99	116	132	149	165	182	198	215	231	248	264	281	297	314	330
12	108	126	144	162	180	198	216	234	252	270	288	306	324	342	360
13	117	137	156	176	195	215	234	254	273	293	312	332	351	371	390
14	126	147	168	189	210	231	252	273	294	315	336	357	378	399	420
15	135	158	180	203	225	248	270	293	315	338	360	383	405	428	450

*Data from *The Criticare Drug Dose and Infusion Calculator Software*, Mt Vernon, Ill, Med-Pharm Information Systems, 1991.
†Infusion rate is found at intersection of "Dose" and Patient's Weight columns.

Bretylium, 2 g in 500 mL
(4 mg/mL)*

mg/min	mL/hr
1	15
1.1	17
1.2	18
1.3	20
1.4	21
1.5	23
1.6	24
1.7	26
1.8	27
1.9	29
2	30

*Data from *The Criticare Drug Dose and Infusion Calculator Software.* Mt Vernon, Ill, Med-Pharm Information Systems, 1991.

Curare, 15 mg in 100 mL (0.15 mg/mL)*†

Dose, µg/kg/min	Patient's Weight (lb/kg)														
	66/30	77/35	88/40	99/45	110/50	121/55	132/60	143/65	154/70	165/75	176/80	187/85	198/90	209/95	220/100
	Infusion Rate, mL/hr														
1	12	14	16	18	20	22	24	26	28	30	32	34	36	38	40
2	24	28	32	36	40	44	48	52	56	60	64	68	72	76	80
3	36	42	48	54	60	66	72	78	84	90	96	102	108	114	120
4	48	56	64	72	80	88	96	104	112	120	128	136	144	152	160
5	60	70	80	90	100	110	120	130	140	150	160	170	180	190	200
6	72	84	96	108	120	132	144	156	168	180	192	204	216	228	240

*Data from *The Criticare Drug Dose and Infusion Calculator Software.* Mt Vernon, Ill, Med-Pharm Information Systems, 1991.
†Infusion rate is found at intersection of "Dose" and Patient's Weight columns.

Dobutamine, 500 mg in 500 mL (1 mg/mL)†

Dose, µg/kg/min	Patient's Weight (lb/kg)														
	66/30	77/35	88/40	99/45	110/50	121/55	132/60	143/65	154/70	165/75	176/80	187/85	198/90	209/95	220/100
	Infusion Rate, mL/hr														
2	4	4	5	5	6	7	7	8	8	9	10	10	11	11	12
4	7	8	10	11	12	13	14	16	17	18	19	20	22	23	24
6	11	13	14	16	18	20	22	23	25	27	29	31	32	34	36
8	14	17	19	22	24	26	29	31	34	36	38	41	43	46	48
10	18	21	24	27	30	33	36	39	42	45	48	51	54	57	60
12	22	25	29	32	36	40	43	47	50	54	58	61	65	68	72
14	25	29	34	38	42	46	50	55	59	63	67	71	76	80	84
16	29	34	38	43	48	53	58	62	67	72	77	82	86	91	96
18	32	38	43	49	54	59	65	70	76	81	86	92	97	103	108
20	36	42	48	54	60	66	72	78	84	90	96	102	108	114	120
22	40	46	53	59	66	73	80	86	92	99	106	112	119	125	132
24	43	50	58	65	72	79	86	94	101	108	115	122	130	137	144
26	47	55	62	70	78	86	94	101	109	117	125	133	140	148	156
28	50	59	67	76	84	92	101	109	118	126	134	143	151	160	168
30	54	63	72	81	90	99	108	117	126	135	144	153	162	171	180
32	58	67	77	86	96	106	115	125	134	144	154	163	173	182	192
34	61	71	82	92	102	112	122	133	143	153	163	173	184	194	204
36	65	76	86	97	108	119	130	140	151	162	173	184	194	205	216
38	68	80	91	103	114	125	137	148	160	171	182	194	205	217	228
40	72	84	96	108	120	132	144	156	168	180	192	204	216	228	240

...line, 400 mg in 250 mL (1600 µg/mL)*†

Dose, µg/kg/min	Patient's Weight (lb/kg)														
	66/30	77/35	88/40	99/45	110/50	121/55	132/60	143/65	154/70	165/75	176/80	187/85	198/90	209/95	220/100
	Infusion Rate, mL/hr														
1	1	1	2	2	2	2	2	2	3	3	3	3	3	4	4
2	2	3	3	3	4	4	5	5	5	6	6	6	7	7	8
3	3	4	5	5	6	6	7	7	8	8	9	10	10	11	11
4	5	5	6	7	8	8	9	10	11	11	12	13	14	14	15
5	6	7	8	8	9	10	11	12	13	14	15	16	17	18	19
6	7	8	9	10	11	12	14	15	16	17	18	19	20	21	23
7	8	9	11	12	13	14	16	17	18	20	21	22	24	25	26
8	9	11	12	14	15	17	18	20	21	23	24	26	27	29	30
9	10	12	14	15	17	19	20	22	24	25	27	29	30	32	34
10	11	13	15	17	19	21	23	24	26	28	30	32	34	36	38
11	12	14	17	19	21	23	25	26	29	31	33	35	37	39	41
12	14	16	18	20	23	25	27	29	32	34	36	38	41	43	45
13	15	17	20	22	24	27	29	32	34	37	39	41	44	46	49
14	16	18	21	24	26	29	32	34	37	39	42	45	47	50	53
15	17	20	23	25	28	31	34	37	39	42	45	48	51	54	56
16	18	21	24	27	30	33	36	39	42	45	48	51	54	57	60
17	19	22	26	29	32	35	38	41	45	48	51	54	57	61	64
18	20	24	27	30	34	37	41	44	47	51	54	57	61	64	68
19	21	25	29	32	36	39	43	46	50	53	57	61	64	68	71
20	23	26	30	34	38	41	45	49	53	56	60	64	68	71	75

*Data from *The Criticare Drug Dose and Infusion Calculator Software.* Mt Vernon, Ill, Med-Pharm Information Systems, 1991.
†Infusion rate is found at intersection of "Dose" and Patient's Weight columns.

Doxapram, 250 mg in 250 mL
(1 mg/mL)*

mg/min	mL/hr
1	60
2	120
3	180
4	240
5	300

*Data from *The Criticare Drug Dose and Infusion Calculator Software*. Mt Vernon, Ill, Med-Pharm Information Systems, 1991.

Epinephrine, 3 mg in 250 mL
(12 μg/mL)*

μg/min	mL/hr
1	5
2	10
3	15
4	20
5	25
6	30
7	35
8	40
9	45
10	50
11	55
12	60
13	65
14	70
15	75
16	80
17	85
18	90
19	95
20	100

*Data from *The Criticare Drug Dose and Infusion Calculator Software*. Mt Vernon, Ill, Med-Pharm Information Systems, 1991.

Esmolol. 5g in 500 mL (10 mg/mL)*†

Dose, µg/kg/min	Patient's Weight (lb/kg)														
	66/30	77/35	88/40	99/45	110/50	121/55	132/60	143/65	154/70	165/75	176/80	187/85	198/90	209/95	220/100
	Infusion Rate, mL/hr														
50	9	11	12	14	15	17	18	20	21	23	24	26	27	29	30
60	11	13	14	16	18	20	22	23	25	27	29	31	32	34	36
70	13	15	17	19	21	23	25	27	29	32	34	36	38	40	42
80	14	17	19	22	24	26	29	31	34	36	38	41	43	46	48
90	16	19	22	24	27	30	32	35	38	41	43	46	49	51	54
100	18	21	24	27	30	33	36	39	42	45	48	51	54	57	60
110	20	23	26	30	33	36	40	43	46	50	53	56	59	63	66
120	22	25	29	32	36	40	43	47	50	54	58	61	65	68	72
130	23	27	31	35	39	43	47	51	55	59	62	66	70	74	78
140	25	29	34	38	42	46	50	55	59	63	67	71	76	80	84
150	27	32	36	41	45	50	54	59	63	68	72	77	81	86	90
160	29	34	38	43	48	53	58	62	67	72	77	82	86	91	96
170	31	36	41	46	51	56	61	66	71	77	82	87	92	97	102
180	32	38	43	49	54	59	65	70	76	81	86	92	97	103	108
190	34	40	46	51	57	63	68	74	80	86	91	97	103	108	114
200	36	42	48	54	60	66	72	78	84	90	96	102	108	114	120
210	38	44	50	57	63	69	76	82	88	95	101	107	113	120	126
220	40	46	53	59	66	73	79	86	92	99	106	112	119	125	132
230	41	48	55	62	69	76	83	90	97	104	110	117	124	131	138
240	43	50	58	65	72	79	86	94	101	108	115	122	130	137	144
250	45	53	60	68	75	83	90	98	105	113	120	128	135	143	150

*Data from *The Criticare Drug Dose and Infusion Calculator Software.* Mt. Vernon, Ill, Med-Pharm Information Systems, 1991.
†Infusion rate is found at intersection of "Dose" and Patient's Weight columns.

Epidural Fentanyl, 500 μg in 100
mL Local Anesthetic (5 μg/mL)*

μg/hr	mL/hr
20	4
25	5
30	6
35	7
40	8
45	9
50	10
55	11
60	12

*Data from *The Criticare Drug Dose and Infusion Calculator Software.* Mt Vernon, Ill, Med-Pharm Information Systems, 1991.

Intravenous Fentanyl, 500 µg in 100 mL (5 µg/mL)*†

Dose, µg/kg/min	Patient's Weight (lb/kg)														
	66/30	77/35	88/40	99/45	110/50	121/55	132/60	143/65	154/70	165/75	176/80	187/85	198/90	209/95	220/100
	Infusion Rate, mL/hr														
0.05	18	21	24	27	30	33	36	39	42	45	48	51	54	57	60
0.06	22	25	29	32	36	40	43	47	50	54	58	61	65	68	72
0.07	25	29	34	38	42	46	50	55	59	63	67	71	76	80	84
0.08	29	34	38	43	48	53	58	62	67	72	77	82	86	91	96
0.09	32	39	43	49	54	59	65	70	76	81	86	92	97	103	108
0.1	36	42	48	54	60	66	72	78	84	90	96	102	108	114	120
0.11	40	46	53	59	66	73	79	86	92	99	106	112	119	125	132
0.12	43	50	58	65	72	79	86	94	101	108	115	122	130	137	144
0.13	47	55	62	70	78	86	94	101	109	117	125	133	140	148	156
0.14	50	59	67	76	84	92	101	109	118	126	134	143	151	160	168
0.15	54	63	72	81	90	99	108	117	126	135	144	153	162	171	180
0.16	58	67	77	86	96	106	115	125	134	144	154	163	173	182	192
0.17	61	71	82	92	102	112	122	133	143	153	163	173	184	194	204
0.18	65	76	86	97	108	119	130	140	151	162	173	184	194	205	216
0.19	68	80	91	103	114	125	137	148	160	171	182	194	205	217	228
0.2	72	84	96	108	120	132	144	156	168	180	192	204	216	228	240

*Data from *The Criticare Drug Dose and Infusion Calculator Software.* Mt Vernon, Ill, Med-Pharm Information Systems, 1991.
†Infusion rate is found at intersection of "Dose" and Patient's Weight columns.

Heparin, 25,000 Units in 250 mL
(100 Units/mL)*

Units/24 hr	Units/hr	mL/hr
19,200	800	8
21,600	900	9
24,000	1000	10
26,400	1100	11
28,800	1200	12
31,200	1300	13
33,600	1400	14
36,000	1500	15
38,400	1600	16
40,800	1700	17

*Data from *The Criticare Drug Dose and Infusion Calculator Software*. Mt Vernon, Ill, Med-Pharm Information Systems, 1991.

Epidural Hydromorphone, 5 mg
in 100 mL Local Anesthetic
(50 µg/mL)*

mg/hr	mL/hr
0.15	3
0.2	4
0.25	5
0.3	6

*Data from *The Criticare Drug Dose and Infusion Calculator Software*. Mt Vernon, Ill, Med-Pharm Information Systems, 1991.

Intravenous Hydromorphone, 5 mg in 100 mL (50 μg/mL)*

mg/hr	mL/hr
0.15	3
0.2	4
0.25	5
0.3	6

*Data from *The Criticare Drug Dose and Infusion Calculator Software.* Mt Vernon, Ill, Med-Pharm Information Systems, 1991.

Isoproterenol, 3 mg in 250 mL (12 μg/mL)*

μg/min	mL/hr
0.5	3
1	5
2	10
3	15
4	20
5	25
6	30
7	35
8	40
9	45
10	50
11	55
12	60
13	65
14	70
15	75
16	80
17	85
18	90
19	95
20	100

*Data from *The Criticare Drug Dose and Infusion Calculator Software.* Mt Vernon, Ill, Med-Pharm Information Systems, 1991.

Ketamine, 250 mg in 250 mL (1 mg/mL)*†

Dose, μg/kg/min	Patient's Weight ($\frac{lb}{kg}$) — Infusion Rate, mL/hr														
	$\frac{56}{30}$	$\frac{77}{35}$	$\frac{88}{40}$	$\frac{99}{45}$	$\frac{110}{50}$	$\frac{121}{55}$	$\frac{132}{60}$	$\frac{143}{65}$	$\frac{154}{70}$	$\frac{165}{75}$	$\frac{176}{80}$	$\frac{187}{85}$	$\frac{198}{90}$	$\frac{209}{95}$	$\frac{220}{100}$
10	18	21	24	27	30	33	36	39	42	45	48	51	54	57	60
20	36	42	48	54	60	66	72	78	84	90	96	102	108	114	120
30	54	63	72	81	90	99	108	117	126	135	144	153	162	171	180
40	72	84	96	108	120	132	144	156	168	180	192	204	216	228	240
50	90	105	120	135	150	165	180	195	210	225	240	255	270	285	300
60	108	126	144	162	180	198	216	234	252	270	288	306	324	342	360
70	126	147	168	189	210	231	252	273	294	315	336	357	378	399	420
80	144	168	192	216	240	264	288	312	336	360	384	408	432	456	480

*Data from *The Criticare Drug Dose and Infusion Calculator Software*. Mt Vernon, Ill, Med-Pharm Information Systems, 1991.
†Infusion rate is found at intersection of "Dose" and Patient's Weight columns.

Labetalol, 200 mg in 200 mL
(1 mg/mL)*

mg/min	mL/hr
0.5	30
0.6	36
0.7	42
0.8	48
0.9	54
1	60
1.1	66
1.2	72
1.3	78
1.4	84
1.5	90
1.6	96
1.7	102
1.8	108
1.9	114
2	120

*Data from *The Criticare Drug Dose and Infusion Calculator Software.* Mt Vernon, Ill, Med-Pharm Information Systems, 1991.

Lidocaine, 2 g in 500 mL
(4 mg/mL)*

mg/min	mL/hr
0.5	8
1	15
1.5	23
2	30
2.5	38
3	45
3.5	53
4	60

*Data from *The Criticare Drug Dose and Infusion Calculator Software.* Mt Vernon, Ill, Med-Pharm Information Systems, 1991.

Magnesium Sulfate, 10 g in 1000
mL (10 mg/mL)*

g/hr	mL/hr
1	100
1.1	110
1.2	120
1.3	130
1.4	140
1.5	150
1.6	160
1.7	170
1.8	180
1.9	190
2	200

*Data from *The Criticare Drug Dose and Infusion Calculator Software*. Mt Vernon, Ill, Med-Pharm Information Systems, 1991.

Epidural Meperidine, 100 mg
in 50 mL Local Anesthetic
(2 mg/mL)*

mg/hr	mL/hr
10	5
12	6
14	7
16	8
18	9
20	10

*Data from *The Criticare Drug Dose and Infusion Calculator Software*. Mt Vernon, Ill, Med-Pharm Information Systems, 1991.

Mephentermine, 250 mg in 250 mL (1 mg/mL)

mg/min	mL/hr
0.25	15
0.5	30
1	60
1.5	90
2	120
2.5	150
3	180
3.5	210
4	240
4.5	270
5	300

*Data from *The Criticare Drug Dose and Infusion Calculator Software.* Mt Vernon, Ill, Med-Pharm Information Systems, 1991.

Methohexital, 500 mg in 50 mL (10 mg/mL)*†

Dose, µg/kg/min	Patient's Weight ($\frac{lb}{kg}$)														
	66/30	77/35	88/40	99/45	110/50	121/55	132/60	143/65	154/70	165/75	176/80	187/85	198/90	209/95	220/100
	Infusion Rate, mL/hr														
50	9	11	12	14	15	17	18	20	21	23	24	26	27	29	30
60	11	13	15	16	18	20	22	23	25	27	29	30	32	34	36
70	13	15	17	19	21	23	25	27	29	32	34	36	38	40	42
80	14	17	19	22	24	26	29	31	34	36	38	41	43	46	48
90	16	19	22	24	27	30	32	35	38	41	43	46	49	51	54
100	18	21	24	27	30	33	36	39	42	45	48	51	54	57	60
110	20	23	26	30	33	36	40	43	46	50	53	56	59	63	66
120	22	25	29	32	36	40	43	47	50	54	58	61	65	68	72
130	23	27	31	35	39	43	47	51	55	59	62	66	70	74	78
140	25	29	34	38	42	46	50	55	59	63	67	71	76	80	84
150	27	32	36	41	45	50	54	59	63	68	72	77	81	86	90

*Data from *The Criticare Drug Dose and Infusion Calculator Software.* Mt Vernon, Ill, Med-Pharm Information Systems, 1991.
†Infusion rate is found at intersection of "Dose" and Patient's Weight columns.

Methohexital, 500 mg in 50 mL (10 mg/mL)*†

Dose, μg/kg/min	Patient's Weight (lb/kg) Infusion Rate, mL/hr														
	66/30	77/35	88/40	99/45	110/50	121/55	132/60	143/65	154/70	165/75	176/80	187/85	198/90	209/95	220/100
50	9	11	12	14	15	17	18	20	21	23	24	26	27	29	30
60	11	13	15	16	18	20	22	23	25	27	29	30	32	34	36
70	13	15	17	19	21	23	25	27	29	32	34	36	38	40	42
80	14	17	19	22	24	26	29	31	34	36	38	41	43	46	48
90	16	19	22	24	27	30	32	35	38	41	43	46	49	51	54
100	18	21	24	27	30	33	36	39	42	45	48	51	54	57	60
110	20	23	26	30	33	36	40	43	46	50	53	56	59	63	66
120	22	25	29	32	36	40	43	47	50	54	58	61	65	68	72
130	23	27	31	35	39	43	47	51	55	59	62	66	70	74	78
140	25	29	34	38	42	46	50	55	59	63	67	71	76	80	84
150	27	32	36	41	45	50	54	59	63	68	72	77	81	86	90

*Data from *The Criticare Drug Dose and Infusion Calculator Software.* Mt Vernon, Ill, Med-Pharm Information Systems, 1991.
†Infusion rate is found at intersection of "Dose" and Patient's Weight columns.

Mivacurium Chloride, 25 mg in 50 mL (0.5 mg/mL)*†

	Patient's Weight $\left(\frac{lb}{kg}\right)$														
Dose, μg/kg/min	$\frac{66}{30}$	$\frac{77}{35}$	$\frac{88}{40}$	$\frac{99}{45}$	$\frac{110}{50}$	$\frac{121}{55}$	$\frac{132}{60}$	$\frac{143}{65}$	$\frac{154}{70}$	$\frac{165}{75}$	$\frac{176}{80}$	$\frac{187}{85}$	$\frac{198}{90}$	$\frac{209}{95}$	$\frac{220}{100}$
	Infusion Rate, mL/hr														
1	4	4	5	5	6	7	7	8	8	9	10	10	11	11	12
2	7	8	10	11	12	13	14	16	17	18	19	20	22	23	24
3	11	13	14	16	18	20	22	23	25	27	29	31	32	34	36
4	14	17	19	22	24	26	29	31	34	36	38	41	43	46	48
5	18	21	24	27	30	33	36	39	42	45	48	51	54	57	60
6	22	25	29	32	36	40	43	47	50	54	58	61	65	68	72
7	25	29	34	38	42	46	50	55	59	63	67	71	76	80	84
8	29	34	38	43	48	53	58	62	67	72	77	82	86	91	96
9	32	38	43	49	54	59	65	70	76	81	86	92	97	103	108
10	36	42	48	54	60	66	72	78	84	90	96	102	108	114	120
11	40	46	53	59	66	73	79	86	92	99	106	112	119	125	132
12	43	50	58	65	72	79	86	94	101	108	115	122	130	137	144
13	47	55	62	70	78	86	94	101	109	117	125	133	140	148	156
14	50	59	67	76	84	92	101	109	118	126	134	143	151	160	168
15	54	63	72	81	90	99	108	117	126	135	144	153	162	171	180

*Data from *The Criticare Drug Dose and Infusion Calculator Software*. Mt Vernon, Ill, Med-Pharm Information Systems, 1991.
†Infusion rate is found at intersection of "Dose" and Patient's Weight columns.

Mivacurium Chloride, 25 mg in 50 mL (0.5 mg/mL)*†

Dose, µg/kg/min	Patient's Weight (lb/kg)																			
	66/30	77/35	88/40	99/45	110/50	121/55	132/60	143/65	154/70	165/75	176/80	187/85	198/90	209/95	220/100
	Infusion Rate, mL/hr														
1	4	4	5	5	6	7	7	8	8	9	10	10	11	11	12
2	7	8	10	11	12	13	14	16	17	18	19	20	22	23	24
3	11	13	14	16	18	20	22	23	25	27	29	31	32	34	36
4	14	17	19	22	24	26	29	31	34	36	38	41	43	46	48
5	18	21	24	27	30	33	36	39	42	45	48	51	54	57	60
6	22	25	29	32	36	40	43	47	50	54	58	61	65	68	72
7	25	29	34	38	42	46	50	55	59	63	67	71	76	80	84
8	29	34	38	43	48	53	58	62	67	72	77	82	86	91	96
9	32	38	43	49	54	59	65	70	76	81	86	92	97	103	108
10	36	42	48	54	60	66	72	78	84	90	96	102	108	114	120
11	40	46	53	59	66	73	79	86	92	99	106	112	119	125	132
12	43	50	58	65	72	79	86	94	101	108	115	122	130	137	144
13	47	55	62	70	78	86	94	101	109	117	125	133	140	148	156
14	50	59	67	76	84	92	101	109	118	126	134	143	151	160	168
15	54	63	72	81	90	99	108	117	126	135	144	153	162	171	180

*Data from *The Criticare Drug Dose and Infusion Calculator Software.* Mt Vernon, Ill, Med-Pharm Information Systems, 1991.
†Infusion rate is found at intersection of 'Dose' and Patient's Weight columns.

Nitroglycerin, 50 mg in 250 mL
(200 μg/mL)*

μg/min	mL/hr
10	3
20	6
30	9
40	12
50	15
60	18
70	21
80	24
90	27
100	30
110	33
120	36
130	39
140	42
150	45
160	48
170	51
180	54
190	57
200	60

*Data from *The Criticare Drug Dose and Infusion Calculator Software*. Mt Vernon, Ill, Med-Pharm Information Systems, 1991.

Norepinephrine, 8 mg in 500 mL
(16 µg/mL)*

µg/min	mL/hr
1	4
2	8
3	11
4	15
5	19
6	23
7	26
8	30
9	34
10	38
11	41
12	45
13	49
14	53
15	56
16	60
17	64
18	68
19	71
20	75

*Data from *The Criticare Drug Dose and Infusion Calculator Software.* Mt Vernon, Ill, Med-Pharm Information Systems, 1991.

Phentolamine, 200 mg in 100 mL
(2 mg/mL)*

mg/min	mL/hr
0.1	3
0.2	6
0.3	9
0.4	12
0.5	15
0.6	18
0.7	21
0.8	24
0.9	27
1	30

*Data from *The Criticare Drug Dose and Infusion Calculator Software.* Mt Vernon, Ill, Med-Pharm Information Systems, 1991.

Phenylephrine, 30 mg in 500 mL
(60 μg/mL)*

μg/min	mL/hr
10	10
20	20
30	30
40	40
50	50
60	60
70	70
80	80
90	90
100	100
110	110
120	120
130	130
140	140
150	150
160	160
170	170
180	180
190	190
200	200

*Data from *The Criticare Drug Dose and Infusion Calculator Software*. Mt Vernon, Ill, Med-Pharm Information Systems, 1991.

Procainamide, 2 g in 500 mL
(4 mg/mL)*

mg/min	mL/hr
0.5	8
1	15
1.5	23
2	30
2.5	38
3	45
3.5	53
4	60
4.5	68
5	75
5.5	83
6	90

*Data from *The Criticare Drug Dose and Infusion Calculator Software.* Mt Vernon, Ill, Med-Pharm Information Systems, 1991.

Propofol, Undiluted (10 mg/mL)†

Dose, µg/kg/min	Patient's Weight (lb/kg) — Infusion Rate, mL/hr														
	65 / 30	77 / 35	88 / 40	99 / 45	110 / 50	121 / 55	132 / 60	143 / 65	154 / 70	165 / 75	176 / 80	187 / 85	198 / 90	209 / 95	220 / 100
100	18	21	24	27	30	33	36	39	42	45	48	51	54	57	60
110	20	23	26	30	33	36	40	43	46	50	53	56	59	63	66
120	22	25	29	32	36	40	43	47	50	54	58	61	65	68	72
130	23	27	31	35	39	43	47	51	55	59	62	66	70	74	78
140	25	29	34	38	42	46	50	55	59	63	67	71	76	80	84
150	27	32	36	41	45	50	54	59	63	68	72	77	81	86	90
160	29	34	38	43	48	53	58	62	67	72	77	82	86	91	96
170	31	36	41	46	51	56	61	66	71	77	82	87	92	97	102
180	32	38	43	49	54	59	65	70	76	81	86	92	97	103	108
190	34	40	46	51	57	63	68	74	80	86	91	97	103	108	114
200	36	42	48	54	60	66	72	78	84	90	96	102	108	114	120

*Data from *The Criticare Drug Dose and Infusion Calculator Software.* Mt Vernon, Ill, Med-Pharm Information Systems, 1991.
†Infusion rate is found at intersection of "Dose" and Patient's Weight columns.

Prostaglandin E₁ in 250 mL (2 µg/mL)*†

Dose, µg/kg/min	Patient's Weight (lb/kg)																	
	2.2/1	4.4/2	6.6/3	8.8/4	11/5	22/10	33/15	44/20	55/25	66/30	77/35	88/40	99/45	110/50	121/55	132/60	143/65	154/70
	Infusion Rate, mL/hr																	
0.05	2	3	5	6	8	15	23	30	38	45	53	60	68	75	83	90	98	105
0.1	3	6	9	12	15	30	45	60	75	90	105	120	135	150	165	180	195	210
0.15	5	9	14	18	23	45	68	90	113	135	158	180	203	225	248	270	293	315
0.2	6	12	18	24	30	60	90	120	150	180	210	240	270	300	330	360	390	420
0.25	8	15	23	30	38	75	113	150	188	225	263	300	338	375	413	450	488	525
0.3	9	18	27	36	45	90	135	180	225	270	315	360	405	450	495	540	585	630
0.35	11	21	32	42	53	105	158	210	263	315	368	420	473	525	578	630	683	735
0.4	12	24	36	48	60	120	180	240	300	360	420	480	540	600	660	720	780	840

*Data from *The Criticare Drug Dose and Infusion Calculator Software*. Mt Vernon, Ill, Med-Pharm Information Systems, 1991.
†Infusion rate is found at intersection of "Dose" and Patient's Weight columns.

Sodium Nitroprusside, 50 mg in 250 mL (200 μg/mL)†

Dose, μg/kg/min	Patient's Weight (lb/kg)														
	66/30	77/35	88/40	99/45	110/50	121/55	132/60	143/65	154/70	165/75	176/80	187/85	198/90	209/95	220/100
	Infusion Rate, mL/hr														
0.1	1	1	1	1	2	2	2	2	2	2	2	3	3	3	3
0.2	2	2	2	3	3	3	4	4	4	5	5	5	5	6	6
0.3	3	3	4	4	5	5	5	6	6	7	7	8	8	9	9
0.4	4	4	5	5	6	7	7	8	8	9	10	10	11	11	12
0.5	5	5	6	7	8	8	9	10	11	11	12	13	14	14	15
0.6	5	6	7	8	9	10	11	12	13	14	14	15	16	17	18
0.7	6	7	8	10	11	12	13	14	15	16	17	18	19	20	21
0.8	7	8	10	11	12	13	14	16	17	18	19	20	22	23	24
0.9	8	10	11	12	14	15	16	18	19	20	22	23	24	26	27
1.0	9	11	12	14	15	17	18	20	21	23	24	26	27	29	30
2.0	18	21	24	27	30	33	36	39	42	45	48	51	54	57	60
3.0	27	32	36	41	45	50	54	59	63	68	72	77	81	86	90
4.0	36	42	48	54	60	66	72	78	84	90	96	102	108	114	120
5.0	45	53	60	68	75	83	90	98	105	113	120	128	135	143	150
6.0	54	63	72	81	90	99	108	117	126	135	144	153	162	171	180
7.0	63	74	84	95	105	116	126	137	147	158	168	179	189	200	210
8.0	72	84	96	108	120	132	144	156	168	180	192	204	216	228	240
9.0	81	95	108	122	135	149	162	176	189	203	216	230	243	257	270
10	90	105	120	135	150	165	180	195	210	225	240	255	270	285	300

*Data from *The Criticare Drug Dose and Infusion Calculator Software.* Mt Vernon, Ill, Med-Pharm Information Systems, 1991.
†Infusion rate is found at intersection of 'Dose' and Patient's Weight columns.

Succinylcholine, 250 mg in 250 mL (1 mg/mL)*

mg/min	mL/hr
0.5	30
1	60
2	120
3	180
4	240
5	300
6	360
7	420
8	480
9	540
10	600

*Data from *The Criticare Drug Dose and Infusion Calculator Software*. Mt Vernon, Ill, Med-Pharm Information Systems, 1991.

Epidural Sufentanil, 100 μg in 100 mL (1 μg/mL)*

μg/hr	mL/hr
5	5
10	10
15	15
20	20
25	25
30	30

*Data from *The Criticare Drug Dose and Infusion Calculator Software*. Mt Vernon, Ill, Med-Pharm Information Systems, 1991.

Intravenous Sufentanil, 500 µg in 100 mL (5 µg/mL)*†

Dose, µg/kg/min	Patient's Weight ($\frac{lb}{kg}$)														
	$\frac{66}{30}$	$\frac{77}{35}$	$\frac{88}{40}$	$\frac{99}{45}$	$\frac{110}{50}$	$\frac{121}{55}$	$\frac{132}{60}$	$\frac{143}{65}$	$\frac{154}{70}$	$\frac{165}{75}$	$\frac{176}{80}$	$\frac{187}{85}$	$\frac{198}{90}$	$\frac{209}{95}$	$\frac{220}{100}$
	Infusion Rate, mL/hr														
0.01	4	4	5	5	6	7	7	8	8	9	10	10	11	11	12
0.02	7	8	10	11	12	13	14	16	17	18	19	20	22	23	24
0.03	11	13	14	16	18	20	22	23	25	27	29	31	32	34	36
0.04	14	17	19	22	24	26	29	31	34	36	38	41	43	46	48
0.05	18	21	24	27	30	33	36	39	42	45	48	51	54	57	60

*Data from *The Criticare Drug Dose and Infusion Calculator Software.* Mt Vernon, Ill, Med-Pharm Information Systems, 1991.
†Infusion rate is found at intersection of "Dose" and "Patient's Weight columns.

Trimetaphan, 1500 mg in 500 mL
(3 mg/mL)*

mg/min	mL/hr
0.3	6
0.4	8
0.5	10
0.6	12
0.7	14
0.8	16
0.9	18
1	20
1.5	30
2	40
2.5	50
3	60
3.5	70
4	80
4.5	90
5	100
5.5	110
6	120

*Data from *The Criticare Drug Dose and Infusion Calculator Software.* Mt Vernon, Ill, Med-Pharm Information Systems, 1991.

Vasopressin, 200 Units in 250 mL
(0.8 Units/mL)*

Units/min	mL/hr
0.2	15
0.3	23
0.4	30
0.5	38
0.6	45
0.7	53
0.8	60
0.9	68
1	75

*Data from *The Criticare Drug Dose and Infusion Calculator Software.* Mt Vernon, Ill, Med-Pharm Information Systems, 1991.

Vecuronium, 20 mg in 100 mL (0.2 mg/mL)*†

Dose, µg/kg/min	Patient's Weight (lb/kg)														
	66/30	77/35	88/40	99/45	110/50	121/55	132/60	143/65	154/70	165/75	176/80	187/85	198/90	209/95	220/100
	Infusion Rate, mL/hr														
1	9	11	12	14	15	17	18	20	21	23	24	26	27	29	30
1.1	10	12	13	15	17	18	20	21	23	25	26	28	30	31	33
1.2	11	13	14	16	18	20	22	23	25	27	29	31	32	34	36
1.3	12	14	16	18	20	21	23	25	27	29	31	33	35	37	39
1.4	13	15	17	19	21	23	25	27	29	32	34	36	38	40	42
1.5	14	16	18	20	23	25	27	29	32	34	36	38	41	43	45
1.6	14	17	19	22	24	26	29	31	33	36	38	41	43	46	48
1.7	15	18	20	23	26	28	31	33	36	38	41	43	46	48	51
1.8	16	19	22	24	27	30	32	35	38	41	43	46	49	51	54
1.9	17	20	23	26	29	31	34	37	40	43	46	48	51	54	57
2	18	21	24	27	30	33	36	39	42	45	48	51	54	57	60

*Data from The Criticare Drug Dose and Infusion Calculator Software. Mt Vernon, Ill, Med-Pharm Information Systems, 1991.
†Infusion rate is found at intersection of "Dose" and Patient's Weight columns.

Appendix 4

TRADE NAME LIST

Trade names listed represent examples chosen by the author and are not complete lists of marketed drugs.

Trade Name	Generic Name
Adalat	Nifedipine
Adenocard	Adenosine
Adrenaline	Epinephrine HCl
Aldomet	Methyldopa
Alfenta	Alfentanil HCl
Americaine	Benzocaine
Amicar	Aminocaproic acid
Amidate	Etomidate
Aminophylline	Aminophylline
Anectine	Succinylcholine chloride
Antilirium	Physostigmine salicylate
Apresoline	Hydralazine HCl
Aquamephyton	Phytonadione-vit k
Aramine	Metaraminol bitartrate
Arduan	Pipecuronium bromide
Arfonad	Trimethaphan camsylate
Astramorph	Morphine sulfate
Ativan	Lorazepam
Atropine sulfate	Atropine sulfate
Benadryl	Diphenhydramine HCl
Bicitra	Sodium citrate
Brethaire	Terbutaline sulfate
Bretylol	Bretylium tosylate
Brevibloc	Esmolol HCl
Brevital	Methohexital sodium
Bricanyl	Terbutaline sulfate
Calan	Verapamil HCl
Calcium chloride	Calcium chloride
Calcium gluconate	Calcium gluconate
Capoten	Captopril
Carbocaine	Mepivacaine HCl
Carfin	Warfarin sodium
Catapres	Clonidine HCl
Citanest	Prilocaine HCl
Cocaine HCl	Cocaine HCl
Compazine	Prochlorperazine
Cordarone	Amiodarone
Coumadin	Warfarin sodium
Dalmane	Flurazepam HCl
Dantrium	Dantrolene sodium
DDAVP	Desmopressin acetate
Decadron	Dexamethasone

Demerol	Meperidine HCl
Dermoplast	Benzocaine
Dilantin	Phenytoin sodium
Dilaudid	Hydromorphone HCl
Dilaudid HP	Hydromorphone HCl
Diprivan	Propofol
Dobutrex	Dobutamine HCl
Dolophine	Methadone HCl
Dopram	Doxapram HCl
Duramorph	Morphine sulfate
Duranest	Etidocaine HCl
Edecrin	Ethacrynic acid
EMLA	Lidocaine and prilocaine
Enlon	Edrophonium chloride
Ephedrine sulfate	Ephedrine sulfate
Epinephrine	Epinephrine HCl
Ergotrate	Ergonovine maleate
Ethrane	Enflurane
Flaxedil	Gallamine triethiodide
Fluothane	Halothane
Forane	Isoflurane
Glucagon	Glucagon
Haldol	Haloperidol
Halperon	Haloperidol
Hemobate	Carboprost tromethamine
Heparin sodium	Heparin sodium
Hespan	Hetastarch
Hexadrol	Dexamethasone
Humulin R	Insulin regular (human)
Hurricaine	Benzocaine
Hydrocortisone acetate	Hydrocortisone
Hydrocortisone cypionate	Hydrocortisone
Hydrocortisone sodium succinate	Hydrocortisone
Hydrocortisone sodium phosphate	Hydrocortisone
Iletin regular	Insulin regular
Inapsine	Droperidol
Inderal	Propranolol HCl
Infumorph	Morphine sulfate
Inocor	Amrinone lactate
Insulin regular	Insulin regular
Intropin	Dopamine HCl
Isoptin	Verapamil HCl
Isuprel	Isoproterenol HCl
Ketalar	Ketamine HCl
Konakion	Phytonadione-vit K

Trade Name	Generic Name
Lanoxin	Digoxin
Lasix	Furosemide
Levophed	Norepinephrine bitartrate
Librium	Chlordiazepoxide hcl
Lopressor	Metoprolol tartrate
Magnesium sulfate	Magnesium sulfate
Marcaine	Bupivacaine HCl
Mazicon	Flumazenil
Medihaler-ISO	Isoproterenol HCl
Medrol	Methylprednisolone
Mestinon	Pyridostigmine bromide
Methergine	Methylergonovine maleate
Methyldopate	Methyldopa
Metubine iodide	Metocurine iodide
Mivacron	Mivacurium chloride
Morphine	Morphine sulfate
MS contin	Morphine sulfate
Narcan	Naloxone HCl
Neo-Synephrine	Phenylephrine HCl
Nesacaine	Chloroprocaine HCl
Nipride	Sodium nitroprusside
Nitro-bid	Nitroglycerin
Nitrocine	Nitroglycerin
Nitrodisc	Nitroglycerin
Nitrogard	Nitroglycerin
Nitroglyn	Nitroglycerin
Nitrol	Nitroglycerin
Nitrolin	Nitroglycerin
Nitrong	Nitroglycerin
Nitropress	Sodium nitroprusside
Nitrostat	Nitroglycerin
Nitrous oxide	Nitrous oxide
Norcuron	Vecuronium bromide
Normodyne	Labetalol HCl
Novocaine	Procaine HCl
Novolin R	Insulin regular (human)
Nubain	Nalbuphine HCl
Nuromax	Doxacurium chloride
Osmitrol	Mannitol
Panwarfin	Warfarin sodium
Pavulon	Pancuronium
Pentothal	Thiopental sodium

Pepcid	Famotidine
Phenergan	Promethazine HCl
Pitocin	Oxytocin
Pitressin	Vasopressin
Polocaine	Mepivacaine HCl
Pontocaine	Tetracaine
Potassium chloride	Potassium chloride
Procan SR	Procainamide HCl
Procardia	Nifedipine
Pronestyl	Procainamide HCl
Prostigmine	Neostigmine
Prostin VR	Prostaglandin E_1—alprostadil
Protamine sulfate	Protamine sulfate
Quelicin	Succinylcholine chloride
Regitine	Phentolamine
Reglan	Metoclopramide
Regonal	Pyridostigmine bromide
Reversol	Edrophonium chloride
Rhulicaine	Benzocaine
Robinul	Glycopyrrolate
Sandimmune	Cyclosporine A
Scopolamine HBr	Scopolamine hydrobromide
Seconal	Secobarbital
Sensorcaine	Bupivacaine HCl
Sevoflurane	Sevoflurane
Shohl's solution	Sodium citrate
Sodium bicarbonate	Sodium bicarbonate
Sofarin	Warfarin sodium
Solarcaine	Benzocaine
Solu-Cortef	Hydrocortisone
Solu-Medrol	Methylprednisolone sodium succinate
Stadol	Butorphanol tartrate
Stimate	Desmopressin acetate
Sublimaze	Fentanyl
Sucostrin	Succinylcholine chloride
Sufenta	Sufentanil citrate
Suprane	Desflurane
Syntocinon	Oxytocin
Tagamet	Cimetidine
Tambocor	Flecainide acetate
Tenormin	Atenolol
Tensilon	Edrophonium chloride
Thorazine	Chlorpromazine HCl
Toradol	Ketorolac

Trade Name	Generic Name
Tracrium	Atracurium besylate
Trandate	Labetalol HCl
Transderm-nitro	Nitroglycerin
Tridil	Nitroglycerin
Tubocurarine chloride	D-Tubocurarine chloride
Urolene blue	Methylene blue
Valium	Diazepam
Vasotec	Enalapril maleate
Vasoxyl	Methoxamine HCl
Versed	Midazolam
Wyamine	Mephentermine sulfate
Xylocaine	Lidocaine HCl
Yutopar	Ritodrine HCl
Zantac	Ranitidine
Zemuron	Rocuronium Bromide
Zofran	Ondansetron HCl

Appendix 5

CPR ALGORITHMS

5-1 Universal Algorithm for Adult*
Emergency Cardiac Care

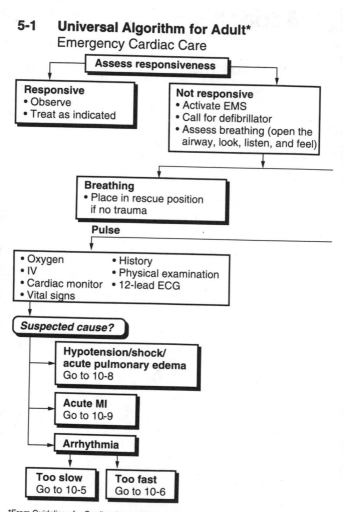

Assess responsiveness

Responsive
- Observe
- Treat as indicated

Not responsive
- Activate EMS
- Call for defibrillator
- Assess breathing (open the airway, look, listen, and feel)

Breathing
- Place in rescue position if no trauma

Pulse

- Oxygen
- IV
- Cardiac monitor
- Vital signs
- History
- Physical examination
- 12-lead ECG

Suspected cause?

Hypotension/shock/ acute pulmonary edema
Go to 10-8

Acute MI
Go to 10-9

Arrhythmia

Too slow
Go to 10-5

Too fast
Go to 10-6

*From Guidelines for Cardiopulmonary Resuscitation and Emergency Cardiac Care, Committee of the American Heart Association, *JAMA* 1992: 268: 2171-2302.

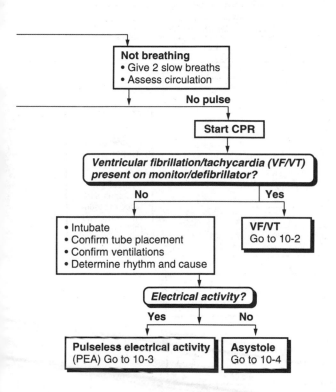

Not breathing
- Give 2 slow breaths
- Assess circulation

No pulse

Start CPR

Ventricular fibrillation/tachycardia (VF/VT) present on monitor/defibrillator?

No **Yes**

- Intubate
- Confirm tube placement
- Confirm ventilations
- Determine rhythm and cause

VF/VT
Go to 10-2

Electrical activity?

Yes **No**

Pulseless electrical activity
(PEA) Go to 10-3

Asystole
Go to 10-4

5-2 Ventricular Fibrillation/Pulseless Ventricular Tachycardia Algorithm (VF/VT)

- ABCs
- Perform CPR until defibrillator attached[a]
- VF/VT present on defibrillator

↓

Defibrillate up to 3 times if needed for persistent VF/VT
(200 J, 200-300 J, 360 J)

↓

Rhythm after the first 3 shocks?[b]

Persistent or recurrent VF/VT	Return of spontaneous circulation
• Continue CPR • Intubate at once • Obtain IV access	• Assess vital signs • Support airway • Support breathing • Provide medications appropriate for blood pressure, heart rate, and rhythm

Persistent or recurrent VF/VT branch:

- *Epinephrine*
  1 mg IV push[c,d]
  repeat every
  3-5 min

↓

- Defibrillate 360 J
  within 30-60 sec[e]

↓

- Administer medications
  of probable benefit (Class IIa)
  in persistent or recurrent VF/VT[f,g]

↓

- Defibrillate 360 J, 30-60 sec
  after each dose of medication[e]
- Pattern should be drug-shock,
  drug-shock

*From Guidelines for Cardiopulmonary Resuscitation and Emergency Cardiac Care, Committee of the American Heart Association. *JAMA* 1992: 268: 2171-2302.

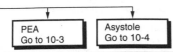

PEA
Go to 10-3

Asystole
Go to 10-4

Class I: definitely helpful
Class IIa: acceptable, probably helpful
Class IIb: acceptable, possibly helpful
Class III: not indicated, may be harmful

(a) Precordial thump is a Class IIb action in witnessed arrest, no pulse, and no defibrillator immediately available.
(b) Hypothermic cardiac arrest is treated differently after this point. *See section on hypothermia.*
(c) The recommended dose of *epinephrine* is 1 mg IV push every 3-5 min.
 If this approach fails, several Class IIb dosing regimens can be considered:
 • Intermediate: *epinephrine* 2-5 mg IV push, every 3-5 min
 • Escalating: *epinephrine* 1 mg-3 mg-5 mg IV push, 3 min apart
 • High: *epinephrine* 0.1 mg/kg IV push, every 3-5 min
(d) *Sodium bicarbonate* (1 mEq/kg) is Class I if patient has known preexisting hyperkalemia.
(e) Multiple sequenced shocks (200, 200-300 J, 360 J) are acceptable here (Class I), especially when medications are delayed.
(f) Medications:
 • *Lidocaine* 1.5 mg/kg IV push. Repeat in 3-5 min to total loading dose of 3 mg/kg; then use
 • *Bretylium* 5 mg/kg IV push. Repeat in 5 min at 10 mg/kg
 • *Magnesium sulfate* 1-2 g IV in torsades de pointes or suspected hypomagnesemic state or severe refractory VF
 • *Procainamide* 30 mg/min in refractory VF (maximum total 17 mg/kg)
(g) *Sodium bicarbonate* (1 mEq/kg IV):
 Class IIa
 • If known preexisting bicarbonate-responsive acidosis
 • If overdose with tricyclic antidepressants
 • To alkalinize the urine in drug overdoses
 Class IIb
 • If intubated and continued long arrest interval
 • Upon return of spontaneous circulation after long arrest interval
 Class III
 • Hypoxic lactic acidosis

5-3 Pulseless Electrical Activity (PEA) Algorithm*
(Electromechanical Dissociation [EMD])

Includes:
- Electromechanical dissociation (EMD)
- Pseudo-EMD
- Idioventricular rhythms
- Ventricular escape rhythms
- Bradyasystolic rhythms
- Postdefibrillation idioventricular rhythms

- Continue CPR
- Intubate at once
- Obtain IV access
- Assess blood flow using Doppler ultrasound

↓

Consider possible causes
(parentheses = possible therapies and treatments)

- Hypovolemia (volume infusion)
- Hypoxia (ventilation)
- Cardiac tamponade (pericardiocentesis)
- Tension pneumothorax (needle decompression)
- Hypothermia (see hypothermia algorithm)

- Massive pulmonary embolism (surgery, *thrombolytics*)
- Drug overdoses such as tricyclics, digitalis, beta-blockers, calcium channel blockers
- Hyperkalemia[a]
- Acidosis[b]
- Massive acute myocardial infarction (go to 10-9)

↓

- *Epinephrine* 1 mg IV push[a,c] repeat every 3-5 min

↓

- If absolute bradycardia (<60 beats/min) or relative bradycardia, give *atropine* 1 mg IV
- Repeat every 3-5 min to a total of 0.04 mg/kg[d]

From Guidelines for Cardiopulmonary Resuscitation and Emergency Cardiac Care, Committee of the American Heart Association. *JAMA* 1992: 268: 2171-2302.

Class I: definitely helpful
Class IIa: acceptable, probably helpful
Class IIb: acceptable, possibly helpful
Class III: not indicated, may be harmful

(a) *Sodium bicarbonate* 1 mEq/kg is Class I if patient has known preexisting hyperkalemia.

(b) *Sodium bicarbonate* (1 mEq/kg):
   Class IIa
   • If known preexisting bicarbonate-responsive acidosis
   • If overdose with tricyclic antidepressants
   • To alkalinize the urine in drug overdoses
   Class IIb
   • If intubated and long arrest interval
   • Upon return of spontaneous circulation after long arrest interval
   Class III
   • Hypoxic lactic acidosis

(c) The recommended dose of *epinephrine* is 1 mg IV push every 3-5 min. If this approach fails, several Class IIb dosing regimens can be considered:
   • Intermediate: *epinephrine* 2-5 mg IV push, every 3-5 min
   • Escalating: *epinephrine* 1 mg-3 mg-5 mg IV push, 3 min apart
   • High: *epinephrine* 0.1 mg/kg IV push, every 3-5 min

(d) Shorter *atropine* dosing intervals are possibly helpful in cardiac arrest (Class IIb).

5-4 Asystole Treatment Algorithm*

- **Continue CPR**
- **Intubate at once**
- **Obtain IV access**
- **Confirm asystole in more than one lead**

↓

Consider possible causes
- Hypoxia
- Hyperkalemia
- Hypokalemia
- Preexisting acidosis
- Drug overdose
- Hypothermia

↓

Consider immediate transcutaneous pacing (TCP)[a]

↓

- ***Epinephrine*** 1 mg IV push[b,c]
  repeat every 3-5 min.

↓

- ***Atropine*** 1 mg IV
  repeat every 3-5 min up to a total of 0.04 mg/kg[d,e]

↓

Consider termination of efforts[f]

Class I: definitely helpful
Class IIa: acceptable, probably helpful
Class IIb: acceptable, possibly helpful
Class III: not indicated, may be harmful

(a) TCP is a Class IIb intervention. Lack of success may be due to delays in pacing. To be effective TCP must be performed early, simultaneously with drugs. Evidence does not support routine use of TCP for asystole.
(b) The recommended dose of ***epinephrine*** is 1 mg IV push every 3-5 min. If this approach fails, several Class IIb dosing regimens can be considered:
- Intermediate: ***epinephrine*** 2-5 mg IV push, every 3-5min
- Escalating: ***epinephrine*** 1 mg-3 mg -5 mg IV push, 3 min apart
- High: ***epinephrine*** 0.1 mg/kg IV push every 3-5 min
(c) **Sodium bicarbonate** 1 mEq/kg is Class I if patient has known preexisting hyperkalemia.
(d) Shorter ***atropine*** dosing intervals are Class IIb in asystolic arrest.
(e) **Sodium bicarbonate** 1 mEq/kg:
Class IIa
- if known preexisting bicarbonate-responsive acidosis
- if overdose with tricyclic anti-depressants
- to alkalinize the urine in drug overdoses
Class IIb
- if intubated and continued long arrest interval
- upon return of spontaneous circulation after long arrest interval
Class III
- hypoxic lactic acidosis
(f) If patient remains in asystole or other agonal rhythms after successful intubation and initial medications and no reversible causes are identified, consider termination of resuscitative efforts by a physician. Consider interval since arrest.

---

*From Guidelines for Cardiopulmonary Resuscitation and Emergency Cardiac Care, Committee of the American Heart Association. *JAMA* 1992: 268: 2171-2302.

5-5 Bradycardia Algorithm*
(Patient is not in cardiac arrest)

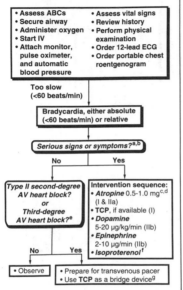

- Assess ABCs
- Secure airway
- Administer oxygen
- Start IV
- Attach monitor, pulse oximeter, and automatic blood pressure

- Assess vital signs
- Review history
- Perform physical examination
- Order 12-lead ECG
- Order portable chest roentgenogram

Too slow (<60 beats/min)

Bradycardia, either absolute (<60 beats/min) or relative

Serious signs or symptoms?[a,b]

No / Yes

Type II second-degree AV heart block? or Third-degree AV heart block?[e]

Intervention sequence:
- *Atropine* 0.5-1.0 mg[c,d] (I & IIa)
- TCP, if available (I)
- *Dopamine* 5-20 µg/kg/min (IIb)
- *Epinephrine* 2-10 µg/min (IIb)
- *Isoproterenol*[f]

No / Yes

- Observe

- Prepare for transvenous pacer
- Use **TCP** as a bridge device[g]

(a) Serious signs or symptoms must be related to the slow rate. Clinical manifestations include:
- symptoms (chest pain, shortness of breath, decreased level of consciousness)
- signs (low BP, shock, pulmonary congestion, CHF, acute MI).

(b) Do not delay TCP while awaiting IV access or for *atropine* to take effect if patient is symptomatic.

(c) Denervated transplanted hearts will not respond to *atropine*. Go at once to pacing, *cactecholamine* infusion, or both.

(d) *Atropine* should be given in repeat doses in 3-5 min up to total of 0.04 mg/kg. Consider shorter dosing intervals in severe clinical conditions. It has been suggested that *atropine* should be used with caution in atrioventricular (AV) block at the His-Purkinje level (type II AV block and new third-degree block with wide QRS complexes) (Class IIb).

(e) Never treat third-degree heart block plus ventricular escape beats with *lidocaine*.

(f) *Isoproterenol* should be used, if at all, with extreme caution. At low doses it is Class IIb (possibly helpful); at higher doses it is Class III (harmful).

(g) Verify patient tolerance and mechanical capture. Use analgesia and sedation as needed.

*From Guidelines for Cardiopulmonary Resuscitation and Emergency Cardiac Care, Committee of the American Heart Association. *JAMA* 1992: 268: 2171-2302.

5-6 Tachycardia Algorithm*

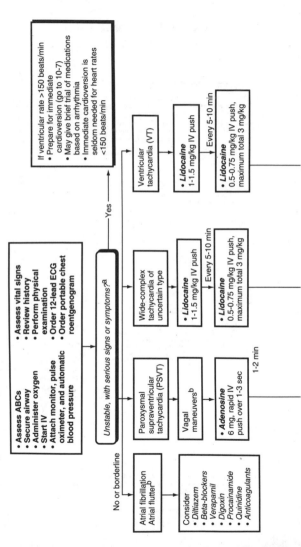

- Assess ABCs
- Secure airway
- Administer oxygen
- Start IV
- Attach monitor, pulse oximeter, and automatic blood pressure
- Assess vital signs
- Review history
- Perform physical examination
- Order 12-lead ECG
- Order portable chest roentgenogram

Unstable, with serious signs or symptoms?[a]

No or borderline

— Yes

If ventricular rate >150 beats/min
- Prepare for immediate cardioversion (go to 10-7)
- May give brief trial of medications based on arrhythmia
- Immediate cardioversion is seldom needed for heart rates <150 beats/min

**Atrial fibrillation
Atrial flutter[b]**

Consider
- *Diltiazem*
- *Beta-blockers*
- *Verapamil*
- *Digoxin*
- *Procainamide*
- *Quinidine*
- *Anticoagulants*

Paroxysmal supraventricular tachycardia (PSVT)

Vagal maneuvers[b]

Adenosine
6 mg, rapid IV push over 1-3 sec

1-2 min

Wide-complex tachycardia of uncertain type

Lidocaine
1-1.5 mg/kg IV push

Every 5-10 min

Lidocaine
0.5-0.75 mg/kg IV push, maximum total 3 mg/kg

Ventricular tachycardia (VT)

Lidocaine
1-1.5 mg/kg IV push

Every 5-10 min

Lidocaine
0.5-0.75 mg/kg IV push, maximum total 3 mg/kg

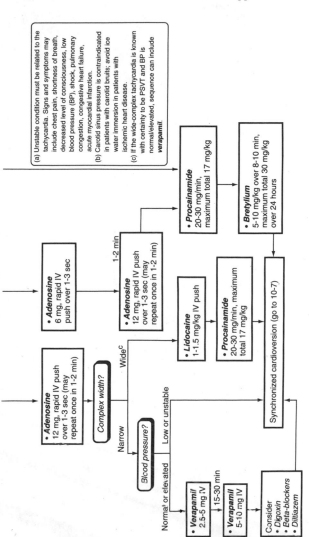

(a) Unstable condition must be related to the tachycardia. Signs and symptoms may include chest pain, shortness of breath, decreased level of consciousness, low blood pressure (BP), shock, pulmonary congestion, congestive heart failure, acute myocardial infarction.

(b) Carotid sinus pressure is contraindicated in patients with carotid bruits; avoid ice water immersion in patients with ischemic heart disease.

(c) If the wide-complex tachycardia is known with certainty to be PSVT and BP is normal/elevated, sequence can include *verapamil*.

• *Adenosine*
6 mg, rapid IV
push over 1-3 sec

1-2 min

• *Adenosine*
12 mg, rapid IV push
over 1-3 sec (may
repeat once in 1-2 min)

• *Procainamide*
20-30 mg/min,
maximum total 17 mg/kg

• *Bretylium*
5-10 mg/kg over 8-10 min,
maximum total 30 mg/kg
over 24 hours

• *Adenosine*
12 mg, rapid IV push
over 1-3 sec (may
repeat once in 1-2 min)

Complex width?

Wide[c]

• *Lidocaine*
1-1.5 mg/kg IV push

• *Procainamide*
20-30 mg/min, maximum
total 17 mg/kg

Narrow

Blood pressure?

Low or unstable

Synchronized cardioversion (go to 10-7)

Normal or elevated

• *Verapamil*
2.5-5 mg IV

15-30 min

• *Verapamil*
5-10 mg IV

Consider
• *Digoxin*
• *Beta-blockers*
• *Diltiazem*

*From Guidelines for Cardiopulmonary Resuscitation and Emergency Cardiac Care, Committee of the American Heart Association. *JAMA* 1992: 268: 2171-2302.

5-7 Electric Cardioversion Algorithm*
(Patient is not in cardiac arrest)

Tachycardia
With serious signs and symptoms
related to the tachycardia

If ventricular rate is >150 beats/min, prepare
for IMMEDIATE CARDIOVERSION. May give
brief trial of medications based on specific
arrhythmias. Immediate cardioversion is
generally not needed for rates <150 beats/min.

Check
- Oxygen saturation
- Suction device
- IV line
- Intubation equipment

Premedicate whenever possible[a]

Synchronized cardioversion[b,c]
VT[d]
PSVT[e] ⎤ 100 J, 200 J
Atrial fibrillation ⎦ 300 J, 360 J
Atrial flutter[e]

(a) Effective regimens have included a sedative (e.g. *diazepam, midazolam, barbiturates, etomidate, ketamine, methohexital*) with or without an analgesic agent (e.g. *fentanyl, morphine, meperidine*). Many experts recommend anesthesia if service is readily available.
(b) Note possible need to resynchronize after each cardioversion.
(c) If delays in synchronization occur and clinical conditions are critical, go to immediate unsynchronized shocks.
(d) Treat polymorphic VT (irregular form and rate) like VF: 200 J, 200-300 J, 360 J.
(e) PSVT and atrial flutter often respond to lower energy levels (start with 50 J).

*From Guidelines for Cardiopulmonary Resuscitation and Emergency Cardiac Care, Committee of the American Heart Association. *JAMA* 1992: 268: 2171-2302.

5-8 Hypotension/Shock/Acute Pulmonary Edema Algorithm*

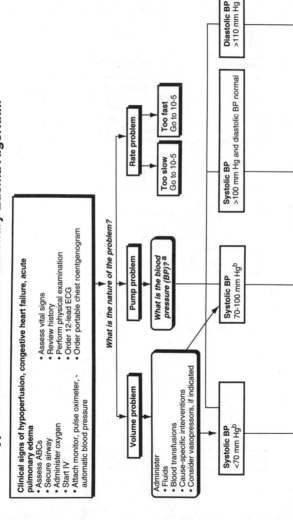

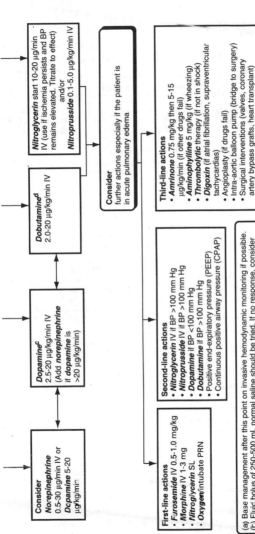

Consider
Norepinephrine 0.5-30 μg/min IV or
Dopamine 5-20 μg/kg/min

*Dopamine*c 2.5-20 μg/kg/min IV
(Add *norepinephrine* if *dopamine* is >20 μg/kg/min IV

*Dobutamine*d 2.0-20 μg/kg/min IV

Nitroglycerin start 10-20 μg/min IV (use if ischemia persists and BP remains elevated. Titrate to effect) and/or *Nitroprusside* 0.1-5.0 μg/kg/min IV

Consider
further actions especially if the patient is in acute pulmonary edema

Third-line actions
• *Amrinone* 0.75 mg/kg then 5-15 μg/kg/min (if other drugs fail)
• *Aminophylline* 5 mg/kg (if wheezing)
• *Thrombolytic* therapy (if not in shock)
• *Digoxin* (if atrial fibrillation, supraventricular tachycardias)
• Angioplasty (if drugs fail)
• Intra-aortic balloon pump (bridge to surgery)
• Surgical interventions (valves, coronary artery bypass grafts, heart transplant)

Second-line actions
• *Nitroglycerin* IV if BP >100 mm Hg
• *Nitroprusside* IV if BP >100 mm Hg
• *Dopamine* if BP <100 mm Hg
• *Dobutamine* if BP >100 mm Hg
• Positive end-expiratory pressure (PEEP)
• Continuous positive airway pressure (CPAP)

First-line actions
• *Furosemide* IV 0.5-1.0 mg/kg
• *Morphine* IV 1-3 mg
• *Nitroglycerin* SL
• *Oxygen*/intubate PRN

(a) Base management after this point on invasive hemodynamic monitoring if possible.
(b) Fluid bolus of 250-500 mL normal saline should be tried. If no response, consider sympathomimetics.
(c) Move to *dobutamine* and stop *norepinephrine* when BP improves.
(d) Add *dopamine* when BP improves. Avoid *dobutamine* when systolic BP <100 mm Hg.

*From Guidelines for Cardiopulmonary Resuscitation and Emergency Cardiac Care, Committee of the American Heart Association. *JAMA* 1992: 268: 2171-2302.

5-9 **Acute Myocardial Infarction Algorithm***

Recommendations for early management of patients with chest pain and possible AMI

| **COMMUNITY** | **Community emphasis on "Call First, Call Fast, Call 911"** |

| **EMS SYSTEM** | EMS system approach that should address
• Oxygen-IV-cardiac monitor-vital signs
• *Nitroglycerin*
• Pain relief with narcotics
• Notification of emergency department
• Rapid transport to emergency department
• Prehospital screening for *thrombolytic* therapy*
• 12-lead ECG, computer analysis, transmission to emergency department*
• Initiation of *thrombolytic* therapy* |

| **EMERGENCY DEPARTMENT** | **"Door-to-drug" team protocol approach**
• Rapid triage of patients with chest pain
• Clinical decision maker established (emergency physician, cardiologist, or other) |

Assessment

Immediate:
  • Vital signs with automatic BP
  • Oxygen saturation
  • Start IV
  • 12-lead ECG (MD review)
  • Brief, targeted history and physical
  • Decide on eligibility for *thrombolytic* therapy

Soon:
  • Chest x-ray
  • Blood studies (electrolytes, enzymes, coagulation studies)

*From Guidelines for Cardiopulmonary Resuscitation and Emergency Cardiac Care, Committee of the American Heart Association. *JAMA* 1992: 268: 2171-2302.
†
‡

†For information on the National Heart Attack Alert Program, contact the National Institutes of Health Information Center, P.O. Box 30105, Bethesda, MD 20824-0105

†Optional guidelines

Time interval in emergency department

Treatments to consider if there is evidence of coronary thrombosis plus no reasons for exclusion:
(some but not all may be appropriate)
- *Oxygen* at 4 L/min
- *Nitroglycerin* SL, paste or spray (if systolic blood pressure >90 mm Hg)
- *Morphine* IV
- *Aspirin* PO
- *Thrombolytic* agents
- *Nitroglycerin* IV (limit systolic BP drop to 10% if normotensive; 30% drop if hypertensive; never drop below 90 mm Hg systolic)
- *Beta-blockers* IV
- *Heparin* IV
- Routine *lidocaine* administration is **NOT** recommended for all patients with AMI
- *Magnesium sulfate* IV
- Percutaneous transluminal coronary angioplasty

30-60 min to *thrombolytic* therapy

Appendix 6

TABLE 6-1 Pediatric CPR Drugs Table

Drug	Concentration	Dose	Frequency	Route/Comments
Atropine	1 mg/ml	0.02 mls/kg IV or ET (0.02 mg/kg)	Every 5 min	Min. dose 0.1 mg. May dilute 1 : 1 with NS if given ET
Bretylium	50 mg/ml	5-10 mg/kg IV	Every 15-30 min	Max dose 30 mg/kg
Calcium Chloride	100 mg/ml (10%)	0.1 ml/kg IV (10 mg/kg)	Every 10 min	Indicated for treatment of hypocalcemia, hyper-magnesemia or hy-pokalemia with cardiac toxicity
Calcium Gluconate	100 mg/ml (10%)	0.3 ml/kg IV (30 mg/kg)	Every 10 min	Indicated for treatment of hypocalcemia, hyper-magnesemia or hy-pokalemia with cardiac toxicity
Cardiover-sion (synchro-nized)	0.5-1 watt/sec/kg	Double dose if necessary. For optimal effect, check oxygeni-zation, acid/base status and correct.		Indicated for ventricular rate >150 beat/min with serious signs and symptoms (not sinus tachycardia). The synchronizer circuit must be activated. On some older models, the QRS complex must be upright for proper acti-vation.
Defibrillation		2 watt/sec/kg	Double dose if necessary. For optimal effect, check acid/base status and correct	Max 4 watt/sec/kg (ven-tricular fibrillation only)
Epinephrine	1 : 10,000	0.1/kg IV or ET (0.01 mg/kg)	Every 5 min	Dilute 1 : 1 with NS if given ET
Glucose	50%	1-2 ml/kg IV		Monitor blood glucose
Lidocaine	10 mg/ml	Loading 1 mg/kg IV or ET (0.01 mls/kg)	Maint. 0.5 mg/kg every 5 min or infusion 20-50 µg/kg/min	May dilute 1 : 1 with NS if given with ET

TABLE 6-1 cont'd

Drug	Concentration	Dose	Frequency	Route/Comments
Naloxone	0.4 mg/ml	0.025-0.25 mls/ kg IV, ET, IM, SQ (0.01-0.1 mg/kg)	Every 2-3 min	Max dosage 10 mg
Sodium Bicarbonate	1 mEq/ml	1-2 mEq/kg IV	Every 10-15 min of arrest	By ABG values
Volume expanders	Whole blood 5% albumin Normal Saline Lactated Ringer's, Hespan	10 mls/kg IV	Give over 5-10 min	Give by syringe or infusion

INFUSIONS*

Drug	Concentration	Dose		
Dobutamine	50 mg/ml	0.5-30 μg/kg/ min		
Dopamine	40 mg/ml	1-50 μg/kg/min		
Isoproterenol	0.2 mg/ml	0.02-0.15 μg/ kg/min		
Norepinephrine	1 mg/ml	0.04-0.4 μ/kg/ min		

*To achieve the desired dose (μg/kg/min) the following amount of drug is added to 100 mls D5W of NS:

$$\text{mg in 100 mls} = \frac{6 \times \text{wt (kg)} \times \text{dose (μg/kg/min)}}{\text{desired infusion rate (ml/hr)}}$$

or

To determine the infusion rate at a desired dose (μg/kg/min) and concentration (mg/ml):

$$\text{infusion rate (mls/hr)} = \frac{\text{wt (kg)} \times 60 \times \text{dose (μg/kg/min)}}{\text{conc (mg/ml)} \times 1000}$$

or

Utilize the infusion table.

Note: ET = Endotracheal Tube
IV = Intravenous
IM = Intramuscular
SQ = Subcutaneous
NS = Normal Saline
ABG= Arterial Blood Gas

Appendix 7

SULFITE-CONTAINING AND NON-SULFITE-CONTAINING ANESTHESIA DRUGS

From Kataria B. Fernandez-Bueno C: Anesthetic management of a patient with sulfite sensitivity, Anesthesiol Rev 18(1): 50-53, 1991.

Table 1. Injectable Drugs Commonly Used During Anesthesia That Contain Sulfite.

Chemical Name	Distributor/ Manufacturer
Amrinone lactate	Winthrop
Bupivacaine HCl with epinephrine	Astra, Winthrop
Chlorpromazine	Smith Kline & French
Dexamethasone	Elkins-Sinn, Merck Sharp & Dohme
Dobutamine HCl	Lilly
Dopamine HCl	Astra, DuPont, Elkins-Sinn, Warner Chilcott
Edrophonium chloride	Organon
Epinephrine	Abbott, Astra, Elkins-Sinn, Parke-Davis
Hydrocortisone sodium phosphate	Merck Sharp & Dohme, Quad
Isoproterenol HCl	Elkins-Sinn, Winthrop
Meperidine HCl	Wyeth-Ayerst
Metaraminol bitartrate	Merck Sharp & Dohme
Nalbuphine HCl	DuPont, Quad
Norepinephrine bitartrate	Winthrop
Prednisolone sodium phosphate	Merck Sharp & Dohme
Phenylephrine	Elkins-Sinn, Quad, Winthrop
Procaine HCl	Winthrop
Procainamide HCl	Elkins-Sinn, Quad, Warner, Chilcott

Chemical Name	Distributor/ Manufacturer
Table 1. (cont'd)	
Promethazine HCl	Wyeth-Ayerst
Tubocuraine	Lilly, Quad

The prescribing physician should always confirm the absence or presence of additives in any product with the package insert or by direct consultation with the manufacturer.

Table 2. Injectable Drugs Commonly Used During Anesthesia That Do Not Contain Sulfite.

Chemical Name	Distributor/ Manufacturer
Acetazolamide sodium	Quad
Alfentanil HCl	Janssen
Aminocaproic acid	Elkins-Sinn, Lederle, Quad
Aminophylline	Abbott, Elkins-Sinn, Lyphomed
Atracurium besylate	Burroughs Wellcome
Atropine sulfate	Abbott, Astra, Elkins-Sinn
Bretylium tosylate	Astra, DuPont, Elkins-Sinn
Bupivacaine HCl without epinephrine	Astra, Winthrop
Bupivacaine in dextrose (spinal)	Astra, Winthrop
Calcium chloride	Abbott, Astra
Calcium gluceptate	Abbott
Chloroprocaine HCl	Astra
Cimetidine	Smith Kline & French
Dantrolene sodium	Norwich Eaton
Diazepam	Elkins-Sinn, Lederle, Roche
Digoxin	Burroughs Wellcome, Elkins-Sinn
Diphenhydramine HCl	Elkins-Sinn, Parke-Davis
Doxapram HCl	Robins
Droperidol	Astra, Janssen, Quad
Ephedrine sulfate	Abbott

Table 2. (cont'd)

Chemical Name	Distributor/ Manufacturer
Esmolol HCl	DuPont
Fentanyl citrate	Astra, Elkins-Sinn, Quad
Furosemide	Astra, Elkins-Sinn, Hoechst-Rousse
Glycopyrrolate	Robins, Quad
Heparin sodium	Elkins-Sinn, Lyphomed, Organon, Upjohn, Wyeth-Ayerst
Hetastarch 6%	DuPont
Hydralazine HCl	CIBA
Hydrocortisone sodium succinate	Abbott, Upjohn
Hydroxyzine HCl	Elkins-Sinn
Ketamine HCl	Parke-Davis, Quad
Labetalol HCl	Allen & Hanburys, Schering
Lorazepam	Wyeth-Ayerst
Magnesium sulfate	Abbott, Astra
Mannitol	Astra, Lyphomed
Meperidine HCl	Astra
Mepivacaine HCl	Astra, Winthrop
Methohexital sodium	Lilly
Methylprednisolone sodium succinate	Upjohn
Metoclopramide HCl	Robins, Quad
Metocurine iodide	Lilly, Quad

Midazolam HCl	Roche
Naloxone HCl	Astra, DuPont, Elkins-Sinn, Quad
Neostigmine methylsulfate	Elkins-Sinn, ICN, Quad
Nitroglycerin IV	DuPont, Parke-Davis, Quad
Oxytocin	Parke-Davis, Sandoz, Wyeth-Ayerst
Pancuronium bromide	Astra, Elkin-Sinn, Organon, Quad
Phentolamine mesylate	CIBA
Phenytoin sodium	Elkins-Sinn, Parke-Davis
Propofol	Stuart
Propranolol HCl	Wyeth-Ayerst
Protamine sulfate	Elkins-Sinn, Lilly, Quad
Pyridostigmine bromide	ICN, Organon
Ranitidine HCl	Glaxo
Scopolamine hydrobromide	Lyphomed
Sodium chloride	Abbott, Elkins-Sinn
Succinylcholine chloride	Burroughs Wellcome
Terbutaline sulfate	Geigy, Lakeside Pharmaceuticals
Thiopental sodium	Abbott
Tolazoline HCl	CIBA
Trimethaphan camsylate	Roche
Vecuronium bromide	Organon
Verapamil HCl	Knoll, Quad

The prescribing physician should always confirm the absence or presence of additives in any product with the package insert or by direct consultation with the manufacturer.

INDEX

Coma—cont'd
  cyclosporine A causing, 69
  insulin regular causing, 168
  potassium chloride causing, 281
Compatibility lists, 400-401
Compazine, 291
Concealed accessory pathways, unmasking, adenosine for, 1
Conduction depression, phenytoin sodium causing, 269
Confusion
  atropine sulfate causing, 22
  chlordiazepoxide HCl causing, 46
  cimetidine causing, 55
  cyclosporine A causing, 69
  diazepam causing, 80
  digoxin causing, 84
  diphenhydramine HCl causing, 86
  esmolol HCl causing, 118
  ethacrynic acid causing, 120
  eutectic mixture of lidocaine and prilocaine causing, 105
  glycopyrrolate causing, 147
  insulin regular causing, 168
  methylene blue causing, 216
  nalbuphine HCl causing, 241
  phenytoin sodium causing, 270
  procainamide HCl causing, 288
  promethazine HCl causing, 296
  propofol causing, 299
  ranitidine causing, 312

Confusion—cont'd
  scopolamine hydrobromide causing, 318
  secobarbital causing, 321
Congenital prolonged-QT syndrome, phenytoin sodium for, 267
Congestion
  chest, nifedipine causing, 250
  nasal
    hydralazine HCl causing, 155
    nifedipine causing, 250
Congestive heart failure
  amiodarone causing, 13
  amrinone for, 13
  captopril for, 40
  clonidine HCl causing, 59
  dexamethasone causing, 77
  enalapril maleate for, 105
  ethacrynic acid for, 119
  flecainide acetate causing, 133
  furosemide for, 138
  hydralazine HCl for, 154
  hydrocortisone causing, 158
  labetalol HCl causing, 179
  methylprednisolone causing, 221
  nitroglycerin for, 250
  propranolol HCl causing, 302
  prostaglandin E_1 causing, 304
Conjunctivitis, cyclosporine A causing, 69
Conscious sedation, midazolam HCl for, 229
Constipation
  cyclosporine A causing, 69
  dantrolene sodium causing, 72

H

560 *Index*